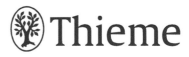

# Endoscopic Surgery of the Orbit

Anatomy, Pathology, and Management

**Benjamin S. Bleier, MD, FACS, FARS**
Associate Professor
Director, Endoscopic Skull Base Surgery
Co-Director, Center for Thyroid Eye Disease and Orbital Surgery
Department of Otolaryngology–Head and Neck Surgery
Massachusetts Eye and Ear Infirmary
Harvard Medical School
Boston, Massachusetts

**Suzanne K. Freitag, MD**
Associate Professor
Director, Ophthalmic Plastic Surgery Service
Co-Director, Center for Thyroid Eye Disease and Orbital Surgery
Department of Ophthalmology
Massachusetts Eye and Ear Infirmary
Harvard Medical School
Boston, Massachusetts

**Raymond Sacks, MBBCH, FRACS, FCS, FARS**
Professor and Chair
Department of Otolaryngology–Head and Neck Surgery
Macquarie University
Clinical Professor and Head of Discipline of Otolaryngology
Sydney University Medical School
Sydney, Australia

Thieme
New York • Stuttgart • Delhi • Rio de Janeiro

Thieme Medical Publishers, Inc.
333 Seventh Avenue
New York, New York 10001

Executive Editor: Timothy Hiscock
Managing Editor: J. Owen Zurhellen
Assistant Managing Editor: Mary Wilson
Director, Editorial Services: Mary Jo Casey
Editorial Director: Sue Hodgson
Production Editor: Sean Woznicki
International Production Director: Andreas Schabert
International Marketing Director: Fiona Henderson
International Sales Director: Louisa Turrell
Director of Institutional Sales: Adam Bernacki
Senior Vice President and Chief Operating Officer: Sarah Vanderbilt
President: Brian D. Scanlan

Library of Congress Cataloging-in-Publication Data
Names: Bleier, Benjamin S., editor. | Freitag, Suzanne K., editor. |
    Sacks, Raymond (Otolaryngologist), editor.
Title: Endoscopic surgery of the orbit : anatomy, pathology, and
    management / [edited by] Benjamin S. Bleier, Suzanne K. Freitag,
    Raymond Sacks.
Description: First edition. | New York : Thieme, [2019] | Includes
    bibliographical references and index. | Identifiers: LCCN
    2018034903 (print) | LCCN 2018037246 (ebook) | ISBN
    9781626235069 (E-book) | ISBN 9781626235052 (hardback)
    | ISBN 9781626235069 (eISBN)
Subjects: | MESH: Orbit–surgery | Paranasal Sinuses–surgery |
    Endoscopy–methods
Classification: LCC RF350 (ebook) | LCC RF350 (print) | NLM WW
    202 | DDC
    617.5/23–dc23
LC record available at https://lccn.loc.gov/2018034903

Thieme Publishers New York
333 Seventh Avenue, New York, NY 10001 USA
+1 800 782 3488, customerservice@thieme.com

Thieme Publishers Stuttgart
Rüdigerstrasse 14, 70469 Stuttgart, Germany
+49 [0]711 8931 421, customerservice@thieme.de

Thieme Publishers Delhi
A-12, Second Floor, Sector-2, Noida-201301
Uttar Pradesh, India
+91 120 45 566 00, customerservice@thieme.in

Thieme Publishers Rio de Janeiro, Thieme Publicações Ltda.
Edifício Rodolpho de Paoli, 25º andar
Av. Nilo Peçanha, 50 – Sala 2508
Rio de Janeiro 20020-906 Brasil
+55 21 3172-2297 / +55 21 3172-1896
www.thiemerevinter.com.br

Cover design: Thieme Publishing Group
Typesetting by Thomson Digital, India

Printed in The United States by King Printing        5 4 3 2 1

ISBN 978-1-62623-505-2

Also available as an e-book:
eISBN 978-1-62623-506-9

**Important note:** Medicine is an ever-changing science undergoing continual development. Research and clinical experience are continually expanding our knowledge, in particular our knowledge of proper treatment and drug therapy. Insofar as this book mentions any dosage or application, readers may rest assured that the authors, editors, and publishers have made every effort to ensure that such references are in accordance with **the state of knowledge at the time of production of the book.**

Nevertheless, this does not involve, imply, or express any guarantee or responsibility on the part of the publishers in respect to any dosage instructions and forms of applications stated in the book. **Every user is requested to examine carefully** the manufacturers' leaflets accompanying each drug and to check, if necessary in consultation with a physician or specialist, whether the dosage schedules mentioned therein or the contraindications stated by the manufacturers differ from the statements made in the present book. Such examination is particularly important with drugs that are either rarely used or have been newly released on the market. Every dosage schedule or every form of application used is entirely at the user's own risk and responsibility. The authors and publishers request every user to report to the publishers any discrepancies or inaccuracies noticed. If errors in this work are found after publication, errata will be posted at www.thieme.com on the product description page.

Some of the product names, patents, and registered designs referred to in this book are in fact registered trademarks or proprietary names even though specific reference to this fact is not always made in the text. Therefore, the appearance of a name without designation as proprietary is not to be construed as a representation by the publisher that it is in the public domain.

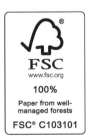

I dedicate this book to my mentors, students, and patients, from whom I continue to learn how to be a better surgeon. Most importantly I dedicate this book to my wife whose love and support form the foundation upon which all my accomplishments rest.

*– BSB*

Dedicated to my mentors with much gratitude: Edward Jaeger, Neil Miller, John Woog, Arthur Grove, Katrinka Heher, and Michael Migliori.

*– SKF*

I dedicate this book to my dear friend, mentor and confidante, Dr Evan Richard Soicher, Ophthalmologist, taken from us in the prime of his life and at the peak of his career. His inspiration and persistent support for me to undertake this project was the driving force behind its publication. He will never be forgotten.

*– RS*

# Contents

Contents

# Menu of Accompanying Videos

# Foreword

Since endoscopic sinus surgery started, the close proximity of the orbit has proved a boon and a danger. The possibility of crossing the sino-orbital interface with excellent visualization and minimal morbidity has opened up a range of opportunities for dealing with a wide variety of intraorbital pathology from abscesses to tumors. Unfortunately, unintentional entry into the orbit has also occurred during sinus surgery, though this is not the exclusive preserve of the endoscopic sinus surgeon. Thus, a knowledge of the detailed anatomy of the area is a prerequisite to surgery in this location as well as a clear understanding of the pathologies that may be encountered. This book which brings together experts from a wide range of disciplines and achieves these objectives admirably by bringing together skull base surgeons, ophthalmologists, reconstructive and rhinologic surgeons under the leadership of Drs. Bleier, Freitag and Sacks. Having worked closely with ophthalmology colleagues all of my career, I can entirely endorse this multi-disciplinary approach which provides fascinating insight into the many conditions that can be managed endoscopically to the benefit of patients.

All aspects are covered, from management of the nasolacrimal system and thyroid eye disease, to trauma and tumors. The role of both endoscopic and open orbital surgery is carefully explored as well as important diagnostic, anesthetic and post-operative aspects of care. Perhaps of greatest interest is the use of transorbital endoscopic approaches to the sinuses, skull base and intracranial compartment to access lesions which were often inaccessible without high potential morbidity. This is a new frontier – and one which will undoubtedly expand – and this is a book for anyone with an interest in the sino-orbital region.

*Valerie J. Lund, CBE*
*London, England, United Kingdom*

Lesions involving the orbit have challenged surgeons for decades. In some cases, the challenges are the lesions themselves, but in many other cases, there are major technical issues related to the location of the lesion and the approach that is required. Thus, many benign neoplasms as well as vascular disorders that occur in the orbit have not been amenable to surgery because of the prohibitive morbidity, particularly permanent visual loss and/or double vision, associated with the procedure used to treat them. During the past several decades, surgery of the orbit has evolved into an interdisciplinary specialty. Surgical teams and referral centers have been formed, and clinical and research interests have accelerated. Improved instruments, microscopes, anesthesia, and imaging all have played a role in the growth of orbital surgery. In particular, endoscopic approaches to orbital lesions have provided surgeons with alternatives to the previously standard open approaches, resulting in less visual morbidity.

The team approach to orbital lesions is beautifully illustrated in this text edited by Dr. Benjamin S. Bleier—a skull base surgeon, Dr. Suzanne K. Freitag—an ophthalmologist and oculoplastic surgeon, and Dr. Raymond Sacks—an otolaryngologist. This triumvirate has assembled chapters for this text from experts throughout the world, many of whom have pioneered this field of special interest. This book thus not only includes standard chapters on orbital anatomy and imaging but also details the state of the art with respect to endoscopic as well as open surgery for lesions that primarily or secondarily involve the orbit. It also provides a benchmark for an evolving surgical discipline that began because of the collegiality and collaboration of experts from various surgical specialties.

*Neil R. Miller, MD FACS*
*Baltimore, Maryland*

# Preface

Endoscopic orbital surgery is one of the most rapidly advancing areas in modern day Rhinology and Ophthalmic Plastic Surgery. While endoscopic techniques have been adapted for lacrimal and orbital decompression surgery for over two decades, advanced endoscopic endonasal and periocular approaches to the orbital apex and skull base have only recently been developed. As a still-nascent field, no single comprehensive compendium of information on these techniques has existed until now. The purpose of this book and its accompanying videos is to bring together the global experience of thought leaders and pioneers in endoscopic orbital surgery to codify the current state of the field and set the stage for future innovations. The multidisciplinary background of the editorship reflects our combined belief that the optimal path forward in the advancement of this field is through the development of strong collaborative orbital teams who can utilize their combined surgical expertise to optimize care for patients with orbital disease.

# Contributors

**Nithin D. Adappa, MD**
Surgical Director, Penn AERD Center
Co-Director, Rhinology and Skull Base Fellowship
Associate Professor
Department of Otorhinolaryngology-Head and Neck
  Surgery
University of Pennsylvania
Philadelphia, Pennsylvania

**Catherine Banks, MbChB, FRACS**
Otolaryngology and Head and Neck Surgeon
Prince of Wales Hospital and Sydney Eye Hospital
University of New South Wales
Sydney, Australia

**Henry P. Barham, MD**
Rhinology and Skull Base Surgery
Sinus and Nasal Specialists of Louisiana
Baton Rouge, Louisiana

**Benjamin S. Bleier, MD, FACS, FARS**
Associate Professor
Director, Endoscopic Skull Base Surgery
Co-Director, Center for Thyroid Eye Disease and Orbital
  Surgery
Department of Otolaryngology–Head and Neck Surgery
Massachusetts Eye and Ear Infirmary
Harvard Medical School
Boston, Massachusetts

**Adam P. Campbell, MD**
Georgia Nasal & Sinus Institute
Savannah, Georgia

**Raewyn Campbell, BMed(Hons), FRACS**
Visiting Medical Officer
Rhinologist and Skull Base Surgeon
Department of Ear, Nose and Throat, Head and Neck Surgery
Royal Prince Alfred Hospital
Sydney, Australia

**Dean M. Cestari, MD**
Assistant Professor of Ophthalmology
Harvard Medical School
Director, Adult Strabismus
Director, Fellowship Education
Massachusetts Eye & Ear Infirmary
Co-Director, Center for Thyroid Eye Disease and Orbital
  Surgery
Boston, Massachusetts

**Catherine J. Choi, MD**
Clinical Instructor, Ophthalmic Plastic and Reconstructive
  Surgery
Department of Ophthalmology
Bascom Palmer Eye Institute
University of Miami Miller School of Medicine
Miami, Florida

**Bo Young Chun, MD, PhD**
Associate Professor
Neuro-Ophthalmology, Pediatric Ophthalmology and
  Strabismus Service
Department of Ophthalmology
Kyungpook National University Hospital
Kyungpook National University School of Medicine
Daegu, Korea

**Hugh Curtin, MD**
Chief of Radiology
Massachusetts Eye and Ear
Harvard Medical School
Boston, Massachusetts

**Lora R. Dagi Glass, MD**
Assistant Professor
Director, Center for Periocular and Facial Dermatitis
Department of Ophthalmology
Edward S. Harkness Eye Institute
Columbia University Medical Center
New York, New York

**Richard Douglas, MD, FRACS**
Rhinologist
Auckland and Gillies Hospitals
Professor
Department of Surgery
The University of Auckland
Auckland, New Zealand

**Suzanne K. Freitag, MD**
Associate Professor
Director, Ophthalmic Plastic Surgery Service
Co-Director, Center for Thyroid Eye Disease and
  Orbital Surgery
Department of Ophthalmology
Massachusetts Eye and Ear Infirmary
Harvard Medical School
Boston, Massachusetts

**Paul A. Gardner, MD**
Associate Professor
Co-Director, Center for Cranial Base Surgery
Departments of Neurological Surgery and Otolaryngology
University of Pittsburgh Medical Center
University of Pittsburgh School of Medicine
Pittsburgh, Pennsylvania

**Jordan T. Glicksman, MD**
Otolaryngology/Ear, Nose & Throat
North Shore Ear, Nose and Throat Associates
Beverly Hospital
Beverly, Massachusetts

**Richard J. Harvey, MD, PhD, FRACS**
Professor and Program Head
Rhinology and Skull Base Research Group
Applied Medical Research Centre
University of New South Wales
Faculty of Medicine and Health Sciences
Macquarie University
Sydney, Australia

**Nahyoung Grace Lee, MD**
Assistant Professor
Ophthalmic Plastic and Reconstructive Surgery
Department of Ophthalmology
Massachusetts Eye and Ear Infirmary
Harvard Medical School
Boston, Massachusetts

**Daniel R. Lefebvre, MD, FACS**
Assistant Professor of Ophthalmology
Harvard Medical School
Ophthalmic Plastic Surgery
Department of Ophthalmology
Massachusetts Eye and Ear Infirmary
Boston, Massachusetts

**Sophie D. Liao, MD**
Assistant Professor, Oculofacial Plastic & Reconstructive
 Surgery
Medical Director, University of Colorado Health Eye Clinics
Department of Ophthalmology
University of Colorado School of Medicine
Aurora, Colorado

**Darlene E. Lubbe, MBChB, FCORL(SA)**
Associate Professor
Division of Otolaryngology–Head and Neck Surgery
Groote Schuur Hospital
University of Cape Town
Cape Town, South Africa

**Valerie J. Lund, CBE**
Professor Emeritus of Rhinology
University College London
Honorary ENT Consultant
Royal National Throat, Nose and Ear Hospital & University
 College London Hospital
London, England, United Kingdom

**Elliott Mappus, MS**
Department of Otolaryngology–Head and Neck Surgery
Medical University of South Carolina
Charleston, South Carolina

**Ralph B. Metson, MD**
Professor
Department of Otolaryngology
Massachusetts Eye and Ear
Harvard Medical School
Boston, Massachusetts

**Kris S. Moe, MD**
Professor and Chief, Division of Facial Plastic Surgery
Departments of Otolaryngology and Neurological Surgery
Chief of Otolaryngology-Head and Neck Surgery,
 Harborview Medical Center
University of Washington School of Medicine
Seattle, Washington

**James N. Palmer, MD**
Professor and Director, Division of Rhinology
Co-Director, Center for Skull Base Surgery
Department of Otorhinolaryngology–Head and
 Neck Surgery
Department of Neurosurgery
University of Pennsylvania
Philadelphia, Pennsylvania

**Alkis J. Psaltis, MBBS, PhD, FRACS**
Associate Professor
Head, Department of Otolaryngology–Head and
 Neck Surgery
The Queen Elizabeth Hospital
Associate Professor, Division of Surgery
University of Adelaide, South Australia
Adelaide, South Australia, Australia

**Saul N. Rajak, PhD, FRCOphth**
Consultant Ophthalmologist and Oculoplastic Surgeon
The Sussex Eye Hospital, Brighton and Sussex University
 Hospital
Honorary Lecturer, Brighton and Sussex Medical School
Brighton, England, United Kingdom

**Vijay R. Ramakrishnan, MD, FARS**
Associate Professor
Co-Director, CU Skull Base Program
Departments of Otolaryngology and Neurosurgery
University of Colorado
Aurora, Colorado

**Katherine L. Reinshagen, MD, FRCPC**
Instructor
Department of Radiology
Massachusetts Eye and Ear Infirmary
Harvard Medical School
Boston, Massachusetts

**Joanne Rimmer, MBBS, FRCS(ORL-HNS), FRACS**
Consultant ENT Surgeon/Rhinologist
Honorary Senior Lecturer
Department of Otolaryngology–Head and Neck Surgery
Monash University
Melbourne, Victoria, Australia

**Jonathan C. P. Roos, MB BChir, PhD (Cantab), FRCOphth**
Director, Polar Skin & Oculoplastics Ltd.
London
Specialist Registrar, National Health Service
Norwich, England, United Kingdom

**Geoffrey E. Rose, MBBS, DSc, MRCP, FRCS, FRCOphth**
Consultant Ophthalmic Surgeon
Adnexal Service, Moorfields Eye Hospital
Honorary Reader in Ophthalmology and Senior Research
  Fellow
NIHR Biomedical Research Centre
UCL Institute of Ophthalmology
Honorary Professor
University of London City University
London, England, United Kingdom

**Raymond Sacks, MBBCH, FRACS, FCS, FARS**
Professor and Chair
Department of Otolaryngology–Head and Neck Surgery
Macquarie University
Clinical Professor and Head of Discipline of Otolaryngology
Sydney University Medical School
Sydney, Australia

**George A. Scangas, MD**
Fellow, Rhinology and Anterior Skull Base Surgery
Department of Otolaryngology–Head and Neck Surgery
Massachusetts Eye and Ear Infirmary
Harvard Medical School
Boston, Massachusetts

**Rodney J. Schlosser, MD**
Professor and Director of Rhinology and Sinus Surgery
Department of Otolaryngology–Head and Neck Surgery
Medical University of South Carolina
Charleston, South Carolina

**Carl H. Snyderman, MD, MBA**
Professor
Co-Director, Center for Cranial Base Surgery
Departments of Otolaryngology and Neurological Surgery
University of Pittsburgh Medical Center
University of Pittsburgh School of Medicine
Pittsburgh, Pennsylvania

**Zachary M. Soler, MD**
Associate Professor
Division of Rhinology and Sinus Surgery
Department of Otolaryngology–Head and Neck Surgery
Medical University of South Carolina
Charleston, South Carolina

**S. Tonya Stefko, MD, FACS**
Associate Professor
Director, Oculoplastic, Aesthetic, and Reconstructive
  Surgery
Departments of Ophthalmology, Otolaryngology,
  and Neurological Surgery
University of Pittsburgh School of Medicine
Pittsburgh, Pennsylvania

**Geoffrey A. Wilcsek, MBBS, FRANZCO**
Director Ocular Plastics Unit
Prince of Wales Hospital
Director Ocular Plastics Unit
Sydney Children's Hospital
Department of Ophthalmology
University of New South Wales
Sydney, Australia

**Natalie Wolkow, MD, PhD**
Fellow, Ophthalmic Plastic and Reconstructive Surgery and
  Ophthalmic Pathology
Department of Ophthalmology
Massachusetts Eye and Ear Infirmary
Harvard Medical School
Boston, Massachusetts

**Michael K. Yoon, MD**
Ophthalmic Plastic Surgery
Department of Ophthalmology
Massachusetts Eye and Ear Infirmary
Harvard Medical School
Boston, Massachusetts

# 1 Anatomy of the Orbit and Paranasal Sinuses

George A. Scangas, Benjamin S. Bleier, and Lora R. Dagi-Glass

## Abstract

The orbit is composed of an array of complex neurovascular and soft-tissue elements that interpolate with a protective bony envelope. The paranasal sinuses further articulate with the bony orbit to form a complex three-dimensional architecture with considerable interpatient variability. The ability to safely address extra- and intraconal pathology is predicated on a deep knowledge of intraorbital anatomy. Similarly, the development of advanced endoscopic approaches to the orbit requires an understanding of the paranasal sinus corridors, which can be exploited to minimize patient morbidity.

*Keywords:* globe, extraocular muscles, ophthalmic artery, optic nerve, eyelid, ethmoid, maxillary, frontal, sphenoid

## 1.1 Anatomy of the Eyelids, Lacrimal System, and Orbit

### 1.1.1 Eyelids

The upper and lower eyelids are anatomically distinct, though analogous. Surgical approaches to the orbit may incorporate various portions of the eyelids, including the upper eyelid crease, lower eyelid conjunctiva, and lateral canthal region (▶ Fig. 1.1).

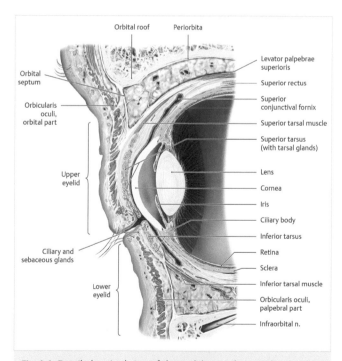

**Fig. 1.1** Detailed sagittal view of the eyelid as it relates to the eye. Note the orbital septum arises from the orbital rim, serving as a landmark dividing the preseptal and orbital space. (Used with permission from Gilroy AM, ed. *Anatomy: An Essential Textbook*. 2nd ed. New York, NY: Thieme; 2017: 485.)

Both the upper and lower eyelids can be conceptually and physically divided into the anterior and posterior lamellae.

### Anterior Lamellae

In both the upper and lower eyelids, the anterior lamellae are composed of skin and orbicularis oculi muscle. Eyelid skin is unique in that there is no underlying subcutaneous fat. The orbicularis muscle is a protractor innervated by cranial nerve VII, allowing for involuntary and voluntary eyelid closure. A continuation of the orbicularis muscle through to the margin of the eyelid is named the muscle of Riolan, more commonly referred to as the "gray line" due to its color.[1]

The eyelid crease is formed from attachments between the anterior and posterior lamellae, namely, fine attachments between the septum, levator aponeurosis, and skin.[1] The varying location of the eyelid crease among ethnic groups is due to differences in anatomic attachment location, but in all cases, an eyelid crease approach is an aesthetically pleasing way to access superior orbital anatomy, including the superomedial orbit.

### Posterior Lamellae

The posterior lamellae differ in the upper and lower eyelids. Both have tarsal plates, a septum, fat pads, retractor muscles that open the eyelids, and conjunctiva. With the exception of the conjunctiva, each of these components is analogous but unique when comparing the upper and lower eyelids.

The tarsus is a dense connective tissue plate, providing structural support to the eyelid. The upper eyelid tarsus measures approximately 10 mm in height, as compared to the lower eyelid tarsus, which is 4 mm. Each tarsal plate is approximately 1 mm thick, and has tapered ends. They are attached to the periorbita through canthal tendons medially and laterally. The medial canthal tendon is split anteriorly and posteriorly to bridge the lacrimal crests, hugging the lacrimal sac, as well as superiorly and inferiorly to reach the respective eyelids. The lateral canthal tendon arises from the lateral orbital tubercle, splitting into superior and inferior components prior to reaching the upper and lower eyelids.[1] Each set of tendons may need to be breached in an external approach to the orbit.

The septum is a thin set of tissue layers arising from the periosteal arcus marginalis at the bony orbital rim. Preservation of the septum prevents fat prolapse into the surgical field. There are two fat pads located between the septum and the levator aponeurosis of the upper eyelid, and three between the septum and the capsulopalpebral fascia of the lower eyelid (▶ Fig. 1.2).[1]

There are two retractor muscles in each of the eyelids. In the upper eyelid, these are the levator palpebrae superioris muscle, including its aponeurotic insertion on the anterior tarsal face, and the more posterior Muller's muscle, also known as the superior tarsal muscle, which inserts at the superior border of the tarsus. Whitnall's ligament is about 4 cm anterior to the orbital apex, and marks the transition of the levator from a horizontal vector posteriorly to a vertical retracting vector

Labels in Fig. 1.1: Orbital roof, Periorbita, Levator palpebrae superioris, Superior rectus, Superior conjunctival fornix, Superior tarsal muscle, Superior tarsus (with tarsal glands), Lens, Cornea, Iris, Ciliary body, Inferior tarsus, Retina, Sclera, Inferior tarsal muscle, Orbicularis oculi, palpebral part, Infraorbital n., Orbital septum, Orbicularis oculi, orbital part, Upper eyelid, Ciliary and sebaceous glands, Lower eyelid

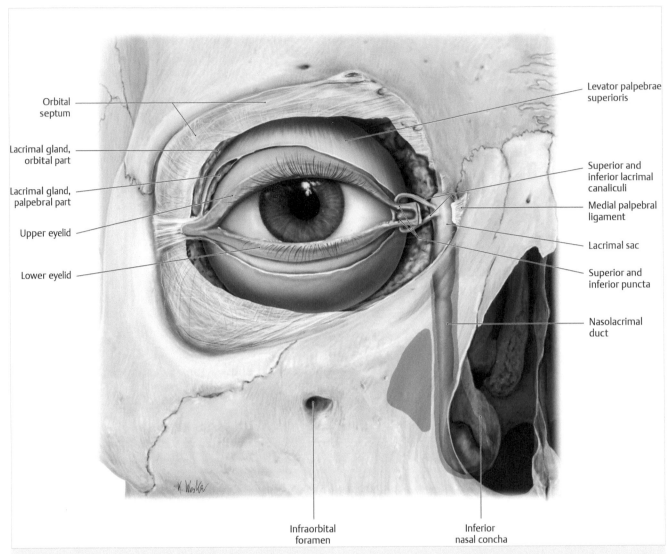

**Fig. 1.2** View of the nasolacrimal system in relation to the eyelids and the nose. While the puncta are located on the medial eyelid margin, the lacrimal sac sits more posteriorly between the split medial canthal tendons. The nasolacrimal duct runs inferiorly in a posteromedial direction, opening in the inferior meatus of the nose. (Used with permission from Gilroy AM, ed. *Anatomy: An Essential Textbook*. 2nd ed. New York, NY: Thieme; 2017: 486.)

anteriorly. Muller's muscle originates around the area of Whitnall's ligament. In the lower eyelid, the retractor muscles are named the capsulopalpebral fascia and the inferior tarsal muscle. The capsulopalpebral fascia originates along the inferior rectus muscle and wraps around the inferior oblique muscle as it is traced anteriorly. As the capsulopalpebral fascial arms fuse anterior to the inferior oblique muscle, they form a fibrous condensation called Lockwood's ligament. Muller's muscle and the inferior tarsal muscle are sympathetically innervated, whereas the levator palpebrae superioris muscle and capsulopalpebral fascia are innervated by cranial nerve III.[1]

The conjunctiva is a nonkeratinizing, squamous epithelial layer coating the most posterior aspect of each eyelid, traveling to create superior and inferior fornices between the eyelids and the globe, and finally covering the ocular surface. The transconjunctival surgical approach in the lower eyelid allows for excellent access to the orbital floor and medial orbital wall.[1]

## Eyelid Margin

The eyelid margin is the terminating platform of the upper and lower eyelids. The anterior and posterior lamellar classification system continues in this region. The gray line denotes the orbicularis muscle, allowing for the anatomic distinction between the lamellae. The cilia, or eyelashes, arise anterior to the gray line and exit along the anterior margin, while the oil-excreting meibomian glands are embedded within the tarsus itself, which is posterior to the gray line.[1] Surgical approaches disrupting the eyelid margin require careful realignment of the margin tissue.

## Vascular System

The eyelids are highly vascular. The arterial supply is indirectly derived from both the internal and external carotid branches. The external carotid artery supplies the angular and temporal arteries, and the internal carotid artery supplies the ophthalmic artery with its multiple branches. The two arterial supplies anastomose via the marginal arcades tracking the eyelid margins, and the upper eyelid peripheral arcade, seated just above the tarsus between the levator aponeurosis and Muller's muscle. Since arterial bleeds can track behind the septum and cause retrobulbar hemorrhage, surgeons must pay close attention to hemostasis during any surgical manipulation behind the septum.[1]

Venous drainage from the anterior lamellae exits along the facial veins, whereas the posterior lamellae drain into the orbital veins. Patterns of lymphatic drainage of the eyelids are variable, but are generally divided into medial and lateral eyelids; the medial eyelids drain into the submandibular lymph nodes, whereas the lateral eyelids drain into the preauricular lymph nodes.[1]

## 1.1.2 Nasolacrimal System

The nasolacrimal system serves to drain the tear film that coats and protects the eye. It has a number of components, each of which must work in order for the system as a whole to function. Disruption or blockage of any component can result in tearing or infection (▶ Fig. 1.2).

### Puncta

In both the upper and lower eyelids, a round hole, the punctum, can be found in the medial-most aspect of the eyelid. Eyelid opening and closing cause both negative and positive pressure forces, pushing tears into the puncta and through the canalicular system. The inferior punctum is believed to allow for the majority of tear drainage.[2] For this reason, surgeons may choose the upper punctum for fiberoptic light source visualization of the lacrimal sac during endoscopic dacryocystorhinostomy.

### Canaliculi

Each punctum is contiguous with a canaliculus, which is lined with nonkeratinized squamous epithelium. The canaliculi first travel vertically for 2 mm prior to an 8-mm horizontal path. Understanding this anatomy is crucial when attempting to intubate the canalicular system so as to prevent false passages. The majority of upper and lower canaliculi meet in a common canaliculus prior to reaching the lacrimal sac. The valve of Rosenmüller helps prevent lacrimal sac reflux at this point.[2] Wide marsupialization of this valve into the nasal cavity is critical to the success of endoscopic dacryocystorhinostomy.

### Lacrimal Sac

The lacrimal sac sits in the orbit between the two arms of the medial canthal tendon, which attach to the anterior and posterior lacrimal crests on either side of the lacrimal sac fossa. The lacrimal sac is approximately 13 to 15 mm in length and is contiguous with the nasolacrimal duct. Its fundus rises approximately 3 to 5 mm above the medial canthal tendon.[2] Dacryocystorhinostomy anastomoses the lacrimal sac with the nasal mucosa of the lateral nasal wall of the middle meatus, bypassing an obstructed nasolacrimal duct.

### Nasolacrimal Duct

The nasolacrimal duct is approximately 15 mm in length and opens into the nose under the inferior turbinate. The valve of Hasner lies at the inferior end and is often a cause of congenital nasolacrimal obstruction.[2]

The lacrimal sac and nasolacrimal duct follow the bony anatomy of their respective sites, traveling inferiorly in a posterolateral direction.[2]

## 1.1.3 Orbit

The orbit is composed of soft tissues and bones. The orbit serves to protect and animate the eye, as well as to provide sensation and vascularity to the periocular tissues.

### Bony Anatomy

The bony orbit is considered to have a floor, roof, medial wall, and lateral wall (▶ Fig. 1.3). The height of the skeletal entrance is 35 mm and the width is 40 mm. The orbital volume is approximately 30 cm³.[3]

The orbital roof is composed of the frontal bone and the lesser wing of the sphenoid bone. It houses the lacrimal gland

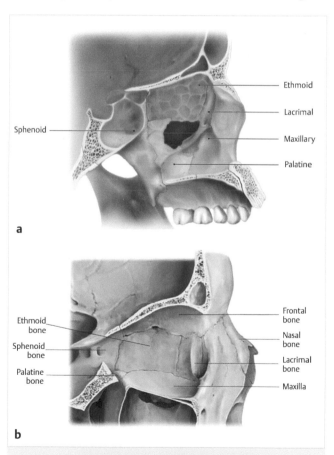

**Fig. 1.3** Medial (**a**) and lateral (**b**) views of the bony orbit. The superior orbital fissure is formed in the space between the greater and lesser wings of the sphenoid. The optic canal lies medial to the superior orbital fissure, in the lesser wing of the sphenoid. (Part **b** used with permission from Schuenke M, Schulte E, Schumacher U, eds. Head and Neuroanatomy: Thieme Atlas of Anatomy. New York, NY: Thieme 2007:14.)

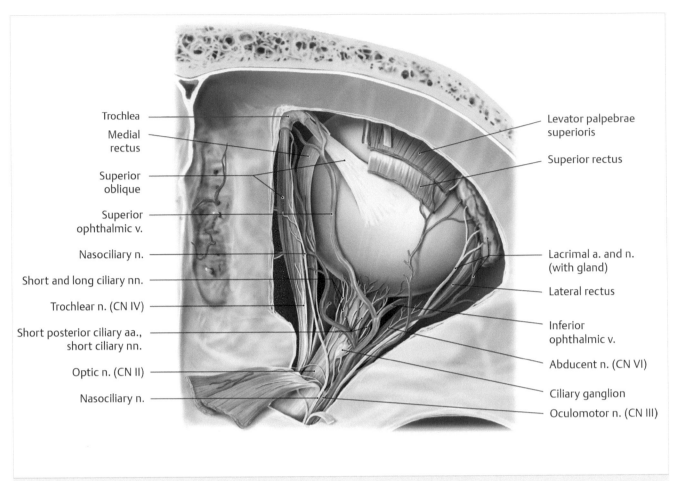

Trochlea

Medial rectus

Superior oblique

Superior ophthalmic v.

Nasociliary n.

Short and long ciliary nn.

Trochlear n. (CN IV)

Short posterior ciliary aa., short ciliary nn.

Optic n. (CN II)

Nasociliary n.

Levator palpebrae superioris

Superior rectus

Lacrimal a. and n. (with gland)

Lateral rectus

Inferior ophthalmic v.

Abducent n. (CN VI)

Ciliary ganglion

Oculomotor n. (CN III)

**Fig. 1.4** A superior view of the orbit, with the roof and periorbita selectively removed, and the levator palpebrae superioris and superior rectus muscles transected and reflected. Note the location of the trochlea in the anterior superomedial orbit, the medial course of the superior oblique and medial rectus muscles, the medial course of the superior ophthalmic vein and branches of the ophthalmic artery, and the ease of accidental approach to the optic nerve in the posteromedial orbit. (Used with permission from Gilroy AM, MacPherson B, Ross L, Atlas of Anatomy. 2nd ed. New York, NY: Thieme; 2012: 543.)

fossa superotemporally. The trochlea is found 5 mm behind the superonasal orbital rim (▶ Fig. 1.4). The superior oblique's mechanism of action is formed through its trochlear attachment at this point. Additionally, the supraorbital notch or foramen can be found superomedially on the orbital rim; the supraorbital neovascular bundle exits the orbit at this point.[3]

The medial wall is composed of the lesser wing of the sphenoid, ethmoid, lacrimal, and maxillary bones, and is 45 mm in anteroposterior length. The frontoethmoidal suture is a landmark for the general region of the cribriform plate. The anterior and posterior ethmoidal arteries are found approximately 25 and 35 mm posterior to the orbital rim, respectively, serving as important landmarks of distance to critical orbital apex structures; additionally, surgical manipulation superior to these arteries may lead to intracranial penetration.[3]

The orbital floor is composed of the zygomatic, maxillary, and palatine bones. As it ends at the pterygopalatine fossa, rather than the orbital apex, it is the shortest of the four walls. The orbital process of the palatine bone may obstruct medial access to the orbital apex and is typically drilled away during an endoscopic approach. The infraorbital groove and canal are found along the medial aspect of the floor and carry cranial nerve V2.[3] This location is of significance in orbital floor fracture repair and decompression surgery.

Finally, the lateral wall is composed of the zygomatic and greater wing of the sphenoid bones.[3] The zygomaticotemporal and zygomaticofacial neurovascular bundles pierce this strongest of the orbital walls and are significant landmarks in lateral orbital wall decompressions.

The superior orbital fissure is found between the greater and lesser wings of the sphenoid bone, and carries cranial nerves III, IV, V1, and VI, sympathetic nerve fibers, and the superior ophthalmic vein. The inferior orbital fissure carries the inferior ophthalmic vein and a branch of cranial nerve V2 (▶ Fig. 1.5).[3]

The optic canal is of significant import, carrying the optic nerve and ophthalmic artery. It is found in the lesser wing of the sphenoid and is 8 to 10 mm in length. The sphenoid sinus lies adjacent to the medial wall of the optic canal.[3]

The periosteum of the orbital bones is called the periorbita. Within the orbital apex, it fuses with the dura of the optic nerve. Anteriorly, it transitions as the arcus marginalis, at the junction with the orbital septum.[3]

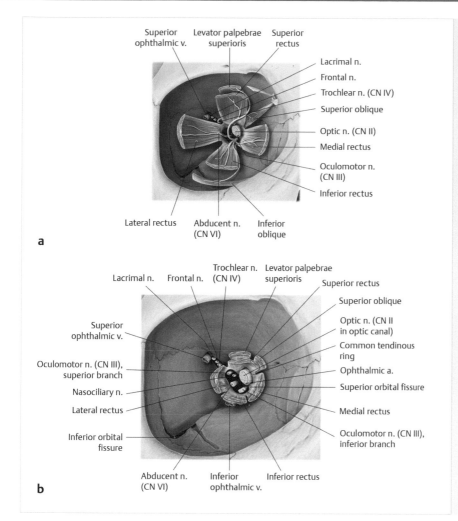

**Fig. 1.5 (a)** The orbital apex and extraocular muscle origins are shown. Note the four rectus muscles, superior oblique muscle, and levator palpebrae superioris muscle arising from the apex; all but the levator palpebrae superioris muscles are attached to the annulus of Zinn. The optic nerve enters the optic canal through the annulus of Zinn. In contrast, the inferior oblique muscle arises from the more anteromedial orbit. **(b)** With further resection of the muscles, the superior and inferior ophthalmic veins are found traversing the superior and inferior orbital fissures, respectively. In the superior orbital fissure region superolateral to the annulus of Zinn, cranial nerve IV and the lacrimal and frontal branches of V1 enter the orbit. Cranial nerves II, III, the nasociliary branch of V1, and VI enter the orbit through the annulus of Zinn. (Used with permission from Gilroy AM, MacPherson B, Ross L, Atlas of Anatomy. 2nd ed. New York, NY: Thieme; 2012: 501, 542).

## Soft Tissues of the Orbit

### Globe

The eyeball, or globe, is found within the central anterior aspect of the orbit. The globe contains approximately 6.5 mL of volume and has an anteroposterior diameter of approximately 25 mm (▶ Fig. 1.4).

### Optic Nerve

The optic nerve is the second cranial nerve, traveling from the globe through the orbit and optic canal to form the chiasm. The orbital segment is approximately 25 to 30 mm in length, with a diameter of 4 mm. Since the distance it travels to the optic canal is 18 mm, the nerve has 7 to 12 mm of redundancy.[3] Knowing the location of the optic nerve in relation to orbital pathology is critical when considering surgical approaches.

### Muscle

Six muscles move each globe. The four rectus muscles are found in the cardinal directions, and are labeled as such: superior, medial, inferior, and lateral. These four originate in the orbital apex in the fibrous annulus of Zinn, a circular structure dividing the superior orbital fissure and encapsulating the entrance of the optic nerve into the optic canal. The remaining two are the inferior and superior oblique muscles. While the superior oblique also originates from the annulus of Zinn, the inferior originates from the anteromedial orbital wall, thus proving important when entering the medial orbit, performing a dacryocystorhinostomy or repairing a medial wall fracture. In addition to the six muscles of movement, the aforementioned levator palpebrae superioris muscle arises above the annulus of Zinn, on the lesser wing of the sphenoid (▶ Fig. 1.5).[3]

### Lacrimal Gland

The lacrimal gland is a bilobed structure split by the levator palpebrae superioris aponeurosis into orbital and palpebral lobes. It lies within the lacrimal gland fossa of the frontal bone, in the superolateral orbit.[3]

### Fat

Orbital fat surrounds the orbital structures.[3] Fine septations divide the orbital fat into compartments. Navigating through orbital fat intraoperatively can be quite challenging. In cases of retrobulbar hemorrhage, a compartment syndrome can result in elevated intraocular pressure and devastating vision loss. ▶ Fig. 1.1 and ▶ Fig. 1.2 demonstrate some orbital fat, but for clarity of view, ▶ Fig. 1.4, ▶ Fig. 1.5, ▶ Fig. 1.6 are shown with orbital fat removed.

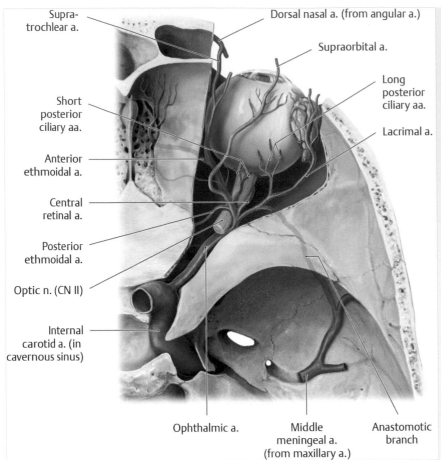

Supra-trochlear a.

Dorsal nasal a. (from angular a.)

Supraorbital a.

Short posterior ciliary aa.

Long posterior ciliary aa.

Lacrimal a.

Anterior ethmoidal a.

Central retinal a.

Posterior ethmoidal a.

Optic n. (CN II)

Internal carotid a. (in cavernous sinus)

Ophthalmic a.

Middle meningeal a. (from maxillary a.)

Anastomotic branch

**Fig. 1.6** A superior view of the arterial orbital anatomy. Note the extensive arterial tree arising from the internal carotid artery, which ultimately anastomoses with branches of the external carotid artery, demonstrated here with the dorsal nasal artery and middle meningeal artery. (Used with permission from Gilroy AM, MacPherson B, Ross L, Atlas of Anatomy. 2nd ed. New York, NY: Thieme; 2012: 540.)

## Nerves

Multiple cranial nerves enter and exit the orbit (► Fig. 1.4 and ► Fig. 1.5). Cranial nerves III (oculomotor nerve), IV (trochlear nerve), V1 (trigeminal nerve), and VI (abducens nerve) enter via the superior orbital fissure; a branch of cranial nerve V2 enters via the inferior orbital fissure. Cranial nerve III divides into superior and inferior branches; the superior branch innervates the superior rectus and levator palpebrae superioris muscles, while the inferior branch innervates the inferior and medial recti and inferior oblique muscles. The innervation pathways of the inferior division of cranial nerve III may lie within the surgical field during an endoscopic approach to the medial intraconal space and will be further discussed in Chapter 14. Cranial nerve IV innervates the superior oblique muscle. Cranial nerve VI innervates the lateral rectus muscle. Cranial nerve V1 splits into three branches: frontal, lacrimal, and nasociliary. The frontal branch gives rise to the supratrochlear and supraorbital nerves, the lacrimal branch provides afferent innervation to the lacrimal gland, and the nasociliary branch innervates the anterior globe structures and the nose. Cranial nerve V2 travels anteriorly, becoming the infraorbital nerve.[3]

Parasympathetic nerves of the orbit travel along cranial nerve III before synapsing in the lateral intraconal ciliary ganglion, ultimately innervating muscles of ocular accommodation and pupillary constriction. Another set of parasympathetic nerves derived from cranial nerve VII provide efferent innervation to the lacrimal gland. The sympathetic nerves enter via the superior orbital fissure and serve to dilate the pupil and innervate smooth muscles of the eyelid and orbit such as Muller's muscle.[4]

## Vascular System

The orbital arterial vascular supply is derived from the ophthalmic artery, which in turn is derived from the internal carotid artery (► Fig. 1.6). The ophthalmic artery branches include the vasculature of the globe (posterior ciliary and central retinal arteries), the extraocular muscles, the anterior and posterior ethmoidal arteries, the lacrimal artery, and the supraorbital and supratrochlear arteries. The inferomedial muscular trunk of the ophthalmic artery generally supplies the inferior rectus, medial rectus, and inferior oblique muscles. Branches of this trunk cross the medial intraconal space dividing it into several zones where tumors may arise and will be discussed in greater detail in Chapter 14. Surgical arterial disruption can cause blinding retrobulbar hemorrhage or ischemic syndromes. There are significant arterial anastomoses with branches of the external carotid artery.[3]

The superior ophthalmic vein travels through the superior orbital fissure, ultimately draining into the cavernous sinus. The inferior ophthalmic vein travels through the inferior orbital fissure, ultimately draining into the pterygopalatine fossa (► Fig. 1.5).[3] Fistulas between the cavernous sinus and the internal carotid artery or its branches may arise sporadically or due to trauma.

# 1.2 Paranasal Sinus Anatomy

## 1.2.1 Embryology

A thorough understanding of embryology is imperative to grasp the complex anatomic relationships between sinonasal structures and the orbit. In the sixth week of gestation, the nasal pits (also known as olfactory pits) become increasingly deepened. Each pit is separated from the oral cavity by the oronasal membrane.[5,6] Gradual breakdown of this oronasal membrane over weeks 6 to 9 leads to the formation of the primitive choanae, which gradually move posterior as the secondary palate develops. The ectodermal epithelium at the roof of the nasal pit thickens and differentiates into the olfactory bulb.[5,6]

Paranasal sinuses develop as diverticula of the lateral nasal wall in utero during primary pneumatization and continue to grow after birth via secondary pneumatization until maximum size is achieved during puberty (▶ Fig. 1.7). Each sinus is derived from an invagination of ciliated, pseudostratified, columnar epithelium, known as a primordium, on the lateral nasal wall. The variable degree of pneumatization results in an irregular collection of spaces that are lined with respiratory mucosa and form physical connections to the nasal cavity.[7]

## 1.2.2 Ethmoid Air Cells

The ethmoids consist of 5 to 15 paired air cells on either side of the septum. The ethmoid bone is often referred to as a labyrinth of a critical collection of cells through which all of the paranasal sinus drainage pathways course.[8] The primary roles of the ethmoids are to increase the surface area of the mucosa and absorb trauma by providing a crush zone, which protects the eyes and the brain.

By the 70th day of gestation, six major furrows and corresponding ridges form in the lateral nasal wall.[7] The ridges, also known as ethmoturbinals as they arise from the ethmoid, are separated into the ramus ascendens and ramus descendens. From the seventh month of gestation to birth, many of the ethmoturbinals either fuse with adjacent ridges or become obliterated, resulting in only two or three persistent ethmoturbinals (middle, superior, and

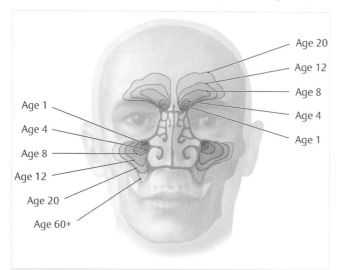

**Fig. 1.7** Paranasal sinus pneumatization with age. (Used with permission from Gilroy AM, MacPherson B, Ross L, Atlas of Anatomy. 2nd ed. New York, NY: Thieme; 2012: 552.)

supreme conchae).[7,9] The ramus descendens and ascendens of the first ethmoturbinal form the uncinate process and the agger nasi cell, respectively. The first furrow (space between the first and second ethmoturbinals) becomes the ethmoid infundibulum and the frontal recess.[6,7] Structures of the ethmoid derived from the ethmoturbinals are attached to the lateral nasal wall via bony partitions known as basal lamellae.[10]

## 1.2.3 Osteomeatal Complex

The osteomeatal complex (OMC) represents the area on the lateral nasal wall that drains the anterior ethmoid cells, frontal sinus, and maxillary sinus. Importantly, it is an anatomically constricted area that can become obstructed, leading to blockage of the natural sinus drainage pathways and chronic rhinosinusitis.[8,10] This anatomic area is bounded by the middle turbinate medially, the lamina papyracea laterally, and the basal lamella superiorly and posteriorly.[8] Individual components of the OMC have important anatomic relationships to the orbit and surrounding sinonasal drainage pathways (▶ Fig. 1.8).

### Uncinate Process

The uncinate process is a thin bony structure that is the most anterior lamellae. It is continuous with the ethmoid bone anteriorly and may have one of three attachment points: the lamina papyracea, the skull base, or the middle turbinate.[11] Close proximity of the uncinate process to the lamina papyracea can predispose to inadvertent orbital injury.[12]

### Ethmoidal Infundibulum and Hiatus Semilunaris

The ethmoidal infundibulum is a three-dimensional space that accepts drainage from the maxillary, anterior ethmoid sinuses, and occasionally the frontal sinus depending on the attachment site of the uncinate process.[10] It is bordered by the uncinate process medially, the medial lamina papyracea laterally, the frontal recess superiorly, and the maxillary sinus ostium inferiorly.[8] The hiatus semilunaris is a two-dimensional space between the lateral/inferior surface of the bulla ethmoidalis and the superior surface of the uncinate, which connects the infundibulum to the middle meatus.[10]

### Bulla Ethmoidalis and Retrobullar Recess

The lateral extension of the second lamellae forms the bulla ethmoidalis,[6] which normally consists of a single, variable air cell that projects over the hiatus semilunaris inferiorly and medially.[13] Often, the ethmoidal bulla has a posterior surface, and in those cases the space between the bulla ethmoidalis and the basal lamella is known as the retrobullar recess or the sinus lateralis. This space can communicate with the suprabullar recess, which is a cleft that is bounded by the superior surface of the ethmoidal bulla inferiorly, the orbit laterally, and the fovea ethmoidalis superiorly.[14]

# 1.3 Basal Lamella

The basal lamella, derived from the third lamella, marks the boundary between the anterior and posterior ethmoid cells. Aside from its clinical significance as a boundary to the spread of infection into

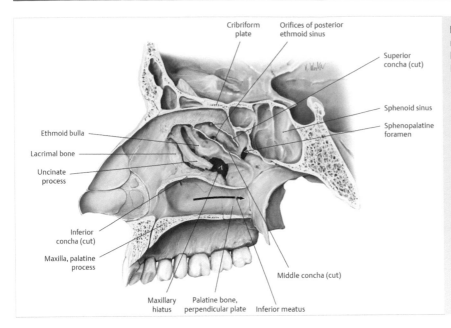

Fig. 1.8 Paranasal sinus anatomy of the lateral nasal wall. (Used with permission from Gilroy AM, MacPherson B, Ross L, Atlas of Anatomy. 2nd ed. New York, NY: Thieme; 2012: 551.)

the posterior ethmoids, the basal lamella attaches to the lateral nasal wall and is an important landmark for posterior ethmoid surgery and access to the lamina papyracea and medial orbit.[15]

## 1.4 Middle Turbinate

The middle turbinate is embryologically derived from the ethmoid bone[5] and can be divided into three segments. The anterior third attaches superiorly at the skull base at the horizontal plate of the ethmoid bone lateral to the cribriform. The middle segment, known as the basal lamella, attaches to the lamina papyracea. The posterior third attaches inferiorly in a horizontal plane onto the palatine bone. This attachment site lies just anterior to the sphenopalatine foramen and serves as a useful anatomic landmark.[16] In addition to the importance of the basal lamella as a landmark for endoscopic orbital surgery, the anterior insertion of the middle turbinate is located just posterior to the lacrimal sac and can help guide the surgeon during endoscopic dacryocystorhinostomy.[17,18]

## 1.5 Superior Turbinate and Sphenoethmoidal Recess

The superior turbinate is situated posterior to the middle turbinate and remains an important anatomic landmark for identification of the sphenoid sinus ostium. The sphenoethmoidal recess is the narrow, vertically oriented space bounded medially by the nasal septum, laterally by the superior turbinate, and superiorly by the cribriform plate, which serves as the natural drainage pathway for both the sphenoid ostium and the posterior ethmoid cells.[10]

## 1.6 Onodi Cell

An Onodi cell is a posterior ethmoidal cell that pneumatizes posterior, lateral, and superior to the sphenoid rostrum and has crucial anatomic implications in endoscopic sinus surgery and orbital surgery.[10] First, the presence of an Onodi cell means that the sphenoid sinus will be in a more inferior and medial position, which increases the risk of skull base injury as normally a surgeon would expect the sphenoid sinus to be behind the last posterior ethmoid cell. Second, the optic nerve can often be dehiscent in a lateral Onodi cell, increasing the chance of injury. Finally, to access the orbital apex, the lateral sphenoid face must be removed up to the lamina papyracea, a task that is rendered more difficult by the anatomic distortion caused by an Onodi cell.[19]

## 1.7 Maxillary Sinus and Haller's Cells

The maxillary sinus lies inferior to the orbit in the maxillary bone and is the largest and first paranasal sinus to develop (▶ Fig. 1.9). It pneumatizes and grows in a biphasic pattern (at years 0–3 and 6–12).[6] The infraorbital nerve runs through the infraorbital canal along the roof of the maxillary sinus, which is also the floor of the orbit. The posterior wall of the maxillary sinus is an important surgical landmark. Just posterior to the wall lies the pterygopalatine fossa. The sphenopalatine artery traverses this fossa and enters the nasal cavity at the sphenopalatine foramen.[8] The Haller cell, or infraorbital cell, is an anterior ethmoid cell located below the inferior orbital wall. A Haller cell can increase the surgical complexity of maxillary antrostomy. Failure to differentiate between a Haller cell and the orbital floor can result in orbital injury.[20]

## 1.8 Sphenoid Sinus

Understanding the anatomy of the lateral wall of the sphenoid sinus remains crucial in endoscopic orbital surgery. From superior to inferior, the lateral wall contains the prominences of the optic nerve, the internal carotid artery, and the maxillary and mandibular divisions of the trigeminal nerve. Between these prominences are bony depressions including the lateral opticocarotid recess, the depression between the cavernous sinus apex and the

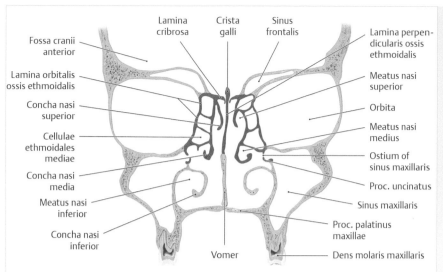

Fossa cranii
anterior

Lamina orbitalis
ossis ethmoidalis

Concha nasi
superior

Cellulae
ethmoidales
mediae

Concha nasi
media

Meatus nasi
inferior

Concha nasi
inferior

Lamina
cribrosa

Crista
galli

Sinus
frontalis

Vomer

Lamina perpen-
dicularis ossis
ethmoidalis

Meatus nasi
superior

Orbita

Meatus nasi
medius

Ostium of
sinus maxillaris

Proc. uncinatus

Sinus maxillaris

Proc. palatinus
maxillae

Dens molaris maxillaris

**Fig. 1.9** Cross sectional bony anatomy of the paranasal sinuses and their relationship to the bony orbit. (Used with permission from Gilroy AM, MacPherson B, Ross L, Atlas of Anatomy. 2nd ed. New York, NY: Thieme; 2012: 553.)

maxillary nerve, and the depression between the maxillary and mandibular divisions of the trigeminal nerve.[21] Up to 25% of patients can have dehiscence over these critical structures in the lateral sphenoid sinus wall.[22] The opticocarotid recess has been labeled the anatomic keyhole in endoscopic skull base surgery.[23]

# 1.9 Arterial Blood Supply and Anatomy

The nasal cavity and sinuses are supplied by both the internal and external carotid arteries. The anterior ethmoidal artery and posterior ethmoidal artery, branches off of the ophthalmic artery, travel across the orbit and enter the nasal cavity through the lamina papyracea. The anterior ethmoidal artery runs across the skull base and branches into smaller arteries to supply the cribriform plate and superior nasal septum. While normally contained within the skull base, in approximately 14 to 43% of cases the artery is dehiscent, rendering it more vulnerable to injury.[24] After piercing the lamina papyracea, the posterior ethmoidal artery courses through the posterior ethmoid cells parallel to the optic nerve as it nears the orbital apex. Vision loss and orbital hematoma can result from damage to either of these vessels. The external carotid artery supplies the nasal cavity via the sphenopalatine artery. This artery passes through the pterygopalatine fossa through the sphenopalatine foramen and into the nasal cavity just posterior to the posterior wall of the maxillary sinus.

# References

[1] Holds JB, Chang WJ, Durairaj VD, et al, eds. Facial and eyelid anatomy. In: Orbit, Eyelids, and Lacrimal System 2. Singapore: American Academy of Ophthalmology; 2011:131–141

[2] Holds JB, Chang WJ, Durairaj VD, et al, eds. Development, anatomy, and physiology of the lacrimal secretory and drainage systems. In: Orbit, Eyelids, and Lacrimal System 2. Singapore: American Academy of Ophthalmology; 2011:243–246

[3] Holds JB, Chang WJ, Durairaj VD, et al, eds. Orbital anatomy. In: Orbit, Eyelids, and Lacrimal System. Singapore: American Academy of Ophthalmology; 2011:5–17

[4] Dutton JJ, ed. Atlas of Clinical and Surgical Orbital Anatomy. Philadelphia, PA: W.B. Saunders Company; 1994

[5] Sadler TW, Langman J. Langman's Medical Embryology. 13th ed. Philadelphia, PA: Wolters Kluwer; 2015

[6] Halewyck S, Louryan S, Van Der Veken P, Gordts F. Craniofacial embryology and postnatal development of relevant parts of the upper respiratory system. B-ENT. 2012; 8 Suppl 19:5–11

[7] Chang C, Incaudo G, Gershwin E. Diseases of the Sinuses. New York, NY: Springer; 2014

[8] Davis WE, Templer J, Parsons DS. Anatomy of the paranasal sinuses. Otolaryngol Clin North Am. 1996; 29(1):57–74

[9] Kainz J, Stammberger H. Danger areas of the posterior nasal base: anatomical, histological and endoscopic findings. Laryngorhinootologie. 1991; 70(9):479–486

[10] Stammberger HR, Kennedy DW, Anatomic Terminology Group. Paranasal sinuses: anatomic terminology and nomenclature. Ann Otol Rhinol Laryngol Suppl. 1995; 167:7–16

[11] Woo KI, Maeng H-S, Kim Y-D. Characteristics of intranasal structures for endonasal dacryocystorhinostomy in Asians. Am J Ophthalmol. 2011; 152(3): 491–498.e1

[12] Vaid S, Vaid N. Normal anatomy and anatomic variants of the paranasal sinuses on computed tomography. Neuroimaging Clin N Am. 2015; 25(4):527–548

[13] Laine FJ, Smoker WR. The ostiomeatal unit and endoscopic surgery: anatomy, variations, and imaging findings in inflammatory diseases. AJR Am J Roentgenol. 1992; 159(4):849–857

[14] Shams PN, Wormald PJ, Selva D. Anatomical landmarks of the lateral nasal wall: implications for endonasal lacrimal surgery. Curr Opin Ophthalmol. 2015; 26(5):408–415

[15] Wang Y, Xiao L, Li Y, Yan H, Yu X, Su F. Endoscopic transethmoidal resection of medial orbital lesions. Zhonghua Yan Ke Za Zhi. 2015; 51(8):569–575

[16] Nurse LA, Duncavage JA. Surgery of the inferior and middle turbinates. Otolaryngol Clin North Am. 2009; 42(2):295–309, ix

[17] Wormald PJ, Kew J, Van Hasselt A. Intranasal anatomy of the nasolacrimal sac in endoscopic dacryocystorhinostomy. Otolaryngol Head Neck Surg. 2000; 123(3):307–310

[18] Rebeiz EE, Shapshay SM, Bowlds JH, Pankratov MM. Anatomic guidelines for dacryocystorhinostomy. Laryngoscope. 1992; 102(10):1181–1184

[19] Kenyon B, Antisdel JL. Anatomic evaluation of endoscopic transnasal transorbital approach to the lateral orbital apex. Am J Rhinol Allergy. 2014; 28(1):82–85

[20] Stackpole SA, Edelstein DR. The anatomic relevance of the Haller cell in sinusitis. Am J Rhinol. 1997; 11(3):219–223

[21] Anusha B, Baharudin A, Philip R, Harvinder S, Shaffie BM. Anatomical variations of the sphenoid sinus and its adjacent structures: a review of existing literature. Surg Radiol Anat. 2014; 36(5):419–427

[22] Anand VK, Schwartz TH. Practical Endoscopic Skull Base Surgery. San Diego, CA: Plural Publishing; 2008

[23] Kassam A, Snyderman CH, Mintz A, Gardner P, Carrau RL. Expanded endonasal approach: the rostrocaudal axis. Part I. Crista galli to the sella turcica. Neurosurg Focus. 2005; 19(1):E3

[24] Moon HJ, Kim HU, Lee JG, Chung IH, Yoon JH. Surgical anatomy of the anterior ethmoidal canal in ethmoid roof. Laryngoscope. 2001; 111(5):900–904

# 2 Anatomy, Physiology, and Treatment of the Tearing Adult

*Natalie Wolkow and Michael K. Yoon*

**Abstract**

Watery and tearing eyes may cause significant interference with activities of daily living and social interactions in adult patients. The causes of watery eyes are many, encompassing dry eyes, eyelid dysfunction, ocular injury, and tear drainage abnormalities. In this chapter, the anatomy and physiology of tear production and tear drainage are reviewed. The signs and symptoms of tearing are discussed, and treatment options are described with an emphasis on endoscopic dacryocystorhinostomy.

*Keywords:* tearing, epiphora, watery eye, dacryocystorhinostomy

## 2.1 Introduction

Tears are essential for normal visual function and the maintenance of a healthy ocular surface. They form a complex liquid layer that coats the ocular mucous membranes and the cornea, contributing to the refractive visual function of the cornea, as well as providing nutrients to the avascular cornea and protection against foreign material. Under ideal circumstances, there is equal production of tears, via the lacrimal glands and accessory lacrimal glands, and elimination of tears, via evaporation and the lacrimal drainage system, maintaining a healthy ocular state. Many factors, however, may tip this balance in one direction or the other, resulting in ocular surface dryness or in excessive tearing and epiphora.

Tearing, when excessive tears pool on the ocular surface, and epiphora, when tears overrun the ocular margin and pour down onto the face, occur if there is either overproduction or insufficient drainage of tears. Although tearing and epiphora may seem trivial, they cause significant morbidity and patient discomfort, interfering with daily activities such as driving and reading, causing periocular skin irritation and infection, as well as disruption in social interactions. Appropriate treatment and

resolution of tearing may be challenging, and determining the appropriate course of action requires a detailed history, careful examination of the eye and lacrimal system, and experience in deciding which medications or procedures will alleviate the problem. In this chapter, we review the normal anatomy and physiology of the lacrimal system, discuss the relevant examination and testing, and conclude with the currently available treatments and their indications.

## 2.2 Anatomy of Tear Production

Tears are produced by both the lacrimal gland and accessory lacrimal glands. There is a basal production rate of approximately 1.2 µL/min, which may increase by over 500% when reflex or emotional tearing are triggered by ocular irritants or emotional states.[1]

### 2.2.1 Lacrimal Gland

The lacrimal gland is responsible for producing over 90% of the tear volume. It is located in the anterior superotemporal orbit and is composed of two lobes: the palpebral lobe (smaller, more anterior and inferior) and the orbital lobe (larger, more posterior and superior; ▶ Fig. 2.1). This gland is composed of secretory acini, which empty tears into 8 to 12 major ducts. The lacrimal gland is innervated by both cranial nerve (CN) V and CN VII, which form part of the reflex tearing arc, as well as by parasympathetic and sympathetic nerve fibers.[2,3]

### 2.2.2 Accessory Lacrimal Glands

The accessory lacrimal glands of Krause and Wolfring are nearly identical in structure to the main lacrimal gland; however, they are smaller and are klocated within the substantia propria of the conjunctiva. There are approximately 20 glands of Krause in the superior conjunctival fornix and 6 to 8 in the lower fornix.

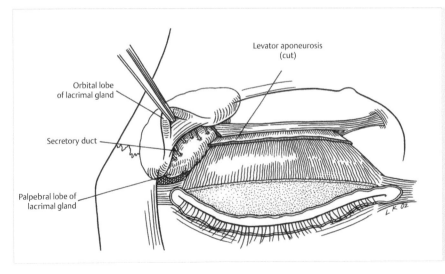

Fig. 2.1 Anatomy of the right lacrimal gland. The accessory lacrimal glands of Krause and Wolfring are not illustrated. (Adapted with permission from Wobig J, Dailey R, eds. *Oculofacial Plastic Surgery*. New York, NY: Thieme; 2004: 131.)

Levator aponeurosis (cut)

Orbital lobe of lacrimal gland

Secretory duct

Palpebral lobe of lacrimal gland

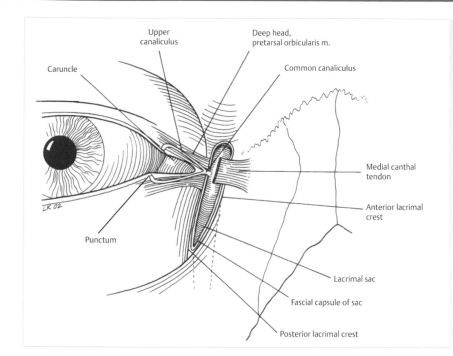

**Fig. 2.2** Anatomy of the right tear drainage system. (Adapted with permission from Wobig J, Dailey R, eds. *Oculofacial Plastic Surgery*. New York, NY: Thieme; 2004: 136.)

Approximately 3 glands of Wolfring are found along the superior border of the upper tarsus.[4]

## 2.2.3 Anatomy of Tear Drainage

Once produced, tears are spread across the ocular surface via the normal blink mechanism. Normal blink and eyelid tension is essential in preventing both dryness of the ocular surface and pooling of tears. Tears then flow toward the medial canthus, where the lacrimal drainage is initiated (▶ Fig. 2.2).[2]

## 2.2.4 Puncta

Each eyelid margin has a small conical protrusion at its medial end, the lacrimal papilla, on which there is a small opening approximately 0.3 mm in diameter, the lacrimal punctum (▶ Fig. 2.2). The normal punctum faces inward toward the globe to be in contact with the tear film. Ectropion of the punctum or stenosis of the punctum prevents the normal outflow of tears and leads to pooling on the ocular surface.[5,6]

## 2.2.5 Canaliculi

From the puncta, the tears enter the canaliculi, which are thin tubes surrounded by fibrous tissue and orbicularis muscle. The canaliculi carry tears medially toward the nasolacrimal sac. There is an upper canaliculus and a lower canaliculus (▶ Fig. 2.2). Both are first oriented vertically for approximately 2 mm, and widen at the base to form an ampulla, and bend medially at a right angle to continue horizontally for 8 mm. In most patients (90%), the upper eyelid and lower eyelid canaliculi join to form a common canaliculus for 1 to 2 mm prior to entering the nasolacrimal sac.[5,6]

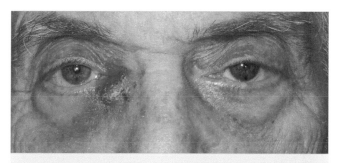

**Fig. 2.3** A patient with right dacryocystitis demonstrating redness and swelling below the level of the medial canthal tendon.

## 2.2.6 Lacrimal sac

The tears pass from the canaliculi into the lacrimal sac. The lacrimal sac sits within the lacrimal sac fossa, formed anteriorly by the frontal process of the maxillary bone and posteriorly by the lacrimal bone, which create the anterior and posterior lacrimal crests, respectively. The lateral and superolateral aspects of the lacrimal sac are not surrounded by bone. Surrounding the lacrimal sac are medial fibers of the orbicularis oculi muscle that become the medial canthal tendon. The anterior fibers are known as the muscle of Riolan, and the posterior fibers (inserting onto the posterior lacrimal crest) are known as Horner's muscle. Due to the strength of the medial canthal tendon, and relative weakness of the fascia inferior to it, enlargement of the lacrimal sac, as in dacryocystitis, typically results in swelling below the medial canthal tendon (▶ Fig. 2.3). The lacrimal sac is approximately 12 to 15 mm in height and about 4 mm in diameter, although it is generally empty and flat.[5]

## 2.2.7 Nasolacrimal Duct

The lacrimal sac narrows and becomes the nasolacrimal duct as it traverses inferiorly in a posterior-inferior-lateral direction. The duct travels through a bony canal in the maxillary bone and narrows to 1 mm in diameter. The duct then empties into the lateral nasal wall of the inferior meatus, below the inferior turbinate. The duct is approximately 18 mm long. At the end of the duct, there is a small flap of valve-like mucosa called the valve of Hasner.[5]

## 2.2.8 Nasal Anatomy

Normally tears exit the nasolacrimal duct into the inferior meatus. However, when a surgical fistula is made, as in dacryocystorhinostomy (DCR) surgery, this occurs in the middle meatus (▶ Fig. 2.4). Protecting this meatus is the middle turbinate, whose anterior end is a key landmark during lacrimal surgery. Other important intranasal landmarks include the maxillary line and the uncinate process. The maxillary line is a vertical elevation of mucosa formed by the underlying frontal process of the maxilla (▶ Fig. 2.5). This generally corresponds to the anterior portion of the nasolacrimal duct. The uncinate process is a smooth mucosal elevation in the anterior middle meatus. Usually, the lacrimal duct is located anterior and lateral to the uncinate process.[3,5]

## 2.3 Physiology of the Lacrimal System

### 2.3.1 Tear Composition

The tear film is composed of three layers. The deepest layer is the mucin layer, which is formed by the goblet cells of the conjunctiva. The mucin acts as a lubricant, a surfactant to stabilize the tear film, and a trap for debris and bacteria. The middle layer of the tear film is the aqueous layer, which is the thickest layer. It contains electrolytes, glucose, oxygen, immunoglobulins (IgA, IgM, IgD, IgE, and IgG), as well as antimicrobial proteins such as lysozyme, lactoferrin, lipocalins and defensins, cytokines, and growth factors. These factors are necessary for maintenance and nutrition of the corneal cells, as well as protection from infectious agents. The most superficial layer is a lipid layer, which is formed by the Meibomian glands. The lipids limit tear evaporation and increase surface tension to retard epiphora.[1]

### 2.3.2 Blink Mechanism

Drainage of tears depends on a normal blink of the eyelids. A combination of positive and negative pressures generated by the contraction of the orbicularis oculi muscle concurrently push the tears from the ocular surface and pull them down the drainage system. Dysfunction of the orbicularis oculi, as in facial nerve palsy, results in poor tear drainage because of absence of this pump function. Closure of the eyelids increases pressure on the lacrimal sac and propels tears down the duct and into the nose. When the eyelids open, negative pressure within the now empty canaliculi draws new fluid into the canaliculi in preparation for the next blink.[2,3,5]

### 2.3.3 Evaporation

Evaporation accounts for approximately 10% of tear loss in the young and up to 20% in the elderly. Abnormal lipid production and insufficient coating of the aqueous layer, low ambient humidity, and air movement/wind can increase the rate of evaporation and dryness on the ocular surface. Excessive dryness leads to ocular irritation, which triggers reflex tearing.[2]

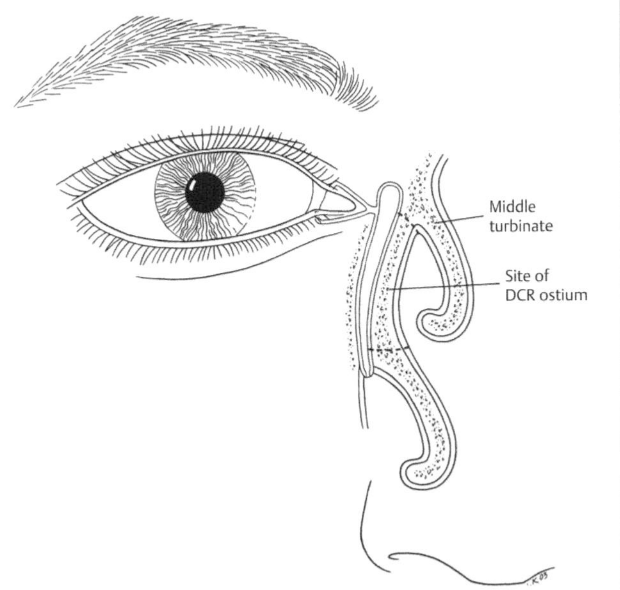

Fig. 2.4 Proposed surgical ostium for dacryocystorhinostomy surgery. (Used with permission from Wobig J, Dailey R, eds. *Oculofacial Plastic Surgery*. New York, NY: Thieme; 2004: 184.)

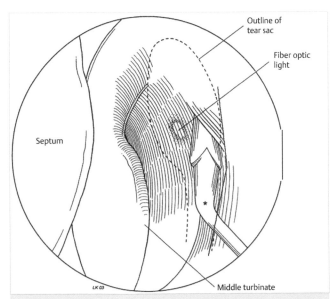

Fig. 2.5 Nasal anatomy relevant for endoscopic dacryocystorhinostomy. (Adapted with permission from Wobig J, Dailey R, eds. *Oculofacial Plastic Surgery*. New York, NY: Thieme; 2004: 179).

## 2.4 Tearing or the Watery Eye

Patients may suffer immensely from tearing or epiphora. They may have almost constant blurry vision, irritation of the eyelid skin or the eye, and embarrassment when other people inquire about their "crying." Although a singular complaint, the etiology of tearing is varied, making the diagnosis challenging and requiring a careful history, detailed examination, and often testing (▶ Table 2.1). One main point to distinguish on history and examination is whether the patient is suffering from epiphora due to obstruction of tear outflow, or from excess tear production (reflex tearing) triggered by dry eye conditions. Patients with tearing may complain of irritation, ocular discomfort, intermittent blurry vision, eye pressure, eye fatigue, and photosensitivity, all symptoms that point toward ocular surface dryness and reflex tearing. Patients may also complain of tears running down their cheeks that require frequent wiping with a tissue, skin irritation, and worsening of tearing in windy conditions, all of which may point to inadequate tear drainage. It is useful to ask patients about the duration of their symptoms, time of day when they occur, exacerbating and alleviating factors, severity of symptoms, and frequency of symptoms. One may gauge the severity of tearing by asking the patient how many times per day he or she needs to wipe the eyes with a tissue. Symptoms produced by various underlying conditions may overlap significantly and therefore a careful history as well as examination is essential (▶ Table 2.1). A baseline slit-lamp examination is critical in this evaluation, and office testing may be useful to further elucidate the underlying etiology.[2,3,5,7,8]

### 2.4.1 Office Testing

The most common office test performed is irrigation of the lacrimal system with saline. Various dye tests have also been described, but are used less frequently in clinical practice than irrigation.

#### Dye Disappearance Testing

This is a simple test to noninvasively assess the functional patency of the nasolacrimal system. One drop of 2% fluorescein is instilled into each inferior conjunctival fornix. The eyes are examined with a cobalt blue light for persistence of dye after 5 to 10 minutes. With normal tear drainage, there should be no detectable dye remaining after 10 minutes. The persistence of dye, sometimes with an elevated tear lake, may suggest either an obstructed drainage system or a functional (physiologic) abnormality limiting flow.[2,3,5]

#### Jones' Testing

Jones' testing involves instillation of 2% fluorescein into the conjunctival fornix and retrieval of fluid from the nose to evaluate for patency of the tear drainage system. While historically noted, this is rarely performed in the modern era.[2,3,5]

#### Irrigation

Nasolacrimal irrigation is perhaps the most important test to evaluate the patency of the nasolacrimal system. It is not a functional test, as nonphysiologic conditions are created by irrigating the system with a cannula. The pressure generated in irrigation may overcome lesser stenoses and blockages that may otherwise cause symptoms. Proparacaine or other topical anesthetic eyedrops are instilled into the eye to be tested. For further anesthesia, a pledget with topical anesthetic is placed over the inferior punctum for several minutes prior to irrigation. The punctum (generally the lower eyelid) is dilated with a punctal dilator, following the natural course of the canaliculus. The punctal dilator is inserted vertically for 2 mm into the punctum, after which the lower lid is distracted laterally and the dilator is rotated 90 degrees into the horizontal position and advanced medially to dilate the punctum. Next, a lacrimal cannula attached to a 3-mL syringe filled with water or saline is used to cannulate the punctum and canaliculus. It is advanced until a hard stop is achieved, that is, a stoppage of the cannula against a rigid structure without movement of the surrounding soft tissues, as in encountering the lacrimal bone. Any stenosis or complete blockage of the punctum or canaliculus should be noted. When these are present, a soft stop is encountered, that is, a stoppage of the cannula that drags the surrounding soft tissue. Then, using minimal force on the plunger, liquid is flushed through. Easy and complete passage of liquid through the system and into the nose without any reflux of liquid out the puncta confirms patency. More difficult passage or reflux suggests stenosis or obstruction. If saline refluxes back through the same canaliculus, a canalicular obstruction or stenosis is present, in which case the upper canaliculus should be tested. If there is an obstruction at the common canaliculus or nasolacrimal duct/sac, reflux through the upper punctum will be seen when irrigation is performed through the lower punctum (▶ Fig. 2.6). If the refluxed fluid is mucoid, it suggests that there is a nasolacrimal duct obstruction (NLDO) below the nasolacrimal sac. If there is partial irrigation through the system and partial reflux through the opposite canaliculus, it suggests partial obstruction.[2,3,5]

#### Nasal Endoscopy

In-office nasal endoscopy may be performed with a topical anesthetic spray and a rigid endoscope with or without a video display. This examination is vital for identifying causes of tearing and for surgical planning. Endoscopy may reveal causes for NLDO, such as tumors, polyps, swollen/edematous mucosa in allergic conditions, or evidence of abnormalities from inflammatory conditions such as sarcoidosis or Wegener's granulomatosis. Additionally, it may reveal abnormal anatomy, such as septal deviation, which may make endoscopic DCR more challenging and may lead one to perform septoplasty concurrently.[2,3,5]

### 2.4.2 Ancillary Testing
#### Computed Tomography

Noncontrast computed tomography (CT) scan of the face may help identify structural abnormalities that contribute to epiphora, as well as other sinonasal abnormalities that may require intervention. If endoscopic DCR is to be performed, image-guidance CT may be obtained, and specific CT sequences should be requested.

**Table 2.1** Causes of tearing: relevant history and examination

| Anatomical location | History | Examination | Diagnoses |
|---|---|---|---|
| • Orbit and lacrimal gland | • Thyroid eye disease<br>• Trauma (orbital/nasal fractures)<br>• Dacryoadenitis<br>• Orbital inflammation | • Proptosis<br>• Eyelid flare<br>• Eyelid retraction<br>• Lagophthalmos<br>• Bony step-offs<br>• Lacrimal gland enlargement | • Thyroid eye disease<br>• Hyperlacrimation<br>• Aberrant reinnervation (crocodile tears)<br>• Sjogren's syndrome<br>• Sarcoidosis<br>• Wegener's granulomatosis |
| • Eyelids | • Eye rubbing<br>• CPAP use (especially if air leakage)<br>• Eyelid surgery<br>• Eyelid trauma (especially marginal or canalicular lacerations)<br>• Facial surgery<br>• Facial skin cancers<br>• Facial burns<br>• Use of glaucoma medications<br>• Facial nerve palsy (traumatic, vascular, viral, idiopathic) | • Eyelid malposition (ectropion, entropion, ptosis, retraction)<br>• Eyelid laxity and degree of recoil<br>• Eyelid closure (lagophthalmos)<br>• Eyelid redness<br>• Eyelid scars<br>• Eyelid margin notching<br>• Punctal ectropion<br>• Symblepharon<br>• Periorbital redness | • Blepharitis<br>• Meibomian gland dysfunction<br>• Floppy eyelid syndrome<br>• Trichiasis<br>• Entropion<br>• Ectropion (mechanical, involutional, cicatricial)<br>• Blepharospasm<br>• Lagophthalmos<br>• Ocular surface toxicity from eyedrops |
| • Puncta | • Treatment for dry eye: punctal plugs, punctal cautery<br>• Prior topical mitomycin C use | • Small puncta<br>• Absent puncta<br>• Scarred puncta<br>• Punctal plugs | • Punctal stenosis<br>• Punctal agenesis |
| • Canaliculi | • Punctal plugs<br>• Chemotherapy (5-fluorouracil, docetaxel)<br>• Marginal eyelid laceration | • Erythema<br>• Inflammation<br>• Pain<br>• Edema along canaliculi | • Canaliculitis<br>• Punctal plug retention<br>• Canalicular stenosis<br>• Canalicular trauma |
| • Conjunctiva | • Itching<br>• Allergy<br>• Contact lens wear<br>• HPV infection<br>• History of ocular surgery (strabismus surgery, glaucoma surgery)<br>• Stevens–Johnson syndrome | • Conjunctival follicles<br>• Conjunctival papillae<br>• Conjunctival injection<br>• Conjunctivochalasis<br>• Conjunctival scar<br>• Conjunctival adhesions (symblepharon) | • Conjunctivochalasis<br>• Allergic conjunctivitis<br>• Conjunctival cyst<br>• Pyogenic granuloma<br>• Papilloma<br>• Symblepharon |
| • Cornea | • Contact lens wear<br>• Artificial tear use<br>• Dry eye syndrome<br>• Refractive surgery (LASIK, PRK)<br>• Graft versus host disease<br>• Sjogren's syndrome<br>• Corneal abrasion<br>• Recurrent corneal erosions<br>• Corneal irregularities and dellen | • Rapid tear film breakup (< 10 s)<br>• Frothy tears<br>• Superficial punctate keratopathy<br>• Corneal pannus<br>• Dellen<br>• Irregular epithelium<br>• LASIK scar<br>• Tear meniscus height | • Evaporative dry eye<br>• Graft versus host disease<br>• Corneal filaments<br>• Corneal dellen<br>• Exposure keratopathy<br>• Superficial punctate keratopathy<br>• Contact lens–related keratitis |
| • Nasolacrimal sac | • Dacryocystitis (swelling, erythema, and pain in nasolacrimal area)<br>• Mucoid discharge<br>• Crusting | • Fluctuance<br>• Inflamed lacrimal sac<br>• Mucus expression out the puncta with pressure over the sac | • Dacryocystitis (acute, chronic)<br>• Dacryolith<br>• Nasolacrimal sac malignancy<br>• Failed DCR |
| • Nasolacrimal duct | • Probing and irrigation for NLDO as a child<br>• Prior DCR surgery | • Obstruction to irrigation<br>• Reflux of mucoid material | • Congenital nasolacrimal duct obstruction<br>• Secondary nasolacrimal duct obstruction |
| • Nasal cavity | • Nasal surgery<br>• Allergic rhinitis<br>• Systemic diseases (Wegener's granulomatosis, sarcoidosis)<br>• Sinonasal cancer | • Endoscopic view: swollen mucosa, tumors, inflammation, scarring | • Allergic rhinitis<br>• Nasal cavity tumor<br>• Granulomatosis with polyangiitis (Wegener's granulomatosis)<br>• Sarcoidosis<br>• Nasal trauma<br>• Deviated septum |

Abbreviations: CPAP, continuous positive airway pressure; DCR, dacryocystorhinostomy; HPV, human papillomavirus; LASIK, laser-assisted in situ keratomileusis; NLDO, nasolacrimal duct obstruction; PRK, photorefractive keratectomy.

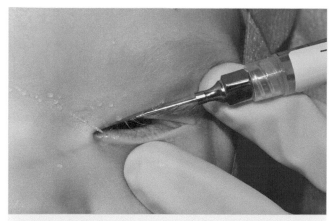

Fig. 2.6 Irrigation of the left upper canaliculus, demonstrating complete reflux through the lower punctum.

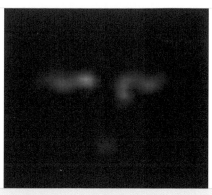

Fig. 2.7 Dacryoscintigraphy. On the right eye, there is minimal entry of the radiolabeled drop into the lacrimal sac. On the left eye, there is entry into the lacrimal sac, but no flow into the lacrimal duct or nose. In this patient, there was a canalicular obstruction on the right and nasolacrimal duct obstruction on the left.

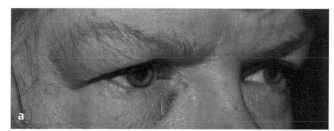
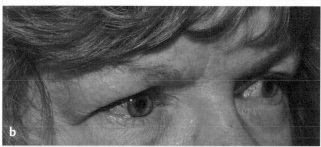

Fig. 2.8 Incision healing after external dacryocystorhinostomy. (a) Postoperative day 8 incision in the lower eyelid tear trough. (b) Three months postoperatively with imperceptible scar.

## Dacryocystography

Dacryocystography (DCG) is useful for visualizing the anatomy of the lacrimal system and in helping localize obstructions or strictures. DCG is helpful in patients who have a blockage on irrigation to identify the location, especially whether it is a pre-sac blockage or postsac blockage. Contrast dye is injected through both puncta concurrently, while X-ray images are obtained. The dye helps localize areas of obstruction, stricture, diverticula, and may also delineate dacryoliths or tumors in the nasolacrimal sac. DCG provides limited functional information as the dye is injected under pressure.[2,5]

## Dacryoscintigraphy

Dacryoscintigraphy (DSG) is a functional study that is useful for better understanding of the function of the lacrimal system, especially useful in patients with tearing or epiphora with normal irrigation findings. The study uses $^{99m}$Tc drops placed in

each conjunctival fornix. A gamma camera acquires images for 30 minutes. The images demonstrate the passage of the labeled drops through the conjunctival sac, nasolacrimal sac, and nasolacrimal duct (▶ Fig. 2.7). While not necessary for most patients with tearing, this test adds valuable information in select cases.[2,5]

# 2.5 Treatment

Once the proper diagnosis is made, a treatment plan can be formulated. The minority of patients who present with complaints of "tearing" will actually have an NLDO. Other causes of tearing far outnumber NLDO, so careful case selection is essential for successful surgical outcomes.

## 2.5.1 Dacryocystorhinostomy

DCR is the definitive surgical procedure to treat NLDO. The purpose of DCR is to create a surgical fistula between the nasolacrimal sac and nasal cavity in order to restore tear flow from the nasolacrimal sac into the nasal cavity.

External DCR has been the standard surgery for treating NLDO for the past 100 years. It has a very high success rate (>90%), with low complications. With the development of improved endonasal endoscopic instrumentation, endoscopic endonasal DCR resurged in popularity starting in the late 1980s. The main advantage of the endoscopic approach was the absence of external scarring, although the rates of unacceptable scar formation are low in external DCR except for darkly pigmented or young patients (▶ Fig. 2.8). Recently, surgeons with extensive experience in endoscopic endonasal DCR have reported almost equal success rates in endoscopic DCR. The decision to proceed with external or endoscopic DCR currently depends on patient factors and surgeon comfort with the technique, and patients should become aware of both surgical approaches before their decision for surgery. Additional considerations in surgical planning include the presence of sinus abnormalities, as these are more easily addressed simultaneously with the endoscopic endonasal DCR than with the external approach.[2,3,6,9,10]

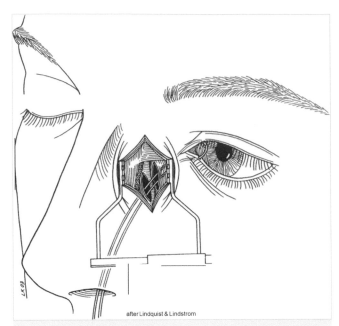

**Fig. 2.9** Schematic of the left external dacryocystorhinostomy. (Used with permission from Wobig J, Dailey R, eds. *Oculofacial Plastic Surgery.* New York, NY: Thieme; 2004: 173.)

## 2.5.2 External Dacryocystorhinostomy

Anesthesia is typically general, although the procedure has been performed under monitored anesthesia care with local anesthetic. The nose is packed with 4% cocaine-soaked pledgets or an alternative vasoconstrictive agent to cause nasal mucosal vasoconstriction and anesthesia. An incision is made either along the tear trough (modern) or the lateral side of the nose (classic). Dissection is carried down to the inferior orbital rim and extended medially to encounter the anterior lacrimal crest (▶ Fig. 2.9). A periosteal elevator is used to elevate the soft tissues of the lacrimal sac fossa and reflected laterally. The lacrimal bone is then infractured with the elevator or small hemostat with gentle pressure. A Kerrison rongeur is used to enlarge the body osteotomy to approximately 10 to 15 mm in diameter, taking care not to injure the nasal mucosa. Then a blade is used to create an incision in the shape of an "H" to form an anterior and posterior nasal mucosal flap. Westcott scissors are used to create mirror image flaps in the medial lacrimal sac. The posterior lacrimal sac flap is then sutured to the posterior nasal mucosal flap with a 4–0 chromic gut sutures. Next, the inferior and superior puncta are intubated with a bicanalicular Crawford tube silicone tubing with the ends tied together and placed in the nose. The anterior lacrimal sac and nasal mucosa flaps are tied together also with 4–0 chronic gut sutures. Finally, the skin incision is closed with a 6–0 fast gut suture.[2,3,5,10]

## 2.5.3 Endoscopic Dacryocystorhinostomy

General anesthesia is induced. The nose is packed with pledgets soaked in a vasoconstrictive agent, such as oxymetazoline,

1:1,000 epinephrine, or 4% cocaine. The face and eyes are prepped and draped and protective corneal shields are placed. With visualization using a 0-degree rigid endoscope, the middle turbinate and nasal sidewall are injected with 1% lidocaine with 1:100,000 epinephrine. The maxillary line, which is a ridge formed by the maxillary process, serves as an important landmark for the nasolacrimal duct. If necessary, the middle turbinate can be infractured to improve visualization of the area. The superior and inferior puncta are dilated with a punctal dilator. A fiberoptic light source, such as the 20-gauge vitrectomy light pipe, is used to cannulate the superior punctum until a hard stop is reached. The light pipe transilluminates the thinner lacrimal bone of the posterior lacrimal sac fossa (▶ Fig. 2.5). With this light as a guide, a crescent blade is used to create a curvilinear incision anterior to the maxillary line. An additional incision is made slightly posterior to it, and the sinus mucosa is elevated with a periosteal elevator. A rectangle of tissue is removed with Blakesley forceps to expose the maxillary and lacrimal bones. A high-speed drill with burr, such as a 2.9-mm diamond burr, or a Kerrison rongeur is used to create an osteotomy in the bone of the anterior lacrimal crest to reveal the lacrimal sac. Additional maxillary bone is removed as needed to adequately expose the sac. The light pipe is used to tent the medial lacrimal sac, while a crescent blade is then used to incise the sac (▶ Fig. 2.10). Endoscopic scissors are used to extend this incision and to create a large anterior mucosal flap. The light pipe is then removed. Crawford silicone tubes are inserted to intubate both the superior and inferior puncta and are tied to each other keeping the knot in the nose. The mucosal flaps are draped in contact with each other.[3,5]

## 2.5.4 Postoperative Care for External and Endoscopic Dacryocystorhinostomy

For external DCR, topical steroid–antibiotic ointment (neomycin and polymyxin B sulfate and dexamethasone) is used on the incision and on the eye three times per day for 5 days. Oral antibiotics are not necessary unless preoperative infection is noted. Nose blowing should be avoided to prevent nasal hemorrhage and early displacement of the lacrimal stent.

For endoscopic DCR patients, a steroid/antibiotic combination drop can be instilled onto the operated eye. Nose blowing should be similarly avoided. Approximately 1 to 2 weeks postoperatively, in-office endoscopy should be performed to evaluate the patency of and to debride material from the ostium.

The silicone tubing is typically left in place for 1 to 3 months, with the longer time period being chosen if there was prior significant inflammation. Tubing is removed in the office. The tubing is cut at the medial canthus and the patient instructed to blow his nose until the tubing comes out. Alternatively, a nasal endoscope may be used to retrieve the cut tubing.[3,5]

## 2.5.5 Postoperative Issues

Patients may report tearing and watering in the early postoperative period while the tubing is in place; this generally resolves once the tubes are removed. Patients should be

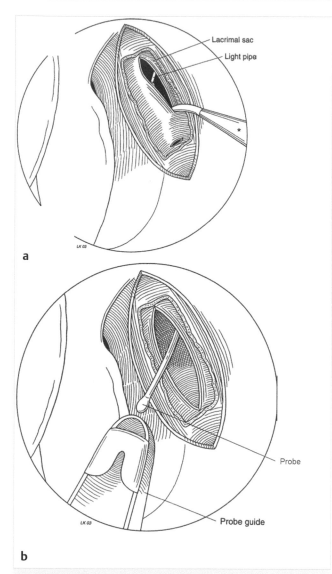

a

b

**Fig. 2.10** Schematic of the left endoscopic dacryocystorhinostomy. (a) Incision of the lacrimal sac. (b) Passage of Crawford tubes. (Used with permission from Wobig J, Dailey R, eds. *Oculofacial Plastic Surgery.* New York, NY: Thieme; 2004: 181-182.)

educated about the silicone tubing, its appearance and function, and to avoid rubbing the eye, which can dislodge it. The silicone tubing may extrude as a loop in the medial canthal area, requiring repositioning with forceps, endoscopy, or early removal.[3,5]

## 2.5.6 Complications of Dacryocystorhinostomy

For both external and endonasal DCR, nasal bleeding remains the most common complication. Other complications to both approaches include wound infection, delayed healing, formation of intranasal synechiae, punctal cheese wiring, formation of granulomata, and lacrimal sump syndrome. For external DCR, complications are generally rare. The risk of wound infection and webbing of skin is very low. For endoscopic DCR, the surgeon who is unfamiliar with endonasal anatomy may inadvertently gain access to an inappropriate location, such as a

sinus or the orbit. This is thankfully rare. Lacrimal sump syndrome is the accumulation of tears and mucoid material within the operated nasolacrimal sac and leads to epiphora, mucoid discharge, and occasionally recurrent infection. This occurs in cases where the ostium is placed too far superiorly or is too small.[3,5,11,12,13]

## 2.6 Other Options for Tearing

### 2.6.1 Endonasal Laser-Assisted Dacryocystorhinostomy

This technique is performed similarly to the above endoscopic endonasal DCR, with a holmium:YAG (yttrium aluminum garnet) or potassium-titanyl-phosphate:neodymium-doped yttrium aluminum garnet (KTP:NdYAG) laser used to create the ostium. Although there is evidence to support this technique, there have been concerns about its safety. Due to the amount of energy delivered in some cases, overlying tissue necrosis has been reported, which can be challenging to repair.[3,5,14]

### 2.6.2 Balloon Dacryoplasty

This technique utilizes catheters with balloons of different sizes to cannulate the lacrimal drainage system and then inflate the balloons for specified durations to dilate the system and overcome stenosis, similar to angioplasty. It has primarily been used in children with congenital NLDO, but has been attempted in adults. In select cases of nasolacrimal duct stenosis without obstruction, dilation with subsequent silicone stent intubation can improve symptoms in up to 73% of patients, although this is not a commonly used technique. Some surgeons have used balloon dacryoplasty to augment endoscopic endonasal DCR or for revision DCR.[5,15]

### 2.6.3 Jones Tube— Conjunctivodacryocystorhinostomy

This technique is used in patients where the proximal lacrimal drainage system (i.e., the puncta or canaliculi) is injured or absent. This procedure is generally the last resort option for patients with drainage abnormalities. A rigid glass hollow bore tube is placed between the ocular surfaces and the nose. Although generally successful, complications may occur, most related to migration, extrusion, and plugging of the tube.[2,3,5,16]

### 2.6.4 Botulinum Toxin

Injection of botulinum toxin has been recently reported as a way to decrease tearing in patients who may not be able to tolerate or may be unwilling to undergo DCR surgery, especially those with medical contraindications to surgery. An absolute contraindication to botulinum toxin injection is dry eye syndrome, and this should be ruled out prior to injection. A transconjunctival injection is placed directly into the palpebral lobe of the lacrimal gland. The treatment lasts on average 10 weeks, and side effects include ptosis, diplopia, and hematoma. Approximately 70% of patients note some degree of improvement in epiphora.[17]

# References

[1] Holland EJ, Mannis MJ, Lee WB. Ocular Surface Disease: Cornea, Conjunctiva and Tear Film. China: Elsevier; 2013

[2] Hornblass A. Oculoplastic, Orbital and Reconstructive Surgery. Vol. 2. Orbit and Lacrimal System. Baltimore, MD: Williams & Wilkins; 1990

[3] Wobig JL, Dailey RA. Oculofacial Plastic Surgery: Face, Lacrimal System, and Orbit. New York, NY: Thieme; 2004

[4] Jakobiec FJ, Iwamoto T. The ocular adnexa: lids, conjunctiva, and orbit. In: Fine BS and Yanoff M, eds. Ocular Histology. 2nd ed. Hagerstown, MD: Harper & Rowe, Publishers, Inc.; 1979:289–342

[5] Olver J. Colour Atlas of Lacrimal Surgery. Oxford, UK: Butterworth-Heinemann; 2002

[6] Kakizaki H, Takahashi Y, Iwaki M, et al. Punctal and canalicular anatomy: implications for canalicular occlusion in severe dry eye. Am J Ophthalmol. 2012; 153(2):229–237.e1

[7] Mansur C, Pfeiffer ML, Esmaeli B. Evaluation and management of chemotherapy-induced epiphora, punctal and canalicular stenosis, and nasolacrimal duct obstruction. Ophthal Plast Reconstr Surg. 2017; 33(1):9–12

[8] Ali MJ, Vyakaranam AR, Rao JE, Prasad G, Reddy PVA. Iodine-131 therapy and lacrimal drainage system toxicity: nasal localization studies using whole body nuclear scintigraphy and SPECT-CT. Ophthal Plast Reconstr Surg. 2017; 33(1):13–16

[9] Grob SR, Campbell A, Lefebvre DR, Yoon MK. External versus endoscopic endonasal dacryocystorhinostomy. Int Ophthalmol Clin. 2015; 55(4):51–62

[10] Dutton JJ. Atlas of Oculoplastics and Orbital Surgery. Philadelphia, PA: Lippincott Williams &Wilkins; 2013

[11] Devoto MH, Zaffaroni MC, Bernardini FP, de Conciliis C. Postoperative evaluation of skin incision in external dacryocystorhinostomy. Ophthal Plast Reconstr Surg. 2004; 20(5):358–361

[12] Castellarin A, Lipskey S, Sternberg P, Jr. Iatrogenic open globe eye injury following sinus surgery. Am J Ophthalmol. 2004; 137(1):175–176

[13] Wu H, Shen T, Chen J, Yan J. Long-term therapeutic outcome of ophthalmic complications following endoscopic sinus surgery. Medicine (Baltimore). 2016; 95(38):e4896

[14] McClintic SM, Yoon MK, Bidar M, Dutton JJ, Vagefi MR, Kersten RC. Tissue necrosis following diode laser-assisted transcanalicular dacryocystorhinostomy. Ophthal Plast Reconstr Surg. 2015; 31(1):e18–e22

[15] Ali MJ, Naik MN, Honavar SG. Balloon dacryoplasty: ushering the new and routine era in minimally invasive lacrimal surgeries. Int Ophthalmol. 2013; 33(2):203–210

[16] Steele EA. Conjunctivodacryocystorhinostomy with Jones tube: a history and update. Curr Opin Ophthalmol. 2016; 27(5):439–442

[17] Ziahosseini K, Al-Abbadi Z, Malhotra R. Botulinum toxin injection for the treatment of epiphora in lacrimal outflow obstruction. Eye (Lond). 2015; 29(5):656–661

# 3 Radiologic Assessment of the Orbit and Lacrimal System

*Katherine L. Reinshagen and Hugh Curtin*

## Abstract

Radiologic assessment of the orbit is helpful for preoperative planning of orbital tumor resection as it can help narrow the differential diagnosis for an orbital mass and assess the surrounding anatomic structures. Computed tomography (CT) and magnetic resonance (MR) can be complementary modalities. CT can help determine osseous landmarks and bone erosion. MR can help assess the extent of soft-tissue abnormality and can be particularly helpful in identifying soft-tissue characteristics that can help determine the identity of a lesion. The presence of orbital fat provides an excellent medium to contrast the extent of tumor involvement. Furthermore, for preoperative assessment for endoscopic approaches to the orbit, MR and CT can help distinguish the lesion in relation to the ophthalmic artery, optic nerve, annulus of Zinn and medial rectus muscle. Additional tests such as dacryocystography can also be considered when assessing for primary nasolacrimal duct lesions.

*Keywords:* magnetic resonance, computed tomography, dacryocystography, anatomy

## 3.1 Introduction

Computed tomography (CT) and magnetic resonance (MR) imaging can be complementary in preoperative imaging of the orbit. CT provides excellent bony detail as well as thin section imaging, which can be used in surgical guidance systems. Normal structures, tumors, and inflammation are contrasted against the orbital fat. MR can provide excellent soft-tissue detail and delineation of orbital masses and infiltrative lesions. In the setting of trauma and possible foreign body, CT is the preferred modality to assess for fractures, globe injury, and retained foreign bodies.

## 3.2 Imaging Techniques

### 3.2.1 Computed Tomography

Modern CT scanners produce high-resolution images that can be reformatted into multiple planes. Intravenously administered nonionic iodinated contrast is primarily used in the setting of infection, inflammatory disease, or tumor. When contrast-enhanced images are required for assessment of infection or tumor, images are typically acquired following a 60-second delay after administration of iodinated contrast. To best delineate the arterial anatomy, a CT angiogram (CTA) can be performed. CTAs are typically acquired following a power injection of intravenous iodinated contrast. Timing of contrast enhancement is usually made following a test bolus injection or using Hounsfield unit timing off the aortic arch. This technique allows for optimized arterial opacification. Typically, images are acquired around 15 to 20 seconds following onset of contrast

injection. Both contrast-enhanced CT and CTAs are acquired with submillimeter slice thickness, which can be reformatted into thicker section imaging for easier viewing or maximum intensity projection (MIP) images. This can be helpful when following the course of the ophthalmic artery.

### 3.2.2 Magnetic Resonance

High-resolution MR imaging of the orbits can be performed when better soft-tissue detail and delineation of surrounding critical anatomic structures is required preoperatively. Images can be obtained at both 1.5 and 3 T and are typically acquired at 2- to 3-mm slice thickness.

Coronal and axial T1-weighted images without fat suppression provide helpful anatomic images delineating the extraocular muscles (EOM), and major neurovascular structures including the course of the optic nerve. Orbital fat is high signal on T1 and provides excellent soft-tissue contrast to help define these small structures.

Coronal short-tau inversion recovery (STIR) and fat-suppressed postcontrast T1-weighted images are helpful for delineating underlying pathology as most abnormalities will appear bright on STIR images and typically demonstrate some degree of contrast enhancement. STIR images or T2-weighted images are also helpful in demonstrating the cerebrospinal fluid (CSF) surrounding the optic nerve as fluid has high signal on these sequences. In addition, signal change in the optic nerve due to mass effect, edema, or injury can best be appreciated on coronal STIR images.

Diffusion-weighted imaging can also be performed in the orbit. Although diffusion-weighted imaging can be distorted at the skull base because of susceptibility artifact due to the presence of multiple soft tissue, bone, and air interfaces, this technique can sometimes be helpful to assess the cellularity of orbital neoplasms.[1] Because hypercellular lesions result in less free movement of water, these lesions typically manifest as dark on the calculated apparent diffusion coefficient (ADC) images and bright on the corresponding diffusion-weighted images. This pattern is commonly referred to as restricted diffusion.

Noncontrast time of flight MR angiogram (MRA) of the circle of Willis can delineate the course of the ophthalmic artery in patients with poor renal function or in young patients to avoid radiation. Occasionally, due to the tortuosity and size of the ophthalmic artery, the anatomy through the optic canal and distally within the orbit may be suboptimal.

### 3.2.3 Dacryocystogram

Fluoroscopic dacryocystogram can be used to delineate the nasolacrimal drainage system. Following intracanalicular administration of nonionic iodinated contrast, the course and caliber of the nasolacrimal duct is followed to the inferior meatus. CT performed shortly after contrast administration can also be acquired to provide adjunctive cross-sectional data.

## 3.3 Imaging of Orbital Anatomy

The orbit is readily divided into multiple compartments: preseptal, postseptal, intraconal, and extraconal. The pre- and postseptal orbit is divided by the thin fibrous orbital septum, which provides a strong barrier to spread of disease. The orbital septum can be seen on high-resolution CT and MR images running parallel to the thicker more superficial orbicularis oculi muscle (▶ Fig. 3.1).

The EOM form the boundary of the intra- and extraconal compartments of the orbit (▶ Fig. 3.2). The extraconal soft tissues contain mostly fat and a few small vessels. The frontal nerve of the V1 division of the trigeminal nerve lies within the extraconal superior orbit above the levator palpebrae muscle. An important landmark to assist in endoscopic planning is the medial rectus muscle separating the medial intra- and extraconal spaces.[2] In the medial extraconal space, there is a medial ethmoidal vein and small ethmoidal vasculature (▶ Fig. 3.2). The intraconal orbit contains critical structures including the optic nerve, ophthalmic artery and branches as well as the superior ophthalmic vein (▶ Fig. 3.2). Smaller vessels and nerves such as the long ciliary artery and nerve, and medial ophthalmic vein are not consistently visualized on standard MR or CT imaging. The ophthalmic artery passes through the optic canal and courses superior and lateral to the optic nerve before giving rise to the lateral lacrimal branch and turning medially and branching into the anterior and posterior ethmoidal branches, which can occasionally be identified (▶ Fig. 3.3, ▶ Fig. 3.4). Occasionally, the ophthalmic artery passes inferior and medial to the optic nerve before coursing superiorly and anteriorly in medial intraconal segment of the orbit, an important variation to note prior to endoscopic surgery.[2] Posteriorly, the intraconal compartment is bounded by the annulus of Zinn, the common tendinous ring from which arise the four rectus EOM. The annulus of Zinn is not readily visible but can be approximated by following the course of the rectus muscles posteriorly to the point at which the rectus muscles become indistinct from the optic nerve (▶ Fig. 3.5). This point is also often located at the boundary of the sphenoid and ethmoid sinuses. The bony orbit posteriorly has three openings: the superior and inferior orbital fissures and the optic canal. These are readily visible on both CT and MR (▶ Fig. 3.5). The cranial nerves III, V1, and V2 are visible on MR with thin section non-fat-suppressed T1-weighted images. These cranial nerves can be identified in the cavernous sinuses and followed into and along the orbit. Cranial nerves IV and VI are less readily visible on conventional MR sequences; however, following the expected course of these cranial nerves is helpful for delineating pathology. Cranial nerves are more readily visible when abnormal, for example, when a schwannoma or perineural tumor spread is present.

The lacrimal gland is readily visible on both CT and MR as an ovoid soft-tissue structure along the superolateral extraconal orbit. On MR, the lacrimal gland is slightly brighter on T1 compared with adjacent EOM (▶ Fig. 3.6), intermediate in signal on T2, and enhances homogeneously. The levator aponeurosis, a T1 hypointense curvilinear band, extends through the lacrimal gland and separates the more superior orbital lobe from the inferior palpebral lobe (▶ Fig. 3.6). The lacrimal outflow apparatus consists of the superior and inferior canaliculi, the common canaliculus, lacrimal sac, and nasolacrimal duct. The nasolacrimal duct passes through the valve of Hasner before draining into the inferior meatus of the nasal cavity (▶ Fig. 3.6). MR is a helpful adjunct to differentiate pathology from surrounding sinonasal secretions and mucosal thickening (▶ Fig. 3.7, ▶ Fig. 3.8, ▶ Fig. 3.9, ▶ Fig. 3.10).

## 3.4 Radiologic Approach to Pathology of the Orbit and Lacrimal Gland

Pathology of the orbit can be approached radiologically with a location-based differential. Lesions may arise from the globe, nerves, EOM, fat, lacrimal gland, and nasolacrimal duct apparatus. Differential diagnosis can be further narrowed based on the

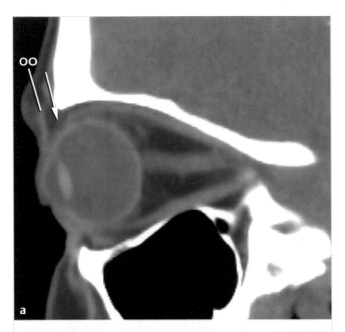

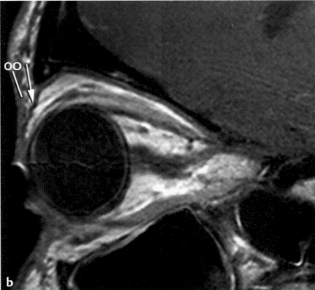

**Fig. 3.1** (a) Orbital septum (*white arrow*) can be seen deep to the orbicularis oculi muscle on computed tomography and (b) MR (magnetic resonance) precontrast T1-weighted images.

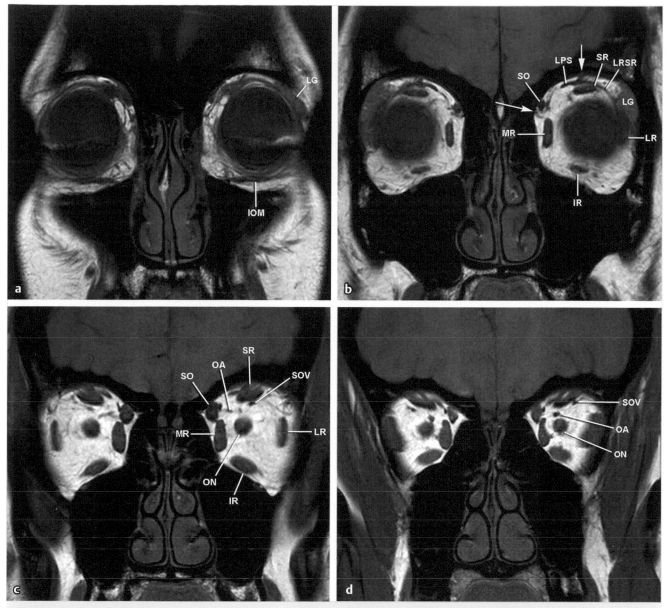

**Fig. 3.2** Coronal T1-weighted MR (magnetic resonance) of a normal orbit. **(a)** IOM, inferior oblique muscle; LG, lacrimal gland. **(b)** SR, superior rectus; LRSR, lateral rectus superior rectus band; LR, lateral rectus.; IR, inferior rectus; MR, medial rectus; SO, superior oblique; LPS, levator palpebrae superioris; *short white arrow*, frontal nerve (V1); *long white arrow*, medial ethmoidal vasculature. **(c, d)** SOV, superior ophthalmic vein; ON, optic nerve; OA, ophthalmic artery.

morphology of the lesion being mass-like or infiltrative. Finally, imaging characteristics can further narrow the diagnosis of an orbital or lacrimal gland lesion. The most common lesions are summarized in ▶ Table 3.1.

The differential for T1 high signal lesions would include melanin containing lesions such as melanoma (▶ Fig. 3.11), proteinaceous contents, fat (dermoid, epidermoid, lipoma), or hemorrhagic lesions (hemorrhage into an existing mass). Assessing for loss of signal on fat-suppressed images is helpful in eliminating fat containing lesions from the differential diagnosis.

Infiltrative or bilateral lesions may be secondary to nonneoplastic entities such as immunoglobulin G4 (IgG4) related orbitopathy (▶ Fig. 3.12), thyroid orbitopathy, sarcoidosis, and granulomatosis with polyangiitis (Wegener's granulomatosis).

Thyroid orbitopathy can be distinguished from other systemic diseases or inflammations by the lack of involvement of the myotendinous junction of the EOM and classic pattern of involvement of the EOM with predilection for the inferior and medial rectus muscles. Differentiation between sarcoidosis, granulomatosis with polyangiitis, and IgG4-related orbital disease can be challenging and may often require histologic diagnosis or a systemic search for the unifying diagnosis. One case series suggests that the finding of an enlarged infraorbital nerve in the setting of orbital inflammatory disease is a specific finding for IgG4-related ophthalmic disease.[9]

Careful assessment of the anatomy is critical to the presurgical planning. In particular, assessment of the optic nerve pathway and annulus of Zinn is important in endoscopic surgical

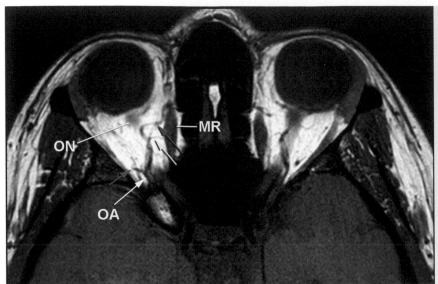

Fig. 3.3 Axial T1-weighted MR (magnetic resonance) of a normal orbit. ON, optic nerve; MR, medial rectus; OA, ophthalmic artery; *blue arrow*, lacrimal branch of the OA; *red arrow*, anterior ethmoidal branch of the OA; *yellow arrow*, posterior ethmoidal branch of the OA.

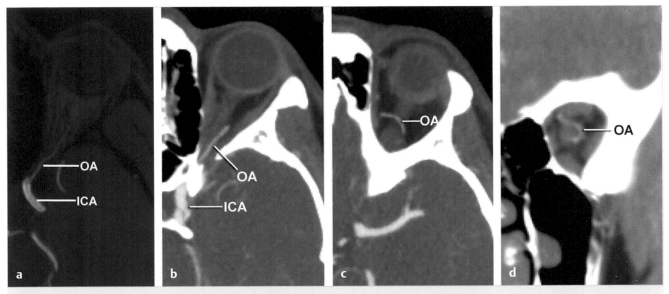

Fig. 3.4 MRA (magnetic resonance angiogram) and CTA (computed tomography angiogram) of the ophthalmic artery (OA) and internal carotid artery (ICA). MR time-of-flight angiography (a) demonstrates the ICA and OA. CT angiogram (b–d) of the ICA and OA. The OA typically courses lateral to the optic nerve (a,b,d) and then courses medially across the superior margin of the optic nerve (c,d).

planning.[2] The optic nerve can best be seen on non-fat-suppressed T1- and T2-weighted images and coronal STIR images (▶ Fig. 3.13). Fat-suppressed images are less helpful due to the absence of soft-tissue contrast between the optic nerve sheath and surrounding intraconal fat; however they can be helpful in the setting of optic nerve sheath pathology such as optic nerve sheath meningiomas. STIR images are fluid sensitive and can assess the degree of CSF effacement in the optic nerve sheath as well as any signal change within the optic nerve itself. While the annulus of Zinn cannot be confidently visualized due to its small nature and location, following the course of the rectus muscles posteriorly to the location where it becomes indistinguishable from the optic nerve canalicular segment can approximate it. Assessing the posterior margin of any tumor to the annulus of Zinn is critical (▶ Fig. 3.13) as it may change the surgical approach.

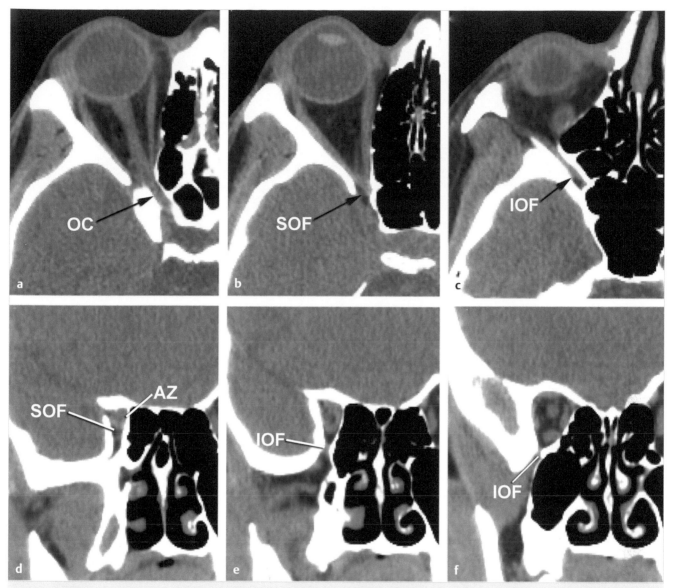

**Fig. 3.5** Orbital fissures and annulus of Zinn on CT (computed tomography). **(a–c)** Axial. **(d–f)** Coronal oblique. **(a)** OC, optic canal; **(b, d)** SOF, superior orbital fissure; **(c, e, f)** IOF, inferior orbital fissure; **(d)** AZ, approximate location of annulus of Zinn.

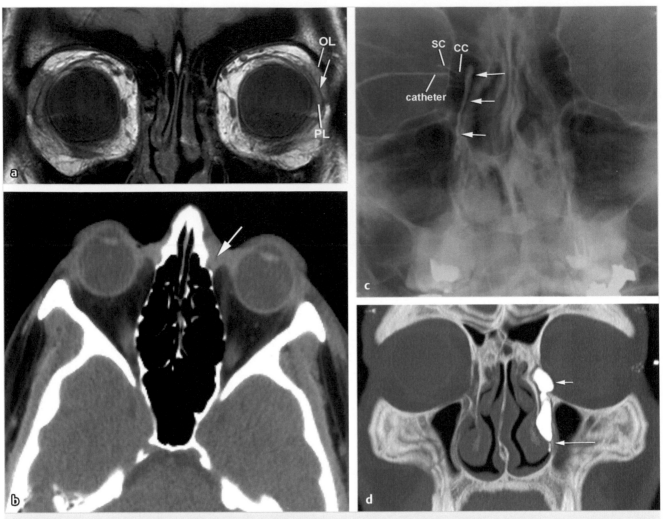

**Fig. 3.6** Lacrimal/nasolacrimal anatomy. **(a)** MR (magnetic resonance) coronal T1-weighted image of the orbit and lacrimal gland (LG). OL, orbital lobe of the LG; PL, palpebral lobe of the LG; *white arrow*, levator aponeurosis. **(b)** Axial CT (computed tomography) of the orbit (*white arrow*: lacrimal gland). **(c)** Dacryocystogram anteroposterior view. SC, superior canaliculus, CC, common canaliculus; *white arrows*, normal lacrimal sac and nasolacrimal duct. **(d)** Abnormal CT dacryocystogram coronal view. Abnormal dilatation of the nasolacrimal duct and lacrimal sac (*short white arrow*) with abrupt narrowing at the valve of Hasner (*long white arrow*) consistent with stenosis.

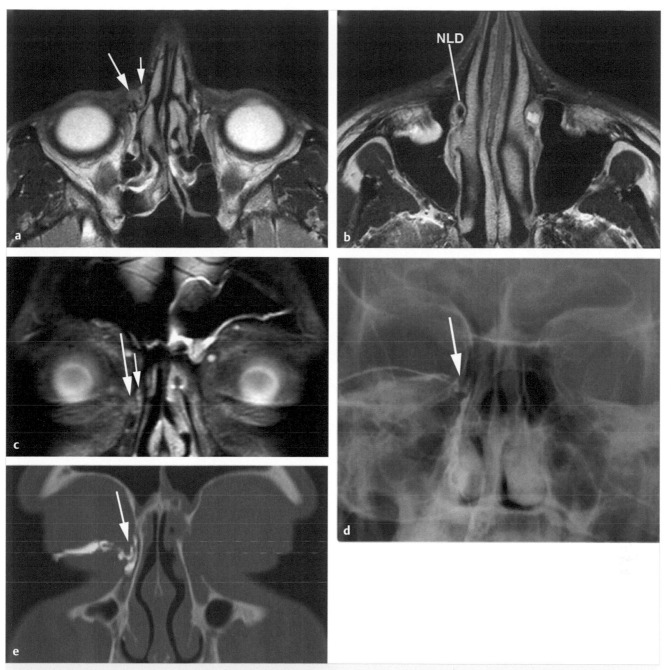

**Fig. 3.7** Nasolacrimal sac squamous cell carcinoma (SCC). **(a,b)** MR (magnetic resonance) axial T2-weighted images. *Long white arrow*, squamous cell carcinoma; *short white arrow*, secretions; NLD, nasolacrimal duct. **(c)** Coronal T2-weighted image demonstrate an intermediate T2 intense lesion (*long white arrow*) along the right medial canthus extending into the lateral wall of the lacrimal sac. MR is able to distinguish surrounding secretions (*short white arrow*) from the mass (*long white arrow*; **a,c**). The remainder of the NLD is normal and air filled **(b)**. **(d)** Dacryocystogram anteroposterior view. **(e)** Computed tomography (CT) dacryocystogram demonstrates a soft-tissue filling defect corresponding with the mass (*long white arrow*). No bony destruction identified on CT.

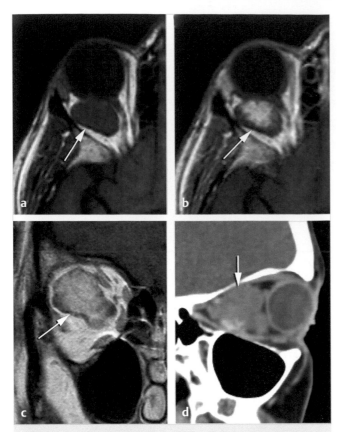

**Fig. 3.8** Enhancement characteristics of a cavernous hemangioma/venous malformation. *White arrow*: cavernous hemangioma. **(a)** Magnetic resonance (MR) precontrast and **(b,c)** postcontrast T1-weighted images of the orbit. Progressive enhancement of the intraconal mass (*white arrow*) can be observed on MR due to the time delay between acquiring sequences (axial image acquired earlier than coronal image). Progressive enhancement can be used as a distinguishing feature from schwannoma. **(d)** Postcontrast sagittal CT. This characteristic enhancement is not typically shown with CT due to single early time point imaging.

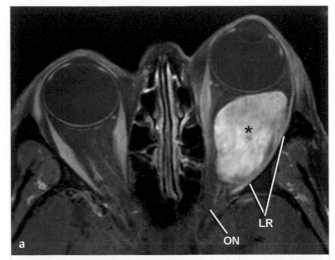

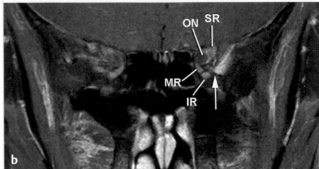

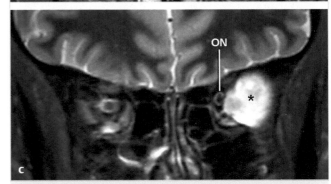

**Fig. 3.9** Schwannoma. *Asterisk*, schwannoma; *white arrow*, posterior margin of schwannoma; ON, optic nerve; LR, lateral rectus; SR, superior rectus; IR, inferior rectus; MR, medial rectus. **(a,b)** Magnetic resonance (MR) postcontrast T1-weighted fat-suppressed images demonstrate a large enhancing mass (*asterisk*) in the lateral intraconal orbit displacing the lateral rectus muscle laterally. The posterior margin of the tumor (*white arrow*) is demonstrated just anterior to the annulus of Zinn, as the rectus muscles and optic nerve are still discernible as separate structures on the coronal image **(b)**. **(c)** MR coronal STIR (short tau inversion recovery) image demonstrates the mass effect on the optic nerve and effacement of the cerebrospinal fluid surrounding the optic nerve from the schwannoma (*asterisk*).

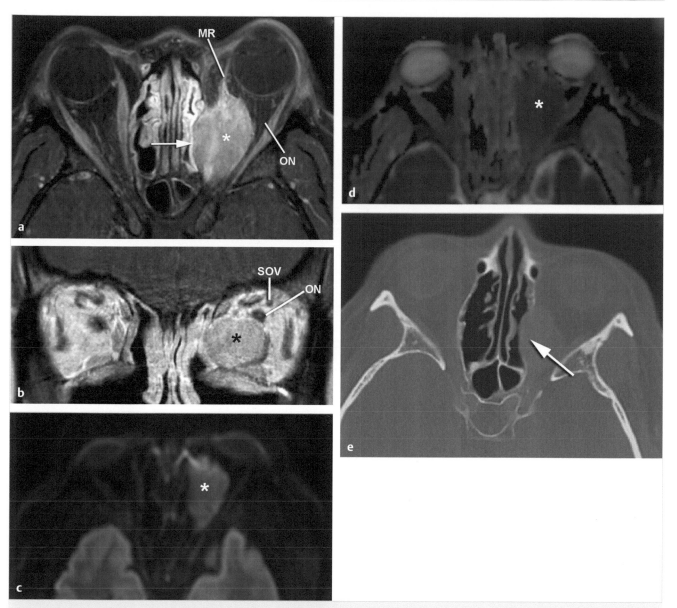

**Fig. 3.10** Rhabdomyosarcoma of the orbit. *Asterisk*, rhabdomyosarcoma; ON, optic nerve; MR, medial rectus; *white arrow*, invasion into ethmoid air cells; SOV, superior ophthalmic vein. **(a)** MR axial postcontrast T1-weighted fat-saturated image demonstrates a large enhancing mass (*asterisk*) encasing the medial rectus muscle and involving the intraconal and extraconal orbit. **(b)** MR (magnetic resonance) coronal postcontrast T1-weighted image demonstrates optic nerve displacement laterally. **(c,d)** MR diffusion weighted imaging with B1000 **(c)** and apparent diffusion coefficient (ADC) map **(d)** demonstrates restricted diffusion (bright on B1000 images; dark on ADC images) consistent with hypercellularity. **(e)** Axial CT (computed tomography) in bone window shows CT is complementary, demonstrating osseous destruction of the ethmoid air cells and lamina papyracea.

**Table 3.1** Common masses of the orbit by location[3,4,5]

| Location | Mass | Imaging characteristics |
|---|---|---|
| Globe | Retinoblastoma | Enhancing mass, commonly calcified |
| | Metastasis | Depends on primary tumor, most common: breast |
| | Primary melanoma | Melanin: T1 high signal, T2 hypointense, most commonly involving the choroid of the uveal tract |
| Fat | Cavernous hemangioma/venous malformation (▶ Fig. 3.8) | T2 hyperintense, T1 isointense to muscle, progressive enhancement,[6] displaces but does not invade |
| | Venolymphatic malformation | Fluid levels seen in lymphatic malformations, may be trans-spatial, heterogeneous enhancement depending on degree of cystic components |
| | Venous varix | Enlarges with dynamic maneuvers |
| | Epidermoid/dermoid cysts | May contain fat and calcifications, no appreciable enhancement, demonstrates restricted diffusion |
| Nerve | Optic nerve glioma | Expansile enlargement of the optic nerve |
| | Optic nerve sheath meningioma | Tram-track enhancement of the optic nerve sheath |
| | Schwannoma (▶ Fig. 3.9) | T2 hyperintense, if large may be heterogeneous in signal, enhancement not progressive as seen in cavernous hemangioma |
| | Neurofibroma | T2 hyperintense, can be indistinguishable from schwannoma |
| Lacrimal Gland | Benign mixed tumor/pleomorphic adenoma | T2 hyperintense, enhancing mass, round mass displaces globe |
| | Lymphoma | Low diffusivity mass, T2 hypointense, molds to globe rather than displaces it |
| | Adenoid cystic carcinoma | Nonspecific imaging characteristics, assess for perineural spread, mass-like rather than infiltrative |
| | Mucoepidermoid carcinoma | Nonspecific imaging characteristics |
| | Metastasis | Mass-like rather than infiltrative typically, depends on primary tumor |
| Lacrimal sac/ nasolacrimal duct apparatus | Dacryocystocele | Smooth, expansion, site of obstruction can be delineated with dacryocystogram if not possible on computed tomography or magnetic resonance |
| | Squamous cell carcinoma (▶ Fig. 3.7) | Lobulated mass, usually involves medial canthus, moderate enhancement, and isointense on T1 and T2, majority expand rather than erode nasolacrimal duct[7] |
| Any space | Fibrous tumor | T2 hypointense, enhancing tumor |
| | Rhabdomyosarcoma (▶ Fig. 3.10) | Isointense to muscle on T1, hyperintense to muscle on T2, low diffusivity, enhancing, adjacent bone destruction[8] |
| | Lymphoma | T2 hypointense, low diffusivity, enhancing, homogeneous |
| | Metastasis (▶ Fig. 3.11) | Dependent on primary tumor, more common in melanoma, breast cancer, lymphoma, and leukemia |

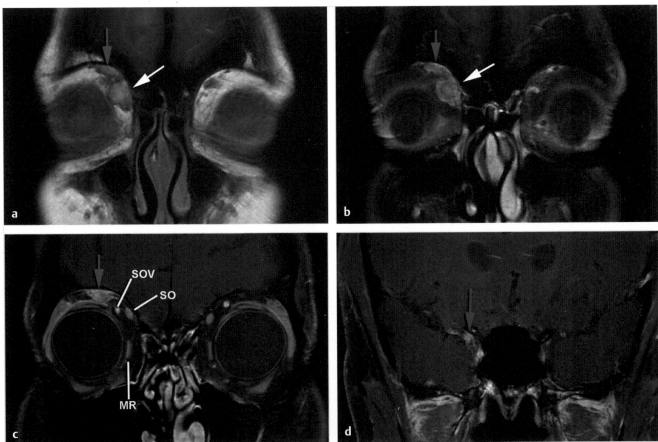

**Fig. 3.11** Metastatic melanoma with perineural spread. *White arrow*: metastatic melanoma; *red arrow*: perineural spread along the frontal nerve (V1). **(a)** MR (magnetic resonance) precontrast coronal T1-weighted image shows tumor (*white arrow*) has high intrinsic signal prior to contrast. **(b,c,d)** MR postcontrast coronal T1-weighted fat-suppressed images show an enhancing lesion in the right superomedial orbit (*white arrow*). Abnormal soft-tissue thickening of similar signal intensity and enhancement demonstrated along the frontal nerve (V1) extending into the superior orbital fissure consistent with perineural spread (*red arrow*).

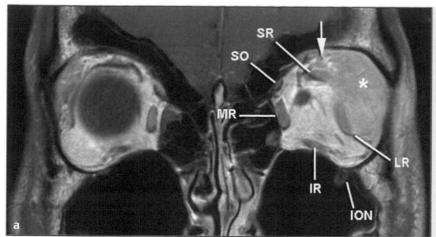

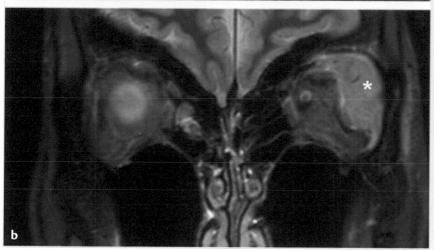

Fig. 3.12 Immunoglobulin G4 (IgG4) related orbitopathy. *Asterisk*, IgG4-related orbitopathy; LR, lateral rectus; ION, infraorbital nerve; IR, inferior rectus; MR, medial rectus; SO, superior oblique; SR, superior rectus; *arrow*, frontal nerve (V1). **(a)** MR (magnetic resonance) postcontrast coronal T1-weighted image demonstrates an infiltrative enhancing mass (*asterisk*) involving the lacrimal gland, lateral rectus muscle as well as intraconal and extraconal fat with enlargement and enhancement of the frontal nerve (V1; *short arrow*) consistent with IgG4-related orbitopathy. **(b)** MR coronal STIR (short tau inversion recovery) image demonstrates a homogeneously low T2/ STIR signal mass, which can be seen in lymphoid lesions such as IgG4 orbitopathy or lymphoma.

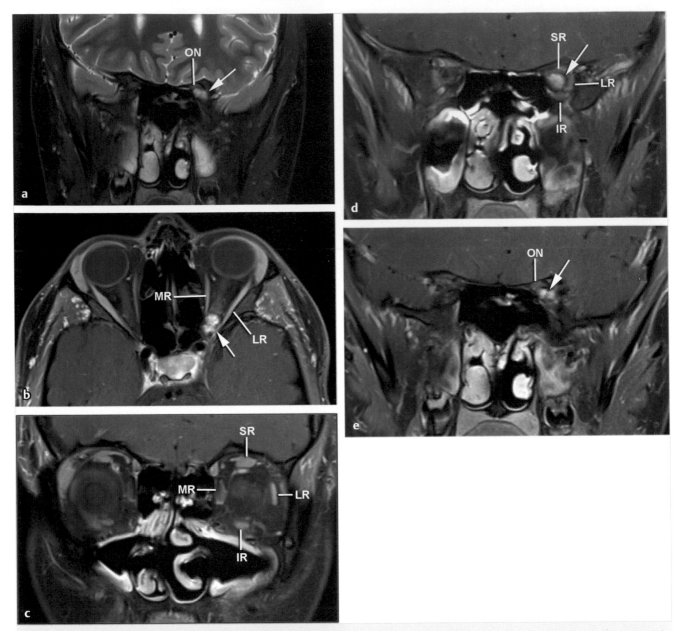

**Fig. 3.13** Cavernous hemangioma/venous malformation at the annulus of Zinn. *White arrow*, cavernous hemangioma; ON, optic nerve; MR, medial rectus; LR, lateral rectus; SR, superior rectus; IR, inferior rectus. **(a)** MR (magnetic resonance) coronal STIR (short tau inversion recovery) images demonstrate a T2 hyperintense lesion (*white arrow*) at the posterior orbital apex extending into the annulus of Zinn and resulting in mass effect on the ON within the optic canal. **(b)** MR axial T1-weighted postcontrast fat-suppressed image shows the enhancing lesion between the medial and lateral rectus muscles. **(c–e)** MR coronal T1-weighted postcontrast fat-suppressed images. Following the rectus muscles on consecutive coronal images to the point at which the rectus muscles are indiscernible from the ON can be used to approximate the location of the annulus of Zinn. In this example, the posterior margin of the lesion (**e**, *white arrow*) is beyond the annulus of Zinn and located close to the optic canal.

# 3.5 Conclusion

Imaging of the sinuses and orbits provides anatomic information and will narrow the list of possible diagnoses. The fat in the orbit is an ideal medium against which abnormalities can be defined. With the advent of endoscopic approaches to the orbit, lesions should be described relative to landmarks important to surgical planning such as the optic nerve, the medial rectus, ophthalmic artery, and annulus of Zinn.

# References

[1] Xu XQ, Hu H, Su GY, Liu H, Shi HB, Wu FY. Diffusion weighted imaging for differentiating benign from malignant orbital tumors: Diagnostic performance of the apparent diffusion coefficient based on region of interest selection method. Korean J Radiol. 2016; 17(5):650–656

[2] Bleier BS, Healy DY, Jr, Chhabra N, Freitag S. Compartmental endoscopic surgical anatomy of the medial intraconal orbital space. Int Forum Allergy Rhinol. 2014; 4(7):587–591

[3] Purohit BS, Vargas MI, Ailianou A, et al. Orbital tumours and tumour-like lesions: exploring the armamentarium of multiparametric imaging. Insights Imaging. 2016; 7(1):43–68

[4] Cunnane MB, Curtin HD. Imaging of orbital disorders. Handb Clin Neurol. 2016; 135:659–672

[5] Tailor TD, Gupta D, Dalley RW, Keene CD, Anzai Y. Orbital neoplasms in adults: clinical, radiologic, and pathologic review. Radiographics. 2013; 33 (6):1739–1758

[6] Tanaka A, Mihara F, Yoshiura T, et al. Differentiation of cavernous hemangioma from schwannoma of the orbit: a dynamic MRI study. AJR Am J Roentgenol. 2004; 183(6):1799–1804

[7] Kumar VA, Esmaeli B, Ahmed S, Gogia B, Debnam JM, Ginsberg LE. Imaging features of malignant lacrimal sac and nasolacrimal duct tumors. AJNR Am J Neuroradiol. 2016

[8] Conneely MF, Mafee MF. Orbital rhabdomyosarcoma and simulating lesions. Neuroimaging Clin N Am. 2005; 15(1):121–136

[9] Soussan JB, Deschamps R, Sadik JC, et al. Infraorbital nerve involvement on magnetic resonance imaging in European patients with IgG4-related ophthalmic disease: a specific sign. Eur Radiol. 2016

# 4 Evaluation and Management of Congenital Lacrimal Obstruction

*Jonathan C. P. Roos and Suzanne K. Freitag*

**Abstract**

This chapter provides a detailed description of the pertinent anatomy and embryology of the lacrimal system, followed by a discussion of the evaluation of the tearing infant. Management recommendations are detailed including the timing of intervention, minimally invasive treatments, and finally surgical management including probing and irrigation, turbinate infracture, and silicone intubation. Adjunctive treatment options including balloon dacryoplasty and nasal endoscopy are also discussed.

*Keywords:* congenital nasolacrimal obstruction, congenital lacrimal obstruction, epiphora, dacryocystitis, dacryocystocele, dacryocele, probing, irrigation, lacrimal intubation

## 4.1 Introduction

Congenital lacrimal obstruction commonly occurs in infants, heralded by symptoms of epiphora and infection including chronic discharge and conjunctivitis or occasionally dacryocystitis. The reported incidence of congenital lacrimal obstruction ranges from 1.2 to 30%.[1,2,3,4,5,6] One of the most commonly quoted incidences is 6%, which arises from a study of 200 consecutive live births in the 1940s in which nasolacrimal patency was assessed by the presence or absence of discharge with pressure on the lacrimal sac.[3] The incidence is known to be higher in children with craniofacial disorders and Down's syndrome.[7,8,9]

The decision-making regarding management of these children is complex for a variety of reasons. First, children are often not bothered by the symptoms, which on the contrary may be quite distressing for parents. Further, congenital nasolacrimal obstruction will resolve in about 96% of children spontaneously before 12 months of age.[4] There are a number of options for management, each with its advantages and disadvantages. Hence, management decisions must be carefully considered in each case and discussed in detail with parents. This chapter will review the thought process as well as procedures required to comprehensively manage the child with congenital lacrimal obstruction.

## 4.2 Anatomy and Embryology

Lacrimal system anatomy is covered in detail in Chapter 1. In brief, the lacrimal drainage system begins proximally with the upper and lower puncta located in the medial aspect of the eyelids. These vertical structures turn horizontally and run medially to form the upper and lower canaliculi, which in about 90% of individuals join to form the common canaliculus (internal common punctum) before entering the lacrimal sac. The lacrimal sac lies within the lacrimal sac fossa formed by the maxilla and lacrimal bone. The medial canthal tendon splits to wrap around the lacrimal sac. This important anatomic landmark provides attachment of the eyelids to the facial bones and must be preserved during lacrimal surgery. The lacrimal sac connects to the nasolacrimal duct, which runs within the maxilla to open into the inferior meatus of the nose, beneath the inferior turbinate. The valve of Hasner lies at the junction of the nasolacrimal duct and the nasal mucosa and is the most common site of congenital nasolacrimal obstruction.[10] There is most often a persistent membrane in this area, which can be disrupted with a probe to eliminate the obstruction. This is in contrast with acquired lacrimal obstruction, in which the site of obstruction is frequently the lacrimal sac or sac–duct junction, and the management paradigm is completely different.

An understanding of the embryology of the lacrimal system is helpful in clinically predicting the anatomy of patients with lacrimal anomalies. The development of the lacrimal system begins with surface ectoderm cells forming a ridge at the naso-optic fissure. These cells, at about 12 weeks' gestation, dive into the nearby mesoderm to form a solid ridge. The cells spread both superiorly toward the puncta and inferiorly toward the nose, while canalization of the solid rod is complete by about 6 months' gestation. The canaliculi become patent in the eyelid margin at about 7 months' gestation, just prior to the eyelids separating.[5]

While canalization of the ectodermal rod should be complete by 6 months' gestation, a persistent membrane often results at the junction with the nose. One study found that more than 70% of stillborn infants have congenital lacrimal obstruction at birth, which is many times higher than that noted in live births.[10] Similarly, infants born via cesarean section have been noted to have an almost double risk of congenital lacrimal obstruction.[11,12] It is thought that perinatal breathing, sucking, and crying likely play a significant role in the rupture of these persistent membranes.

Other less common lacrimal anomalies may occur as a result of embryologic dysgenesis at any stage of development. If portions of surface ectoderm fail to invaginate, agenesis of this section of the lacrimal system will result. Incomplete separation of the ectoderm from the surface may result in lacrimal fistulas or supernumerary puncta (▶ Fig. 4.1). These are rare and may be treated, if symptomatic, with excision or ablation. Incomplete ridge canalization may result in stenosis in any affected portion of the lacrimal outflow system.

## 4.3 Evaluation and Considerations in the Tearing Infant

Congenital lacrimal obstruction may be unilateral or bilateral, and parents may not recognize the problem until the child is a few weeks of age. Observations often include epiphora, elevated tear lake, mucopurulent discharge, and occasionally a visibly swollen lacrimal sac. Symptoms may not be present at birth since tear production in infants is not fully operational until about 3 weeks of age.

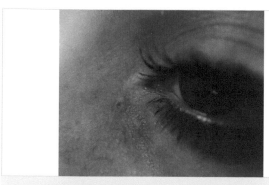

Fig. 4.1 External photograph of a young woman with a supranumerary punctum in a typical location inferior to the medial commissure of the eyelids.

It is important during the examination to keep in mind other possible etiologies of tearing in infants. The first distinction is to determine if there is overproduction of tears versus obstruction of outflow. Hypersecretion in infants may be a result of trichiasis, entropion, foreign body, corneal abrasion, congenital glaucoma, or other anterior segment pathology. Careful evaluation and consultation with a pediatric ophthalmologist is indicated if there are any concerns, as these etiologies may affect visual development, resulting in amblyopia.

Lacrimal system patency in infants is evaluated in several ways. First, the tear film is observed for elevation and presence of mucopurulent discharge. The eyelid skin and lashes are examined for erythema and crusting from chronic epiphora. The lacrimal sac is palpated for fullness and ability to express discharge through the puncta. Next a modified fluorescein dye disappearance test is performed. Fluorescein with topical anesthetic solution is placed into the inferior fornix of both eyes and the excess liquid is blotted. After 5 minutes, involving minimal manipulation of the eyes and eyelids, a cobalt blue filtered light is used to assess for presence of dye. In cases of normal lacrimal outflow, there should be no residual fluorescein present at 5 minutes.[13] A prospective study of 80 infants concluded that this test is 90% sensitive and 100% specific in the presence of nasolacrimal obstruction.[14] The presence of residual fluorescein is suggestive of lacrimal obstruction, although it does not specify which anatomic portion of the lacrimal system is affected. Hence, the history is important, as most parents can report when the obstruction began. Some children will have acquired lacrimal obstruction, which may occur after an episode of conjunctivitis, for example. The obstruction in this situation is likely to involve the canaliculi or lacrimal sac and is managed in a different manner than the child thought to have a persistent congenital membrane at the valve of Hasner. See Chapter 5 for a discussion of acquired lacrimal obstruction.

Infants may also present with a mass in the lacrimal sac area suggestive of dacryocele, also known as dacryocystocele or amniotocele when thought to be filled with amniotic fluid.[15] This dilatation of the lacrimal sac results from an obstruction not only distally at the valve of Hasner, but also proximally at the valve of Rosenmüller, creating a closed system. This condition is more common in females (78%)[16,17] and unilateral in 84 to 100% of cases.[16,17,18,19] If large, these masses can result in astigmatism and amblyopia.[16] Conservative treatment with warm compresses and massage has reported success rates of 17 to 80%.[16,17,19]

The trapped fluid is often sterile in young children, but there is a reported 14 to 75% risk of infection resulting in dacryocystitis with surrounding erythema and tenderness.[16,17,18,19] This preseptal cellulitis can spread to involve the orbit and other structures; hence, close monitoring is indicated. Hospital admission with intravenous antibiotics should be considered in cases of fever, orbital cellulitis, or severe preseptal cellulitis. Culture of the infectious material may be beneficial in selecting antimicrobial coverage, as is consultation with an infectious disease specialist. The most common organisms include *Staphylococcus aureus*, *Streptococcus pneumoniae*, and *Haemophilus influenza*.[20] Once the acute infection is improved with systemic antibiotic therapy, a definitive procedure such as probing should be performed, as will be discussed later in this chapter.

Care must be taken to identify other potential causes of medial canthal masses in children. Concern should be especially high in those masses that are centered above the medial canthal tendon. Such etiologies include meningoencephalocele, capillary hemangioma, dermoid cyst, pneumatocele, lymphangioma, primary lacrimal sac tumor, rhabdomyosarcoma, and nasal glioma.[21,22,23,24,25,26,27,28,29] If there are findings on examination causing concern about a diagnosis other than lacrimal obstruction, then imaging should be considered prior to surgical exploration so that there are proper expectations and planning. Radiographic imaging is discussed in Chapter 3.

It is important to be aware of the entity of congenital nasolacrimal obstruction associated with intranasal cyst formation, first described by Raflo et al in 1982.[30] This is most often recognized in the neonatal period when infants show signs of respiratory obstruction and distress, as they are obligate nose breathers. This rare entity requires a high level of suspicion and rapid intervention with nasal endoscopy and definitive treatment to rupture or marsupialize the cysts.[31,32,33,34,35,36]

## 4.4 Treatment

### 4.4.1 Conservative Management: Crigler's Massage

A conservative approach to the young infant with congenital lacrimal obstruction is often appropriate, as the majority of these obstructions will resolve spontaneously or with minimally invasive measures. The mainstays of conservative management are topical antibiotic as needed for discharge and lacrimal sac massage. Crigler described a technique for lacrimal sac massage in 1923 that involves placing a finger over the common canaliculus to block upward flow of contents and then stroking downward along the lacrimal sac in an effort to increase hydrostatic pressure to rupture the membrane at the junction of the nasolacrimal duct and nasal mucosa.[37] Parents may report a popping sensation if the massage is successful, followed by resolution of symptoms. Several reports show high success rates ranging from 85 to 94.7%, especially in very young patients.[19,38,39,40]

### 4.4.2 Probing and Irrigation

If conservative measures fail and the child is approaching 1 year of age, consideration must be given to more aggressive intervention. Most clinicians and investigators recommend lacrimal probing and irrigation as the next intervention.

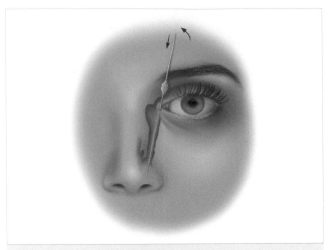

**Fig. 4.2** Probing of the nasolacrimal system. A lacrimal probe has been placed through the inferior punctum and canaliculus and then rotated vertically to traverse the lacrimal sac and nasolacrimal duct. The probe enters the nose in the inferior meatus where it will disrupt persistent membranes in cases of congenital lacrimal obstruction.

**Table 4.1** Success rate of probing for congenital nasolacrimal duct obstruction by age

| Study | No. of subjects | Success rate by age (%) | |
|---|---|---|---|
| Stager et al[42] | 2,369 | < 9 mo. = 94 | > 9 mo. = 84 |
| Katowitz and Welsh[45] | 572 | < 13 mo. = 97 | > 13 mo. = 55 |
| Mannor et al[46] | 142 | < 13 mo. = 92 | < 24 mo. = 89 |
| Zwaan[47] | 110 | < 12 mo. = 97 | < 24 mo. = 88 |
| Perveen et al[49] | 100 | < 12 mo = 94 | < 18 mo. = 84<br>< 24 mo. = 83<br>< 36 mo. = 62 |
| Robb[48] | 303 | | > 12 mo. = 92 |
| Le Garrec et al[51] | 329 | < 11mo. = 77 | |
| Rajabi et al[50] | 343 | | < 36 mo = 85<br>< 48 mo = 63<br>< 60 mo = 50 |

Probing may be performed either in the office setting in very young infants using a papoose device or at any age in the operating room under general anesthesia. The procedure begins with inspection of the anatomy including the puncta, medial canthus, and nasal cavity. Irrigation is performed next, prior to placement of probes in the lacrimal system, to confirm impatency of the system. Next, a punctal dilator is used to enlarge the lower punctum. A lacrimal probe is placed vertically into the punctum and then turned horizontally and advanced through the canaliculus until the "hard stop" of the lacrimal sac fossa bone is felt. The probe is then turned 90 degrees inferiorly and very slightly posteriorly to advance through the nasolacrimal duct into the inferior meatus of the nose (▶ Fig. 4.2). Occasionally, a popping sensation may be noted as the obstructing membrane is ruptured. Irrigation is repeated to confirm patency of the system. The same procedure should then be performed via the upper punctum and canaliculus. Some experts advocate using progressively larger probes to dilate the system.

The most common complication of nasolacrimal probing is creation of a false passage. The surgeon must exercise caution by passing the probe slowly and stop the procedure if a "soft stop" is encountered, suggesting that there is a proximal obstructive problem in the common canaliculus or lacrimal sac.

Because of the high rate of spontaneous resolution of lacrimal obstruction, often quoted at 96% by 1 year of age,[4] there has been much discussion in the literature regarding the optimal time for surgical intervention. Arguments for early intervention include early relief of symptoms (although these are usually more bothersome to the parent than the child) and avoidance of complications of lacrimal obstruction such as conjunctivitis, dacryocystitis, and cellulitis as well as chronic fibrosis of the lacrimal system. In addition, early probing may be performed in the office without the need for general anesthesia. This may be somewhat traumatic to parent and child, but one survey showed that 95% of parents found the procedure to be easier than expected and 81% were happy with their decision for early intervention.[41,42] The disadvantage of early probing is

that there is a high chance of resolution over time without surgical intervention.

Many experts strike a balance by advocating for probing under general anesthesia as soon as the child reaches 1 year of age. Anesthesia is thought to be safest by this age[43,44] and numerous studies have shown a decreasing rate of success of probing with increasing age after 1 year. ▶ Table 4.1 lists studies with 50 or more patients, showing various rates of decline.[42,45,46,47,48,49,50,51] It is logical that the more complex anatomic problems persist without spontaneous improvement and therefore older children have lower success rates with probing.

When probing and irrigation fail to resolve symptoms of lacrimal obstruction, many advocate a second probing and irrigation. Reported success rates for repeated probing procedures are variable, with one study of 1,748 patients up to 4 years of age showing 100% success,[52] while other studies are more typical of the Katowitz and Welsh report showing 54% success for second probing in 18- to 24-month-old children and 33% success in those older than 2 years.[45] Adjunctive procedures that may be beneficial at the time of the second probing include silicone bicanalicular intubation, infracture of the inferior turbinate, balloon catheter dilation, and nasal endoscopic evaluation.

## 4.5 Silicone Bicanalicular Intubation

Placement of silicone tubing in the lacrimal system at the time of probing is common practice, particularly after one failed probing. The tubing stents and dilates the newly opened lacrimal passage to prevent adhesion and restenosis. This procedure preserves the normal anatomy and is typically performed before other more invasive surgeries are considered. Quickert and Dryden first described this technique in 1970.[53] Under general anesthesia, a vasoconstricting agent such as oxymetazoline is placed in the inferior meatus of the nose. A silicone tube with metal probes at both ends is fed first through one punctum and

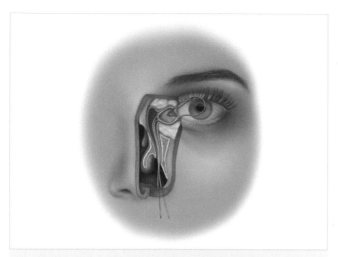

**Fig. 4.3** Silicone bicanalicular intubation of the nasolacrimal system. A silicone tube with both ends attached to metal probes is passed horizontally through the upper and lower puncta and canaliculi and then turned inferiorly through the lacrimal sac and nasolacrimal duct into the inferior meatus of the nose. The metal probe ends are retrieved and externalized through the nostril. Subsequently, the metal probe tips are removed and the tube tensioned appropriately.

canaliculus to the hard-stop, turned inferiorly and directed into the inferior meatus of the nose. A second probe is similarly placed through the ipsilateral punctum. The probes are retrieved from the nose with a hook and fixated at a tension that allows for some tube movement but not significant tube prolapse (▶ Fig. 4.3). Fixation may be via a foam bolster, a series of knots, or suture fixation to nasal wall.

The tube is generally well tolerated with only a small portion visible in the middle commissure of the eyelids. The optimal time for tube removal is controversial. It should be soon enough to avoid changes from chronic irritation such as pyogenic granuloma formation or slit puncta. Most advocate leaving tubes in place for 3 to 6 months,[54,55,56,57,58] but success has been reported with removal as early as 6 weeks.[59] Depending on the method of tube fixation and the cooperation of the patient, tube removal may require a general anesthetic. The overall success rate reported for silicone intubation in congenital lacrimal obstruction ranges from 77 to 100%.[42,46,47,48,53,54,60,61] Similar alternative techniques have proposed double bicanalicular intubation for wider dilation[62] and monocanalicular intubation, which has the disadvantage of poor stability and falling out in children.[63]

## 4.6 Infracture of the Inferior Turbinate

Infracture of the inferior turbinate stretches and moves the nasal mucosa away from the inferior meatus and ostium of the nasolacrimal duct. If there is any persistent membrane tissue, this procedure may relieve the physical obstruction and preserve the patency of a newly opened duct. This technique, described by Jones and Wobig in the 1970s,[64] is performed by placing an instrument such as a Freer elevator under the inferior turbinate and pushing medially until a sense of movement or give is felt (▶ Fig. 4.4). Havins and Wilkins reported an 88% success for this procedure combined with a second probing after failure of a first probing.[65]

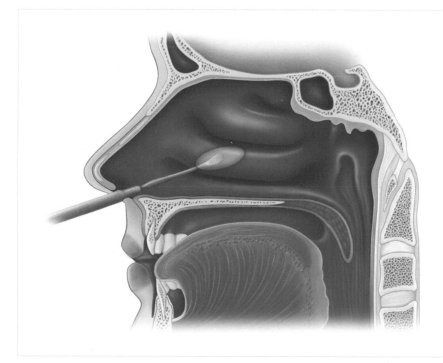

**Fig. 4.4** Infracture of the inferior turbinate is performed by placing an instrument such as a Freer elevator under the inferior turbinate and pushing medially until there is movement and slight inward dislocation of the turbinate.

## 4.7 Balloon Catheter Dilation

This procedure involving placement of a specially designed balloon within the lacrimal system and inflating it for dilation was first described by Becker et al in 1996.[66] Their original investigation reported a 95% success rate in 34 lacrimal systems with failed previous procedures. A meta-analysis of seven other studies suggested an 80% success rate in more heterogeneous groups of patients.[67] However, this procedure has fallen out of favor in recent years, likely due to the realization that other less expensive and less equipment-intensive techniques offer similar results.

## 4.8 Nasal Endoscopy

Viewing the inferior meatus of the nose endoscopically for purposes of inspection for physical obstructions as well as verification of probe placement during probing and irrigation may be useful. Probing failure rates due to false passage may be higher than realized. Choi et al reported visualization of a false passage in 5 of 11 probings, which were thought, based on surgeons' tactile feedback, to be in the correct location. Redirection of the probe in four of these five cases resulted in anatomic and functional success.[68] A similar study by MacEwen et al in 52 probings found false passage in 15% that were thought to be anatomically accurate.[69] Hence, endoscopic visualization of lacrimal procedures may help verify proper anatomic placement of instrumentation.

## 4.9 Dacryocystorhinostomy

Dacryocystorhinostomy (DCR) is a surgical procedure that creates a bypass fistula between the lacrimal sac and the nasal mucosa in the middle meatus of the nose. The procedure may be performed either endoscopically or externally. DCR is indicated in children in the following situations: congenital obstruction with failed previous procedures, congenital obstruction with dacryocystitis not resolved with antibiotics and probing, and traumatic or acquired nasolacrimal obstruction.

External DCR was first described in adults in 1904 by Toti.[70] The procedure involves creation of a skin incision in the area of the tear trough. Dissection is carried down to the anterior lacrimal crest periosteum, which is elevated with a periosteal elevator. A rongeur is used to create an osteotomy in this area to expose the underlying nasal mucosa in the middle meatus of the nose. The lacrimal sac is opened and anterior and posterior flaps are created. The nasal mucosa is similarly incised with creation of anterior and posterior flaps. Bicanalicular silicone tubes are passed through the upper lacrimal system and into the lacrimal sac. They are then directed through the ostium and fixated at the correct tension in the nose. The lacrimal sac flaps are anastomosed to the nasal mucosa flaps to allow for epithelialization of this new tract. Additional details about DCR surgery are found in Chapter 5.

Overall, the success rate for DCR in children is similar to that in adults, with reports ranging from 84 to 96%. Several studies that calculate DCR success rates based on various indications show that success is slightly higher for DCR performed in children for congenital obstruction (88–96%) than for other reasons (83–88%).[7,8,71,72,73]

Improvements in endoscopic equipment have led to a revival of the endonasal DCR approach, even for small pediatric noses. The endoscopic technique is described in Chapter 7. In 1998, Cunningham and Woog first reported endoscopic DCR in children with all four patients having a successful outcome.[74] Other reported success rates for pediatric endoscopic DCR range from 82 to 88%.[75,76,77] The main advantage of endoscopic DCR over external DCR is the absence of a cutaneous incision. Studies of adult patient satisfaction with external DCR incision scars suggest that most patients (67–79%) heal in a satisfactory manner.[78] However, there was a trend toward dissatisfaction in younger patients, and no data exist on pediatric external DCR scar acceptance. Hence, endoscopic DCR provides an excellent alternative, except for patients with congenital craniofacial abnormalities or syndromes in whom only 10% experienced complete resolution.[79]

## 4.10 Upper Lacrimal System Surgery

When congenital anomalies of the upper lacrimal system occur, it is important to attempt to delineate the anatomic abnormality. If there is focal canalicular obstruction, options include excision of the stenotic area with re-anastomosis, canalicular trephination with silicone intubation,[80] or holmium laser-assisted canaliculotomy with intubation.[81] However, most traditionally and for larger or unknown length segments of canalicular stenosis, conjunctivodacryocystorhinostomy (CDCR) is the procedure of choice.[82] This involves placement of a Pyrex glass tube from the medial canthus of the ocular surface to the middle meatus of the nose for direct drainage of tears. This is also useful in cases of agenesis of the upper lacrimal system, multiple failed DCRs, and common canalicular stenosis. Endoscopic guidance may be used to assure proper tube length and placement, so that a short tube is not occluded by the lateral nasal wall and a long tube is not occluded by the nasal septum or turbinate. Tube variants with bends, frosted glass, and rubber parasol flanges exist with the aim to reduce tube loss.

However, experience with CDCR in children is limited. In a recent review of 15 pediatric CDCR cases in children aged 9 to 14 years, Komínek et al, found a high level of success (14/15), but also a high rate of complication. These included tube malposition and tube extrusion requiring additional general anesthesia for reinsertion.[83] Although CDCR can be a successful procedure in children, parents and patients must be counseled that they are likely to require more than one surgery as well as frequent tube maintenance for life. For this reason, CDCR is usually delayed until a child is older and more able to tolerate tube manipulation in the office setting.

## References

[1] Cassady JV. Dacryocystitis of infancy. Am J Ophthalmol. 1948; 31(7):773–780, 875–877

[2] Ffooks OO. Dacryocystitis in infancy. Br J Ophthalmol. 1962; 46(7):422–434

[3] Guerry D, III, Kendig EL, Jr. Congenital impatency of the nasolacrimal duct. Arch Ophthal. 1948; 39(2):193–204

[4] MacEwen CJ, Young JDH. Epiphora during the first year of life. Eye (Lond). 1991; 5(Pt 5):596–600

[5] Sevel D. Development and congenital abnormalities of the nasolacrimal apparatus. J Pediatr Ophthalmol Strabismus. 1981; 18(5):13–19

[6] Stephenson S. A preliminary communication on the affections of the tear passages in newly born infants. M Press and Circ. 1899; 119:103–104

[7] Hakin KN, Sullivan TJ, Sharma A, Welham RA. Paediatric dacryocystorhinostomy. Aust N Z J Ophthalmol. 1994; 22(4):231–235

[8] Welham RA, Hughes SM. Lacrimal surgery in children. Am J Ophthalmol. 1985; 99(1):27–34

[9] Berk AT, Saatci AO, Erçal MD, Tunç M, Ergin M. Ocular findings in 55 patients with Down's syndrome. Ophthalmic Genet. 1996; 17(1):15–19

[10] Cassady JV. Developmental anatomy of nasolacrimal duct. AMA Arch Opthalmol. 1952; 47(2):141–158

[11] Kuhli-Hattenbach C, Lüchtenberg M, Hofmann C, Kohnen T. Increased prevalence of congenital dacryostenosis following cesarean section. Ophthalmologe. 2016; 113(8):675–683

[12] Spaniol K, Stupp T, Melcher C, Beheiri N, Eter N, Prokosch V. Association between congenital nasolacrimal duct obstruction and delivery by cesarean section. Am J Perinatol. 2015; 32(3):271–276

[13] Zappia RJ, Milder B. Lacrimal drainage function. 2. The fluorescein dye disappearance test. Am J Ophthalmol. 1972; 74(1):160–162

[14] MacEwen CJ, Young JDH. The fluorescein disappearance test (FDT): an evaluation of its use in infants. J Pediatr Ophthalmol Strabismus. 1991; 28(6): 302–305

[15] Jones LT, Wobig JL. The lacrimal system. Am Acad Ophthalmol Otolaryngol. 1977; 83:603–616

[16] Mansour AM, Cheng KP, Mumma JV, et al. Congenital dacryocele. A collaborative review. Ophthalmology. 1991; 98(11):1744–1751

[17] Sullivan TJ, Clarke MP, Morin JD, Pashby RC. Management of congenital dacryocystocoele. Aust N Z J Ophthalmol. 1992; 20(2):105–108

[18] Boynton JR, Drucker DN. Distention of the lacrimal sac in neonates. Ophthalmic Surg. 1989; 20(2):103–107

[19] Petersen RA, Robb RM. The natural course of congenital obstruction of the nasolacrimal duct. J Pediatr Ophthalmol Strabismus. 1978; 15(4):246–250

[20] MacEwen CJ, Phillips MG, Young JD. Value of bacterial culturing in the course of congenital nasolacrimal duct (NLD) obstruction. J Pediatr Ophthalmol Strabismus. 1994; 31(4):246–250

[21] Baron EM, Kersten RC, Kulwin DR. Rhabdomyosarcoma manifesting as acquired nasolacrimal duct obstruction. Am J Ophthalmol. 1993; 115(2):239–242

[22] Brownstein MH, Helwig EB. Subcutaneous dermoid cysts. Arch Dermatol. 1973; 107(2):237–239

[23] Dayal Y, Hameed S. Periorbital dermoid. Am J Ophthalmol. 1962; 53:1013–1016

[24] Hurwitz JJ, Rodgers J, Doucet TW. Dermoid tumor involving the lacrimal drainage pathway: a case report. Ophthalmic Surg. 1982; 13(5):377–379

[25] Lampertico P, Ibanez ML. Nasal glioma (encephalochoristoma nasofrontalis). Arch Otolaryngol. 1964; 79:628–631

[26] Mims J, Rodrigues M, Calhoun J. Sudoriferous cyst of the orbit. Can J Ophthalmol. 1977; 12(2):155–156

[27] Rashid ER, Bergstrom TJ, Evans RM, Arnold AC. Anterior encephalocele presenting as nasolacrimal obstruction. Ann Ophthalmol. 1986; 18(4):132–136, 134–136

[28] Remulla HD, Rubin PA, Shore JW, Cunningham MJ. Pseudodacryocystitis arising from anterior ethmoiditis. Ophthal Plast Reconstr Surg. 1995; 11(3):165–168

[29] Saunders JF. Congenital sudoriferous cyst of the orbit. Arch Ophthalmol. 1973; 89(3):205–206

[30] Raflo GT, Horton JA, Sprinkle PM. An unusual intranasal anomaly of the lacrimal drainage system. Ophthalmic Surg. 1982; 13(9):741–744

[31] Calcaterra VE, Annino DJ, Carter BL, Woog JJ. Congenital nasolacrimal duct cysts with nasal obstruction. Otolaryngol Head Neck Surg. 1995; 113(4):481–484

[32] Denis D, Saracco JB, Triglia JM. Nasolacrimal duct cysts in congenital dacryocystocele. Graefes Arch Clin Exp Ophthalmol. 1994; 232(4):252–254

[33] Divine RD, Anderson RL, Bumsted RM. Bilateral congenital lacrimal sac mucoceles with nasal extension and drainage. Arch Ophthalmol. 1983; 101 (2):246–248

[34] Grin TR, Mertz JS, Stass-Isern M. Congenital nasolacrimal duct cysts in dacryocystocele. Ophthalmology. 1991; 98(8):1238–1242

[35] Righi PD, Hubbell RN, Lawlor PP, Jr. Respiratory distress associated with bilateral nasolacrimal duct cysts. Int J Pediatr Otorhinolaryngol. 1993; 26(2): 199–203

[36] Yee SW, Seibert RW, Bower CM, Glasier CM. Congenital nasolacrimal duct mucocele: a cause of respiratory distress. Int J Pediatr Otorhinolaryngol. 1994; 29(2):151–158

[37] Crigler LW. The treatment of congenital dacryocystitis. JAMA. 1923; 81:21–24

[38] Nelson LR, Calhoun JH, Menduke H. Medical management of congenital nasolacrimal duct obstruction. Ophthalmology. 1985; 92(9):1187–1190

[39] Paul TO. Medical management of congenital nasolacrimal duct obstruction. J Pediatr Ophthalmol Strabismus. 1985; 22(2):68–70

[40] Nucci P, Capoferri C, Alfarano R, Brancato R. Conservative management of congenital nasolacrimal duct obstruction. J Pediatr Ophthalmol Strabismus. 1989; 26(1):39–43

[41] Goldblum TA, Summers CG, Egbert JE, Letson RD. Office probing for congenital nasolacrimal duct obstruction: a study of parental satisfaction. J Pediatr Ophthalmol Strabismus. 1996; 33(4):244–247

[42] Stager D, Baker JD, Frey T, Weakley DR, Jr, Birch EE. Office probing of congenital nasolacrimal duct obstruction. Ophthalmic Surg. 1992; 23(7):482–484

[43] Backeljauw B, Holland SK, Altaye M, Loepke AW. Cognition and brain structure following early childhood surgery with anesthesia. Pediatrics. 2015; 136(1):e1–e12

[44] Sun L. Early childhood general anaesthesia exposure and neurocognitive development. Br J Anaesth. 2010; 105 Suppl 1:i61–i68

[45] Katowitz JA, Welsh MG. Timing of initial probing and irrigation in congenital nasolacrimal duct obstruction. Ophthalmology. 1987; 94(6):698–705

[46] Mannor GE, Rose GE, Frimpong-Ansah K, Ezra E. Factors affecting the success of nasolacrimal duct probing for congenital nasolacrimal duct obstruction. Am J Ophthalmol. 1999; 127(5):616–617

[47] Zwaan J. Treatment of congenital nasolacrimal duct obstruction before and after the age of 1 year. Ophthalmic Surg Lasers. 1997; 28(11):932–936

[48] Robb RM. Success rates of nasolacrimal duct probing at time intervals after 1 year of age. Ophthalmology. 1998; 105(7):1307–1309, discussion 1309–1310

[49] Perveen S, Sufi AR, Rashid S, Khan A. Success rate of probing for congenital nasolacrimal duct obstruction at various ages. J Ophthalmic Vis Res. 2014; 9 (1):60–69

[50] Rajabi MT, Abrishami Y, Hosseini SS, Tabatabaee SZ, Rajabi MB, Hurwitz JJ. Success rate of late primary probing in congenital nasolacrimal duct obstruction. J Pediatr Ophthalmol Strabismus. 2014; 51(6):360–362

[51] Le Garrec J, Abadie-Koebele C, Parienti JJ, Molgat Y, Degoumois A, Mouriaux F. Nasolacrimal duct office probing in children under the age of 12 months: cure rate and cost evaluation. J Fr Ophtalmol. 2016; 39(2):171–177

[52] Singh Bhinder G, Singh Bhinder H. Repeated probing results in the treatment of congenital nasolacrimal duct obstruction. Eur J Ophthalmol. 2004; 14(3): 185–192

[53] Quickert MH, Dryden RM. Probes for intubation in lacrimal drainage. Trans Am Acad Ophthalmol Otolaryngol. 1970; 74(2):431–433

[54] al-Hussain H, Nasr AM. Silastic intubation in congenital nasolacrimal duct obstruction: a study of 129 eyes. Ophthal Plast Reconstr Surg. 1993; 9(1):32–37

[55] Dortzbach RK, France TD, Kushner BJ, Gonnering RS. Silicone intubation for obstruction of the nasolacrimal duct in children. Am J Ophthalmol. 1982; 94 (5):585–590

[56] Leone CR, Jr, Van Gemert JV. The success rate of silicone intubation in congenital lacrimal obstruction. Ophthalmic Surg. 1990; 21(2):90–92

[57] Welsh MG, Katowitz JA. Timing of Silastic tubing removal after intubation for congenital nasolacrimal duct obstruction. Ophthal Plast Reconstr Surg. 1989; 5(1):43–48

[58] Durso F, Hand SI, Jr, Ellis FD, Helveston EM. Silicone intubation in children with nasolacrimal obstruction. J Pediatr Ophthalmol Strabismus. 1980; 17(6): 389–393

[59] Migliori ME, Putterman AM. Silicone intubation for the treatment of congenital lacrimal duct obstruction: successful results removing the tubes after six weeks. Ophthalmology. 1988; 95(6):792–795

[60] Honavar SG, Prakash VE, Rao GN. Outcome of probing for congenital nasolacrimal duct obstruction in older children. Am J Ophthalmol. 2000; 130 (1):42–48

[61] Kashkouli MB, Kassaee A, Tabatabaee Z. Initial nasolacrimal duct probing in children under age 5: cure rate and factors affecting success. J AAPOS. 2002; 6(6):360–363

[62] Mauffray RO, Hassan AS, Elner VM. Double silicone intubation as treatment for persistent congenital nasolacrimal duct obstruction. Ophthal Plast Reconstr Surg. 2004; 20(1):44–49

[63] Kaufman LM, Guay-Bhatia LA. Monocanalicular intubation with Monoka tubes for the treatment of congenital nasolacrimal duct obstruction. Ophthalmology. 1998; 105(2):336–341

[64] Jones LT, Wobig JL. The Wendell L. Hughes Lecture. Newer concepts of tear duct and eyelid anatomy and treatment. Trans Sect Ophthalmol Am Acad Ophthalmol Otolaryngol. 1977; 83(4, Pt 1):603–616

[65] Havins WE, Wilkins RB. A useful alternative to silicone intubation in congenital nasolacrimal duct obstructions. Ophthalmic Surg. 1983; 14(8): 666–670

[66] Becker BB, Berry FD, Koller H. Balloon catheter dilatation for treatment of congenital nasolacrimal duct obstruction. Am J Ophthalmol. 1996; 121(3): 304–309

[67] Lin AE, Chang YC, Lin MY, Tam KW, Shen YD. Comparison of treatment for congenital nasolacrimal duct obstruction: a systematic review and meta-analysis. Can J Ophthalmol. 2016; 51(1):34–40

[68] Choi WC, Kim KS, Park TK, Chung CS. Intranasal endoscopic diagnosis and treatment in congenital nasolacrimal duct obstruction. Ophthalmic Surg Lasers. 2002; 33(4):288–292

[69] MacEwen CJ, Young JD, Barras CW, Ram B, White PS. Value of nasal endoscopy and probing in the diagnosis and management of children with congenital epiphora. Br J Ophthalmol. 2001; 85(3):314–318

[70] Toti A. Nuovo metodo conservatore dicura radicale delle sopperazioni croniche del sacco lacrimale (dacriocistorinostomia). Clin Moderna. 1904; 10:385–387

[71] Nowinski TS, Flanagan JC, Mauriello J. Pediatric dacryocystorhinostomy. Arch Ophthalmol. 1985; 103(8):1226–1228

[72] Becker BB. Dacryocystorhinostomy without flaps. Ophthalmic Surg. 1988; 19 (6):419–427

[73] Rosen N, Sharir M, Moverman DC, Rosner M. Dacryocystorhinostomy with silicone tubes: evaluation of 253 cases. Ophthalmic Surg. 1989; 20(2):115–119

[74] Cunningham MJ, Woog JJ. Endonasal endoscopic dacryocystorhinostomy in children. Arch Otolaryngol Head Neck Surg. 1998; 124(3):328–333

[75] Wong JF, Woog JJ, Cunningham MJ, Rubin PA, Curtin HD, Carter BL. A multidisciplinary approach to atypical lacrimal obstruction in childhood. Ophthal Plast Reconstr Surg. 1999; 15(4):293–298

[76] Komínek P, Cervenka S. Pediatric endonasal dacryocystorhinostomy: a report of 34 cases. Laryngoscope. 2005; 115(10):1800–1803

[77] Vanderveen DK, Jones DT, Tan H, Petersen RA. Endoscopic dacryocystorhino-stomy in children. J AAPOS. 2001; 5(3):143–147

[78] Caesar RH, Fernando G, Scott K, McNab AA. Scarring in external dacryocystorhinostomy: fact or fiction? Orbit. 2005; 24(2):83–86

[79] Jones DT, Fajardo NF, Petersen RA, VanderVeen DK. Pediatric endoscopic dacryocystorhinostomy failures: who and why? Laryngoscope. 2007; 117(2): 323–327

[80] Sisler HA, Allarakhia L. New minitrephine makes lacrimal canalicular rehabilitation an office procedure. Ophthal Plast Reconstr Surg. 1990; 6(3): 203–206

[81] Dutton JJ, Holck DE. Holmium laser canaliculoplasty. Ophthal Plast Reconstr Surg. 1996; 12(3):211–217

[82] Jones LT. The cure of epiphora due to canalicular disorders, trauma and surgical failures on the lacrimal passages. Trans Am Acad Ophthalmol Otolaryngol. 1962; 66:506–524

[83] Komínek P, Cervenka S, Matousek P, Pniak T, Zeleník K. Conjunctivocysto-rhinostomy with Jones tube: is it the surgery for children? Graefes Arch Clin Exp Ophthalmol. 2010; 248(9):1339–1343

# 5 Evaluation and Management of Acquired Lacrimal Obstruction

Catherine Banks, Raymond Sacks, and Geoffrey Wilcsek

**Abstract**

The evaluation and management of the tearing patient requires a systematic approach to avoid incorrect diagnosis and treatment. This chapter demonstrates the essential features of history and examination in patients with epiphora. By understanding the basic etiology of tearing, identifying key questions on history, and appropriate functional clinical tests on examination, informed decisions can be made utilizing the treatment pathways for the tearing patient. The clinician cannot assess acquired nasolacrimal duct obstruction (ANLDO) in isolation. Understanding the range of issues that can cause epiphora in patients is essential in order to adequately manage patients with ANLDO. If the clinician treats all tearing patients as NLDO requiring nasolacrimal drainage surgery, some patients will not improve and other patients will suffer increased symptoms based on ocular surface issues, leaving the patient injured and the surgeon frustrated.

*Keywords:* epiphora, acquired nasolacrimal duct obstruction, dye disappearance test, Jones 1, Jones 2, sac washout, dacryocystorhinostomy, punctal, canalicular, treatment pathways

## 5.1 Introduction

Epiphora is the presence of a watering eye with overflow on to the cheek. Its impact on quality of life (QOL) should not be trivialized and is often underestimated by those who do not suffer from epiphora.

Symptomatic epiphora can affect vision and activities of daily living, including reading, driving, an ability to work, and an ability to enjoy outdoor activities. Patients suffer from social embarrassment and a reduction in overall vision-related QOL.[1,2,3,4]

When evaluating epiphora, it is helpful to think in terms of either an overproduction or an underdrainage of tears, although in reality etiology is often multifactorial. The goal of management and the decision to operate is dependent on the relative component of overproduction and underdrainage and the presence of intercurrent dry eye, acknowledging they are often mixed.

This chapter presents a systematic approach to the patient with epiphora to better identify and treat those patients with acquired lacrimal obstruction. The fundamental principles of this chapter have been conceptualized and are represented as two flow diagrams (▶ Fig. 5.1 and ▶ Fig. 5.2) to permit a clear framework for the reader to base decision-making and treatment strategies.

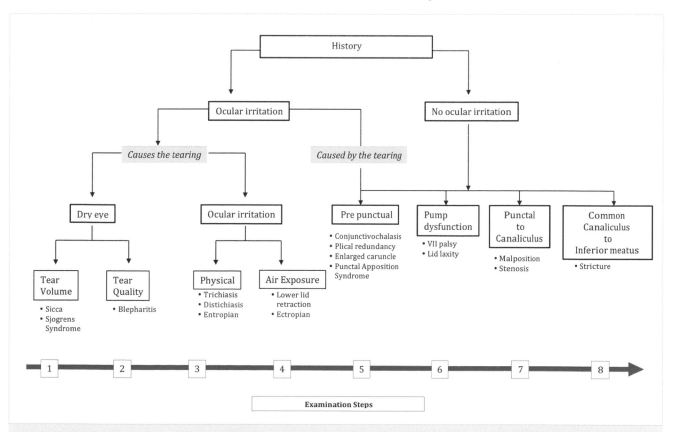

**Fig. 5.1** Treatment pathway: history and examination steps. Summary of evaluation of acquired nasolacrimal obstruction. Essential steps in history and the sequential examination steps proceeding from left to right beginning with tear volume and ending with inferior meatus.

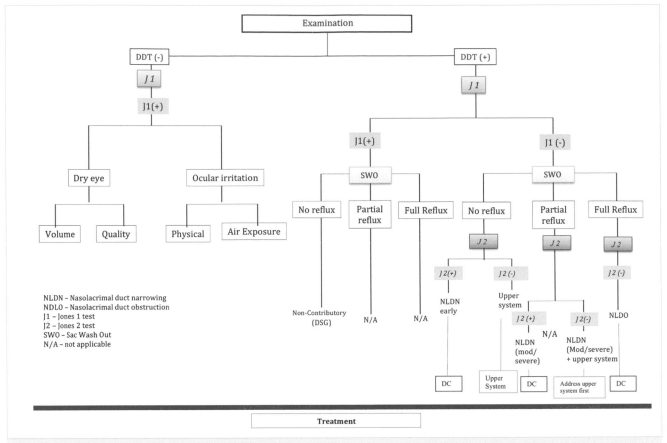

**Fig. 5.2** Treatment pathway: examination and treatment. Summary of examination and treatment of acquired nasolacrimal obstruction. No reflux: fluid is forced into the nose with no reflux into the upper lid. Partial reflux: saline fluid is forced out the fellow ipsilateral canaliculus with some fluid in the nose. Full reflux: all the normal saline refluxes out of the ipsilateral companion punctum with no fluid forced into the nose.

# 5.2 Evaluation of Patients with Epiphora: History

The critical goal is to establish if a patient has overproduction or underdrainage of tears. This process can be simplified by a series of sequential steps on history and examination as shown in ▶ Fig. 5.1.

## 5.2.1 Does the Patient Have Ocular Irritation or Not? If So, Are Tears the Cause or the Result of the Ocular Irritation?

The afferent arm of the tearing reflex originates as trigeminal nerve endings within the cornea.[5] Hence, anything that causes corneal irritation and therefore pain stimulates tear production. Conversely, reduced drainage of tears from the conjunctival sac with resultant stasis of tears on the cornea will irritate the cornea and cause a foreign body sensation and irritation. It is therefore critical to delineate on history whether the patient feels that the irritation precedes (causes) the epiphora and is likely to be due to irritation of the cornea.

In this case, the corneal irritation is due to either dry patches developing on the cornea in dry eye or ocular exposure, or a physical irritation such as lash-to-cornea touch.

If, however, the patient feels that the ocular irritative symptoms are secondary to (occur after) the epiphora, then the foreign body sensation is more likely due to stasis of tears on the cornea secondary to reduced lacrimal drainage.

The tear film is a complex trilamellar structure of mucus, aqueous, and lipid layers that should be produced in an adequate volume and function. An important function of tears is to adhere to the cornea for the period between blinks when the corneal tear film is again replenished. As such, dry eye can be divided into sicca, which is a reduction in volume of tears within the tear film, and quality issues that are often due to abnormalities of the lipid layer, associated with meibomian gland dysfunction (MGD).

### For the Dry Eye: Is the Tear Volume Inadequate or Is Tear Quality Reduced?

#### Tear Volume

Causes of reduced tear volume include sicca. The dry eye is a multifactorial disease of the tears and ocular surface that results in symptoms of discomfort, visual disturbance, and tear film instability with potential damage to the ocular surface. Sjögren's syndrome should also be considered in the differential of the dry eye.

When there are symptoms with tearing secondary to dry eye, these patients will have irritation or stinging causing the tearing or preceding the tearing. They tend to get more issues toward the end of the day and complain of the eyes feeling heavy and tired. It is worse when exposed to a dry environment or performing visual tasks, such as driving or reading, as the blink rate is reduced undertaking these tasks.

## Tear Quality

Blepharitis is often associated with dysfunction of the meibomian glands. The meibomian glands produce the lipid layer of tears. Blepharitis is a common condition and a cause of poor tear quality. These patients tend to note crusting of the eyelids on waking associated with discharge and often describe a burning sensation associated with red eyelid rims. They also tend to get the progression of symptoms throughout the day, especially when undertaking visual tasks when the blink rate reduces. On further questioning, they have a history of rosacea, acne type symptoms, and facial flushing, which can be associated with alcohol consumption.

If ocular irritation is not due to a dry eye, the focus of our attention becomes the following.

## 5.2.2 Is the Cause of the Tearing due to Ocular Irritation? If So, Is It Related to Physical Trauma or Air Exposure?

The other cohort of patients that will have irritation causing the tearing. They are further divided into either physical or air exposure groups.

## For Ocular Irritation, Is the Ocular Irritation Secondary to Physical Irritation or Air Exposure?

### Physical

Physical causes of stimulation/irritation of the cornea include trichiasis (follicles in a normal position but lashes misdirected toward the cornea), distichiasis (lash follicles originate in an abnormally posterior position at the lid margin emerging from the meibomian glands) and entropion (the entire lid turns in causing normal lashes and skin to irritate the cornea). These conditions stimulate the corneal nerve endings causing pain and stimulating lacrimation. Patients with trichiasis and distichiasis tend to have a history of epilation by an eye care physician. Entropion or spastic entropion tends to be episodic; during episodes of spastic entropion, there is a lot of irritation and tearing. This will settle for hours to days, only to recur. Over time, this will progressively get worse until it becomes constant.

### Air Exposure

The normal palpebral aperture (distance between the upper and lower eyelid) is 7 to 10 mm; thus, lower lid retraction or ectropion causing only a 1-mm lowering of the lid margin will increase ocular exposure by a minimum of 10%. Other less common causes of ocular exposure include upper lid retraction

(most commonly thyroid orbitopathy), proptosis, and facial nerve palsy.

Patients with lower lid retraction and ectropion tend to have similar symptoms to the sicca and dry eye patients, except the former present red eye and inflamed tarsal conjunctiva of ectropion and associated mucus discharge in the mornings and throughout the day. The mucus produced overnight by the irritated tarsal conjunctiva dries during sleep as the aqueous solution of the tear film reduces overnight and the eyelids are glued together on waking.

## Now Consider the Following: Is Ocular Irritation Caused by Tearing?

If the patient notes that their epiphora is not preceded by ocular irritation but rather follows or is caused by the tearing, "underdrainage" is considered. Tears are a dilute protein solution made up of lysozymes, lactoferrin, secretory immunoglobulin A, serum albumin, lipocalin and lipophilin, and electrolytes. A study comparing the composition of normal tears to those with acquired lacrimal duct obstruction found patients with acquired lacrimal duct obstruction had more alkaline tears, higher calcium concentration, and unstable proportion of tear proteins compared with normal persons.[6] Irritation results from stasis of tears.

The lacrimal drainage apparatus is divided into the proximal and distal sections. The proximal section includes the punctum, canaliculus, and the common canaliculus. The distal lacrimal section consists of the lacrimal sac and the nasolacrimal duct that opens into inferior meatus of the nose.

Once underdrainage is presumed, our approach is to classify ocular irritation caused by tearing into four key groups. It is worth noting that the four key groups are also to be considered for epiphora with absence of ocular irritation (▶ Fig. 5.1):
- Prepunctal.
- Pump dysfunction.
- Punctal to canaliculus.
- Common canaliculus to inferior meatus.

### Prepunctal

Any condition that blocks access to the punctum is considered prepunctal. This includes conjunctivochalasis, redundant plica, and lateralized or enlarged caruncle abutting the puncta. Conjunctivochalasis is redundant, loose, nonedematous bulbar conjunctival folds over the lid margin that affect the flow of tears along the lower lid tear meniscus. Similarly redundancy of the plica semilunaris overlying the lower lid punctum can abut and occlude the punctum. Punctal apposition syndrome occurs when laxity of the lateral canthal tendon allows medialization of the lower punctum (normally sits medial to the upper punctum) such that it lines up with the upper punctum. With blinking, the upper and lower puncta "kiss" occluding each other during the active phase of the blink.

History is usually noncontributory in diagnosing prepunctal issues, and they are much better diagnosed on examination. Patients with conjunctivochalasis may comment on a foreign body sensation in the eye.

### Pump Dysfunction

During active phase of blinking, tears are actively driven via the upper and lower canaliculi into the sac. The orbicularis, along with its attachment around the lacrimal sac and bony attachment at the medial and lateral canthal tendons, plays a crucial role in a dynamic pump mechanism. If these muscles or tendons are compromised in any way, such as facial nerve palsy, underdrainage can occur.[7]

Medical history will entail a facial nerve injury or operations involving the facial nerve, parotid surgery, or Bell's palsy. It is in examination as described below that pump dysfunction is most effectively diagnosed.

### Punctal to Canaliculus

Stenosis of the punctum can be defined as inability to pass a 26-gauge lacrimal cannula.[8] Chronic blepharitis is widely associated with punctal stenosis secondary to the development of fibrotic change within the ostium. Topical and systemic medications and numerous systemic diseases have also been implicated. Eyelid malposition, due to either localized inflammation or underuse, may also cause punctal stenosis. Canalicular obstruction can be anatomically classified as proximal with involvement of the proximal 2 to 3 mm, mid-canalicular obstructions 3 to 8 mm from the punctum, and distal obstructions as defined by a membrane at the opening of the common canaliculus to the lacrimal sac.[9]

A history of chronic use of preserved eye drops, certain chemotherapeutics (e.g., docetaxel), and significant episode of conjunctivitis preceding the tearing should raise a suspicion of canalicular stenosis. History of any surgery to punctum, punctal snips or canaliculi or any trauma should be elicited.

### Common Canaliculus to the Inferior Meatus

Stricture formation or obstruction secondary to trauma, infections, prior surgery, postradiation, chronic sinus disease, or neoplasms can affect and obstruct any portion of the nasolacrimal system.

For common canaliculus to inferior meatus, you might ask for a history of use of punctal plugs, as these can migrate and cause a stricture.

## 5.3 Evaluation of Patient with Epiphora: Examination

The flow diagram in ▶ Fig. 5.2 allows for a systematic approach to examination and subsequent treatment, which is outlined in the following section.

### 5.3.1 Dye Disappearance Test

On examination, the fluorescein dye disappearance test (DDT) is the most important functional test in deciding whether epiphora is likely secondary to overproduction or underdrainage. At the start of the consultation, two drops of either 1 or 2% fluorescein solution is instilled into each conjunctival sac. After 5 minutes of history taking, a fluorescein stain tear meniscus that remains high is considered delayed DDT and would be due to outflow obstruction (▶ Fig. 5.3). A normal or negative DDT (DDT−) is defined as having fluorescein cleared from the meniscus over a 5-minute period.[10]

A DDT− indicates that the epiphora is likely due to dry eye with reflex dumping of tears or ocular irritation as per ▶ Fig. 5.2.

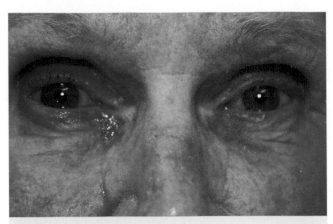

Fig. 5.3 Dye disappearance test. A positive dye disappearance test in the right eye. Note the fluorescein stain tear meniscus remains high compared to the left eye.

### 5.3.2 The Jones 1 and 2 Tests

In a patient with a delayed DDT (positive DDT), a Jones test under nasal endoscopic control is the next important functional test. Two sprays of Co-Phenylcaine intranasally at the start of the consultation will decongest the nose and allow a more efficient endoscopic examination. A Jones test is aimed at detecting any fluorescein egress at the distal end of the nasolacrimal duct within the inferior meatus. Jones initially described this by placing a cotton tip within the inferior meatus.[11] It is much more effectively done using an endoscope (▶ Fig. 5.4a). A Jones 2 test is performed when the Jones test is repeated after flushing the lacrimal system with normal saline via the upper or lower canaliculus (▶ Fig. 5.4b).

### 5.3.3 Sac Washout

The next important functional test is a sac washout (SWO). We use a saline-filled 3-mL syringe with a 26-gauge lacrimal cannula. With the lower lid on stretch, the cannula is placed through the punctum and the plunger depressed (▶ Fig. 5.5a, b). In patients with patent ducts or ducts with early narrowing, fluid is forced into the nose with no reflux into the upper lid. In patients with narrowing severe enough to cause back pressure within the duct, saline fluid is forced out the fellow ipsilateral canaliculus in a retrograde fashion. In patients with complete nasolacrimal duct obstruction, the entire volume of normal saline will reflux back out of the ipsilateral companion punctum. In patients with enough narrowing of the nasolacrimal duct to stop the passage of fluorescein-stained tears, the Jones 1 test will be negative. Then given the force of the plunger pushing saline through the system, any fluorescein that has been held up at the nasolacrimal duct narrowing will be pushed through, resulting in a positive Jones 2 test. Patients who have a completely obstructed nasolacrimal duct will not have any fluid that would be passed into the nose and as such the Jones 2 test will remain negative.

The Jones test is a qualitative, not quantitative, test and so it is difficult to tell a small versus a large amount of dye and, by the same logic, even a small narrowing that may cause epiphora in a patient with robust tear production may still allow some passage of fluorescein-stained tears. It is important to understand that patients with early narrowing of the nasolacrimal duct may cause a mismatch between the amount of tears

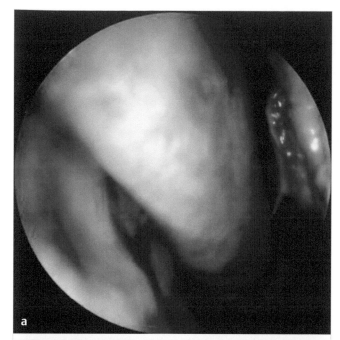

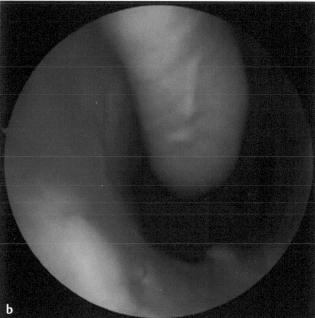

**Fig. 5.4** **(a)** The Jones 1 test. A positive Jones 1 test with visible fluorescein seen in the right inferior meatus. **(b)** The Jones 2 test. The Jones test is repeated after flushing the lacrimal system with normal saline via the upper or lower canaliculus.

could have either early nasolacrimal duct narrowing (NLDN) or a delay in tears reaching the sac. If the anatomy of the lid (punctal position, caliber, etc.) is normal on inspection, then lacrimal pump dysfunction is considered. DSG can demonstrate abnormalities in 80 to 95% of symptomatic patients with a patent lacrimal system on syringing; however, it cannot reliably distinguish between these two conditions. The absence of anatomical detail on the scintigraphy often prevents localization of the delay site.[12] In the authors' experience, it is a reasonable test to differentiate upper versus lower system issues in these patients and therefore can help prognosticate the likelihood of a successful dacryocystorhinostomy (DCR) resulting in an improvement in the patient's epiphora.

## 5.3.5 Treatment

Knowing which way to treat a tearing patient is dependent on the examination, given that the Jones test and SWO are functional tests. The interpretation of the results is influenced by the history, but history is more important in guiding the clinician on which part of the examination to pay extra attention to.

The following is a summary based on ▶ Fig. 5.2. For those patients with a positive Jones 1 test, history and examination as outlined earlier will allow the patient to decide whether the causative issue is dry eye or whether the dry eye is a volume or quality issue. It cannot be overemphasized how important it is to identify these patients. Performing a DCR successfully on a patient with dry eye problems, due to either volume or quality deficiency of the tear film, will result in increased egress of tears away from the conjunctival sac, further drying of the ocular surface, an increase in patient symptoms and potentially corneal decompensation. For those patients with a Jones 1 positive test and ocular irritation due to either physical disruption of the cornea such as in entropion or purely air exposure such as lid retraction, treatment of these conditions are beyond the remit of this chapter.

For those patients that are DDT +, these patients have an underdrainage issue. Those patients who have a Jones 1 positive test will be followed by SWO. If the SWO reveals no reflux into the ipsilateral companion punctum, then the function tests are not contributory and a DSG is indicated as this scenario can equally be caused by very early nasolacrimal duct narrowing or an upper system or lacrimal pump issue.

In those patients with a DDT + and a negative Jones 1 test, the next step would be an SWO. Should there be no reflux into the companion punctum and the Jones 2 test becomes positive, this indicates an early nasolacrimal duct narrowing and DCR is indicated. If, however, the Jones 2 test remains negative, then an upper system issue will be the rate-limiting step and the clinician must again look for punctal malposition or a stenosis. If no anatomical problem can be found, then lacrimal pump dysfunction should be entertained and potentially a Jones tube is indicated.

In those patients with a DDT + and a negative Jones 1, where on SWO there is partial reflux resulting in a positive Jones 2 test, again this indicates a more significant narrowing of the nasolacrimal duct and DCR is indicated. If the Jones 2 test remains negative, then although the SWO indicates a moderate nasolacrimal duct narrowing, the rate-limiting step must still be in the upper system and therefore either lid surgery or lid canalicular or lid and canalicular surgery or Jones tube would be required depending on the underlying cause.

produced and the amount of tears that can be drained through the slightly narrowed duct. In these patients, if there is not enough narrowing to cause a backflow pressure and reflux at the upper canaliculus, they will have a positive Jones 1 test, normal SWO, and positive Jones 2 test. It is in these patients that a dacryoscintigraphy (DSG) may be helpful.

## 5.3.4 Dacryoscintigraphy

DSG can be utilized in patients who appear to have a patent system on SWO and yet have a delayed DDT (see ▶ Fig. 5.2). These patients

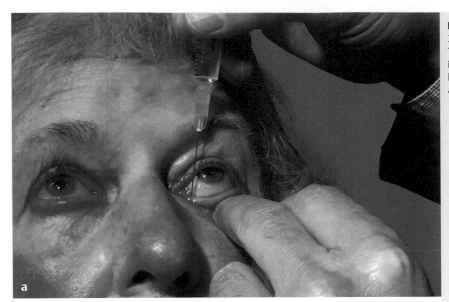

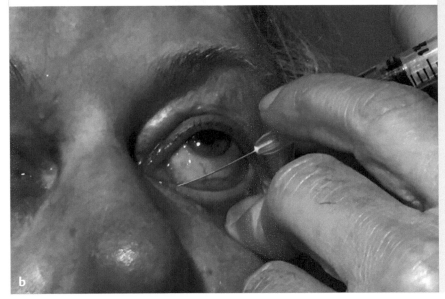

**Fig. 5.5** **(a)** The sac washout test. A saline-filled 3-mL syringe with a 26-g lacrimal cannula is used. The lower lid on stretch, the cannula is placed initially vertically through the punctum. **(b)** The lacrimal cannula is then angulated horizontally and the plunger is depressed.

In a patient with a DDT + and a negative Jones 1 test with the subsequent SWO showing full reflux into the companion punctum, the Jones 2 test will remain negative, confirming the nasolacrimal duct obstruction suspected on full reflux from SWO and a DCR is indicated.

## 5.4 Surgical Treatment of the Lower System

Critics of the endoscopic approach argued that external outcomes were superior to endonasal outcomes. Since Wormald et al's anatomic study and a better description of the endonasal anatomy of the nasolacrimal sac, with an appreciation for the location of the common canaliculus, the outcomes in endoscopic DCR have been steadily improving (▸ Fig. 5.6a).[13] It is, however, important to note that while the anatomical location of the sac and duct as described by Wormald et al is fairly consistent, the exact relationship of the lacrimal apparatus to the middle turbinate and in particular the axilla of the middle turbinate does vary according to the variable pneumatization of both the turbinate itself and the agger nasi cell. This should be assessed on preoperative endoscopy, although preoperative CT (computed tomography) is potentially helpful.[14] We do not advocate this as standard practice unless there are other indications such as prior surgery or regarding the local anatomy such as suspicion of congenital anatomic abnormalities. Similarly, the position of the common canaliculus ostium can be extremely variable in relation to the axilla to the middle turbinate. The age of the patient also has a significant impact upon the variability of the sac and common canaliculus with the pediatric patient typically demonstrating a position more posterior and superior to that described in the adult literature.

However, all endoscopic methods are not equal; some endonasal techniques use a multidiode laser to create a simple fistulous tract, while others are using both powered and cold instrumentation to remove bone and marsupialize the lacrimal sac, similar to that performed externally. The utilization of

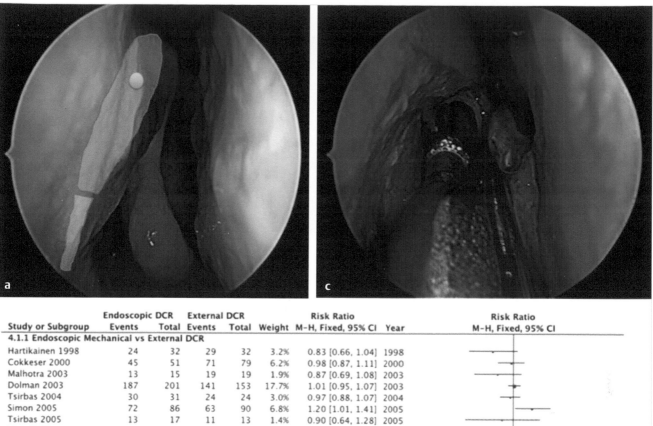

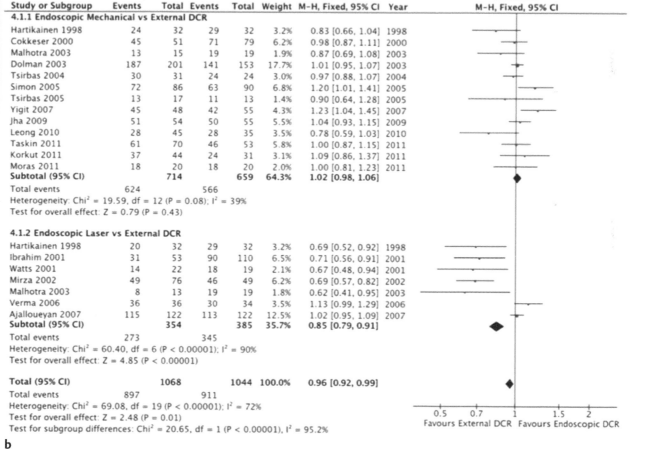

| Study or Subgroup | Endoscopic DCR Events | Total | External DCR Events | Total | Weight | Risk Ratio M-H, Fixed, 95% CI | Year |
|---|---|---|---|---|---|---|---|
| **4.1.1 Endoscopic Mechanical vs External DCR** | | | | | | | |
| Hartikainen 1998 | 24 | 32 | 29 | 32 | 3.2% | 0.83 [0.66, 1.04] | 1998 |
| Cokkeser 2000 | 45 | 51 | 71 | 79 | 6.2% | 0.98 [0.87, 1.11] | 2000 |
| Malhotra 2003 | 13 | 15 | 19 | 19 | 1.9% | 0.87 [0.69, 1.08] | 2003 |
| Dolman 2003 | 187 | 201 | 141 | 153 | 17.7% | 1.01 [0.95, 1.07] | 2003 |
| Tsirbas 2004 | 30 | 31 | 24 | 24 | 3.0% | 0.97 [0.88, 1.07] | 2004 |
| Simon 2005 | 72 | 86 | 63 | 90 | 6.8% | 1.20 [1.01, 1.41] | 2005 |
| Tsirbas 2005 | 13 | 17 | 11 | 13 | 1.4% | 0.90 [0.64, 1.28] | 2005 |
| Yigit 2007 | 45 | 48 | 42 | 55 | 4.3% | 1.23 [1.04, 1.45] | 2007 |
| Jha 2009 | 51 | 54 | 50 | 55 | 5.5% | 1.04 [0.93, 1.15] | 2009 |
| Leong 2010 | 28 | 45 | 28 | 35 | 3.5% | 0.78 [0.59, 1.03] | 2010 |
| Taskin 2011 | 61 | 70 | 46 | 53 | 5.8% | 1.00 [0.87, 1.15] | 2011 |
| Korkut 2011 | 37 | 44 | 24 | 31 | 3.1% | 1.09 [0.86, 1.37] | 2011 |
| Moras 2011 | 18 | 20 | 18 | 20 | 2.0% | 1.00 [0.81, 1.23] | 2011 |
| **Subtotal (95% CI)** | | 714 | | 659 | 64.3% | 1.02 [0.98, 1.06] | |
| Total events | 624 | | 566 | | | | |

Heterogeneity: Chi² = 19.59, df = 12 (P = 0.08); I² = 39%
Test for overall effect: Z = 0.79 (P = 0.43)

| Study or Subgroup | Endoscopic DCR Events | Total | External DCR Events | Total | Weight | Risk Ratio M-H, Fixed, 95% CI | Year |
|---|---|---|---|---|---|---|---|
| **4.1.2 Endoscopic Laser vs External DCR** | | | | | | | |
| Hartikainen 1998 | 20 | 32 | 29 | 32 | 3.2% | 0.69 [0.52, 0.92] | 1998 |
| Ibrahim 2001 | 31 | 53 | 90 | 110 | 6.5% | 0.71 [0.56, 0.91] | 2001 |
| Watts 2001 | 14 | 22 | 18 | 19 | 2.1% | 0.67 [0.48, 0.94] | 2001 |
| Mirza 2002 | 49 | 76 | 46 | 49 | 6.2% | 0.69 [0.57, 0.82] | 2002 |
| Malhotra 2003 | 8 | 13 | 19 | 19 | 1.8% | 0.62 [0.41, 0.95] | 2003 |
| Verma 2006 | 36 | 36 | 30 | 34 | 3.5% | 1.13 [0.99, 1.29] | 2006 |
| Ajalloueyan 2007 | 115 | 122 | 113 | 122 | 12.5% | 1.02 [0.95, 1.09] | 2007 |
| **Subtotal (95% CI)** | | 354 | | 385 | 35.7% | 0.85 [0.79, 0.91] | |
| Total events | 273 | | 345 | | | | |

Heterogeneity: Chi² = 60.40, df = 6 (P < 0.00001); I² = 90%
Test for overall effect: Z = 4.85 (P < 0.00001)

| | | | | | | | |
|---|---|---|---|---|---|---|---|
| **Total (95% CI)** | | 1068 | | 1044 | 100.0% | 0.96 [0.92, 0.99] | |
| Total events | 897 | | 911 | | | | |

Heterogeneity: Chi² = 69.08, df = 19 (P < 0.00001); I² = 72%
Test for overall effect: Z = 2.48 (P = 0.01)
Test for subgroup differences: Chi² = 20.65, df = 1 (P < 0.00001), I² = 95.2%

Favours External DCR    Favours Endoscopic DCR

**Fig. 5.6** (a) The endoscopic location of the lacrimal sac. The exact relationship of the lacrimal apparatus to the middle turbinate and in particular the axilla of the middle turbinate does vary according to the variable pneumatization of both the turbinate itself and the agger nasi cell. (b) A forest plot comparing the different dacryocystorhinostomy (DCR) techniques. (Adapted from Huang et al.[16]) (c) Right endoscopic DCR. Endoscopic drill exposing superior sac and agger nasi cell.

powered endoscopic drills have enabled access to the bone superior to the region of the common canaliculus and complete exposure of the sac.[15] A systematic review and meta-analysis by Huang et al proved the endoscopic mechanical DCR technique to be equitable if not superior to the external approach in terms of success and both short- and long-term sequelae and complications[16] (▶ Fig. 5.6b).

## 5.5 The Endoscopic Dacryocystorhinostomy Technique

Endoscopic DCR as described by Wormald has analogous bony goals to that of the external DCR. Clearance of the bone superior to the common canaliculus and down to the nasolacrimal duct allows complete marsupialization of the lacrimal sac with mucosal to mucosal apposition and avoidance of a sump syndrome.[17] With adequate bone removal and marsupialization of the sac, the common canaliculus is effectively incorporated directly onto the lateral nasal wall, rather than the simple creation of a fistulous tract between the lacrimal sac and lateral wall of the nose as originally described.

The nasal mucosal flaps are elevated in a subperiosteal fashion with two horizontal incisions joined by an anterior vertical incision to create a posteriorly based U-shaped flap. The initial incision runs approximately 10 to 12 mm above the axilla of the middle turbinate and extends from 3 mm posterior to the axilla to about 10 mm anterior to the axilla. The inferior incision is made close to the medial flare of the superior border of the inferior turbinate with the aim of then including the superior duct into the marsupialization of the sac. The anterior ends of each incision are then joined by a single vertical incision and the mucoperiosteal flap elevated to expose the underlying bone. A 2-mm Kerrison punch is then utilized to remove as much of the thinner bone overlying the lacrimal duct and inferior aspect of the sac. A 2.5-mm Diamond DCR burr is then used to remove the superior thicker bone of the frontal process of the maxilla in order to fully expose the entire lacrimal sac (▶ Fig. 5.6c); the agger nasi cell is then opened to allow the complete opening of the posterior lacrimal sac flap. The medial wall of the lacrimal sac is tented medially with a Bowman probe inserted through either the upper or lower punctum; the lacrimal sac mucosa is then opened and a larger anteriorly based lacrimal mucosal flap opposes the nasal mucosa with a smaller posteriorly based flap to oppose the exposed mucosa of the agger nasi cell. This will result in exposure of the common canaliculus to the nasal cavity. Mucosal preservation and limitation of exposed bone cannot be overemphasized and is key for optimal results. The initial nasal mucoperiosteal flap is then fashioned to create mucosal apposition and bony covering. Silicon stents are threaded through the upper and lower canaliculi and a Gelfoam pledget (Pfizer, New York, NY) is railroaded over the stents stabilizing the placement of the Gelfoam, which in turn maintains flap position.

The decision to place stents or not is very controversial. The authors utilize a Crawford stent for a 3- to 4-week period for the following purposes:
- To hold the surgical dressing in place to maintain flap position.
- To promote capillary drainage along the tube.
- To dilate possibly initially edematous common canaliculus.

It must, however, be noted that there is no evidence to support the need for stenting, and Liang and Lane showed comparable results both with and without stenting in their publication.[18]

## 5.6 Surgical Treatment of the Upper System

The treatment of obstruction of the upper system can be more complex than that of the lower system. The surgical approach is divided based on level of obstruction within the system as follows:
- Punctal stenosis:
  - Punctal stenosis.
  - Punctal obstruction.
- Canalicular stenosis:
  - Proximal.
  - Distal.

## 5.7 Common Canalicular Stenosis/ Obstruction + Valve of Rosenmüller

### 5.7.1 Punctal Stenosis

Punctal stenosis is defined as the inability to pass a 26-gauge lacrimal cannula. Numerous studies report equal tear flow between the upper and lower canalicular systems, contrary to previous reports identifying the greatest drainage via the lower canalicular system.[19,20]

### Punctal Stenosis Treatment

Punctal stenosis is treated in rooms with the aid of magnification under loupes by excising a small (~1 mm) segment of the posterior margin of the punctum. It is vital that only a small portion is removed. The incision must never reach the ampulla, which is at the junction of the vertical and horizontal portion of the canaliculus. Overzealous removal of the canalicular tissue will damage the lacrimal pump function.
- Initially the punctum is dilated with a lacrimal dilator.
- A small "U" is removed from the posterior lip of the punctum using 0.12-mm-toothed forceps and a sharp-tipped Vannas scissors.
- Postoperatively topical antibiotic and steroid drops are used for 7 to 10 days. (It is important to note that steroids are contraindicated in some patients.)

### Punctal Obstruction

This requires sequential slivers of tissue to be cut down in a plane tangential to the line of the punctum. This is performed under binocular operating microscope magnification to locate the distal end of the obstruction. Once located, the canaliculus can be reconstructed around a mini-Monoka stent (FCI Ophthalmics Inc., Pembroke, MA) using 7.0 or 8.0 Vicryl. The stent is left in situ for 4 months. The Vicryl suture passes through the adventitia of the canaliculus and does not transgress the endothelium lining the canaliculus.

## 5.7.2 Canalicular Stenosis

### Proximal

Stenosis of the proximal 2 to 3 mm of canaliculus is carried out in a similar fashion to a punctal obstruction; however, the exploratory incision is parallel to the line of the canaliculus. The occluded segment is excised and an end-to-end anastomosis around a Monoka stent is performed. In our experience, reconstruction of an occlusion of greater than approximately 3 mm is likely to fail. The stent is left in situ for a minimum of 6 months.

### Distal

It is generally accepted without a clear proximal 8 mm of patent canaliculus preceding the obstruction; then a bypass tube is indicated.[21] A canaliculodacryocystorhinostomy (CDCR) can be performed externally or endoscopically.

### External Canaliculodacryocystorhinostomy

A standard dissection for an external DCR is commenced; then using a Bowman lacrimal probe to delineate the distal obstruction, the canaliculus is transected and silicone stents passed. The lacrimal sac is opened at the junction of the lacrimal sac and periosteum of the anterior lacrimal crest. The nasal mucosa is then incised and then the posterior lacrimal sac sutured to the posterior nasal mucosal flap incorporating the transected canaliculi. Finally, the anterior nasal and lacrimal sac flaps are sutured to form the anterior bridge.[21]

### Endoscopic Canaliculodacryocystorhinostomy

Endoscopic DCR is as described earlier. Once the lacrimal sac has been opened to expose the medial wall of the lacrimal sac so that the common canaliculus is on show, its position is verified with the assistance of a dental Burnisher double-ended ostium seeker (Hu-Friedy, Chicago, IL). This allows trephination of the stenosed segment using a Sisler lacrimal trephine (Visitec, Sarasota, FL) to be performed under direct endoscopic vision. The trephine is passed from the punctum; the direction of trephination is controlled under nasal endoscopic vision to ensure the trephine exits the natural common canalicular opening. Crawford's stents are inserted under endoscopic control to ensure exit via the common canaliculus. A 0.03% solution of mitomycin C (MMC) in a 2-mL syringe with a 26-gauge lacrimal cannula (BD Visitec, Franklin Lakes, NJ) is used to irrigate the newly trephined canaliculus via the punctum into the nose, with the stents in place. A Codman neurosurgical patty (Johnson & Johnson, Raynham, MA) is preplaced in the nose to soak up any excess MMC. The conjunctival sac is immediately irrigated with normal saline.[22]

Since the publication of the article,[22] we have generally omitted the use of MMC to the above-mentioned technique and in as yet unpublished data we have not noted a significant deterioration in success rate.

### Jones Tube Placement

A standard DCR either externally or endoscopically is performed. The superficial conjunctival covering of the caruncle with approximately 30% of the caruncle is amputated. A 0.8-mm K-wire is passed through the center of the caruncle in plane of the iris and an approximately 30-degree angle toward the lateral wall of the nose, exiting the inferior half of the bony ostium. A 2-mm trephine is the railroaded over the K-wire. The position of the distal end of the K-wire should clear the nasal mucosa by about 4 mm. The trephine is removed and a surgical marker is used to mark the level of the caruncle on the K-wire. The trephine is then again railroaded and the K-wire removed and measured to the mark in order to choose the Jones tube length. The K-wire is then reinserted through the trephine, the trephine removed, and the Jones tube railroaded over the K-wire and pushed into place. The distal end of the tube is clear of the nasal mucosa of the lateral wall of the nose, the middle turbinate, and septum. If this is not the case, a turbinoplasty or septoplasty is indicated.

Using a 7.0 Vicryl suture through the remaining carbuncular tissue and lassoing it around the proximal flange of the Jones tube will stabilize the position until the tissue around the tube fibroses

## 5.8 Conclusion

The evaluation and management of acquired lacrimal obstruction requires an understanding of the basic etiology of tearing. The history and examination remain the critical components to correctly diagnose and manage patients with tearing. The implementation of treatment pathways outlined in this chapter provides a guide to simplify the evaluation and management of a complex condition. Understanding the range of issues that can cause epiphora in patients is essential in order to adequately manage patients with acquired nasolacrimal duct obstruction.

## References

[1] Cheung LM, Francis IC, Stapleton F, Wilcsek G. Symptom assessment in patients with functional and primary acquired nasolacrimal duct obstruction before and after successful dacryocystorhinostomy surgery: a prospective study. Br J Ophthalmol. 2007; 91(12):1671–1674

[2] Shin JH, Kim YD, Woo KI, Korean Society of Ophthalmic Plastic and Reconstructive Surgery (KSOPRS). Impact of epiphora on vision-related quality of life. BMC Ophthalmol. 2015; 15:6

[3] Deschamps N, Ricaud X, Rabut G, Labbé A, Baudouin C, Denoyer A. The impact of dry eye disease on visual performance while driving. Am J Ophthalmol. 2013; 156(1):184–189.e3

[4] Vitale S, Goodman LA, Reed GF, Smith JA. Comparison of the NEI-VFQ and OSDI questionnaires in patients with Sjögren's syndrome-related dry eye. Health Qual Life Outcomes. 2004; 2:44

[5] Meng ID, Kurose M. The role of corneal afferent neurons in regulating tears under normal and dry eye conditions. Exp Eye Res. 2013; 117:79–87

[6] Lew H, Yun YS, Lee SY. Electrolytes and electrophoretic studies of tear proteins in tears of patients with nasolacrimal duct obstruction. Ophthalmologica. 2005; 219(3):142–146

[7] Tucker SM, Linberg JV, Nguyen LL, Viti AJ, Tucker WJ. Measurement of the resistance to fluid flow within the lacrimal outflow system. Ophthalmology. 1995; 102(11):1639–1645

[8] Soiberman U, Kakizaki H, Selva D, Leibovitch I. Punctal stenosis: definition, diagnosis, and treatment. Clin Ophthalmol. 2012; 6:1011–1018

[9] Liarakos VS, Boboridis KG, Mavrikakis E, Mavrikakis I. Management of canalicular obstructions. Curr Opin Ophthalmol. 2009; 20(5):395–400

[10] Hatton MP, Rubin PAD. Evaluation of the tearing patient. In: Albert DM, ed. Albert & Jakobiec's Principles and Practice of Ophthalmology. Philadelphia, PA: Saunders; 2008

[11] Zappia RJ, Milder B. Lacrimal drainage function. 1. The Jones fluorescein test. Am J Ophthalmol. 1972; 74(1):154–159

[12] Sagili S, Selva D, Malhotra R. Lacrimal scintigraphy: "interpretation more art than science.". Orbit. 2012; 31(2):77–85

[13] Wormald PJ, Kew J, Van Hasselt A. Intranasal anatomy of the nasolacrimal sac in endoscopic dacryocystorhinostomy. Otolaryngol Head Neck Surg. 2000; 123(3):307–310

[14] Francis IC, Kappagoda MB, Cole IE, Bank L, Dunn GD. Computed tomography of the lacrimal drainage system: retrospective study of 107 cases of dacryostenosis. Ophthal Plast Reconstr Surg. 1999; 15(3):217–226

[15] Knisely A, Harvey R, Sacks R. Long-term outcomes in endoscopic dacryocystorhinostomy. Curr Opin Otolaryngol Head Neck Surg. 2015; 23(1):53–58

[16] Huang J, Malek J, Chin D, et al. Systematic review and meta-analysis on outcomes for endoscopic versus external dacryocystorhinostomy. Orbit. 2014; 33(2):81–90

[17] Jordan DR, McDonald H. Failed dacryocystorhinostomy: the sump syndrome. Ophthalmic Surg. 1993; 24(10):692–693

[18] Liang J, Lane A. Is postoperative stenting necessary in endoscopic dacryocystorhinostomy? Laryngoscope. 2013; 123(11):2589–2590

[19] White WL, Glover AT, Buckner AB, Hartshorne MF. Relative canalicular tear flow as assessed by dacryoscintigraphy. Ophthalmology. 1989; 96(2):167–169

[20] Meyer DR, Antonello A, Linberg JV. Assessment of tear drainage after canalicular obstruction using fluorescein dye disappearance. Ophthalmology. 1990; 97(10):1370–1374

[21] McNab AA. Manual of Orbital and Lacrimal Surgery. 2nd ed. Oxford, UK: Butterworth-Heinemann; 1998

[22] Nemet AY, Wilcsek G, Francis IC. Endoscopic dacryocystorhinostomy with adjunctive mitomycin C for canalicular obstruction. Orbit. 2007; 26(2):97–100

# 6 Pathogenesis of Thyroid Eye Disease

*Catherine J. Choi and Nahyoung Grace Lee*

## Abstract

The pathogenesis of thyroid eye disease is poorly understood. It is known to be an autoimmune, inflammatory condition that peaks in severity within the first 1.5 years of diagnosis with subsequent varying degrees of recovery. The clinical manifestations of thyroid eye disease include exophthalmos, strabismus, eyelid retraction, as well as optic neuropathy in severe cases. The medical gold standard therapy of severe thyroid eye disease consists of intravenous or oral steroids. However, this may not be enough to halt or prevent permanent vision loss. Therefore, it is of utmost importance to be able to clinically judge when a patient must undergo urgent surgery versus watchful waiting until the disease stabilizes. This chapter highlights the pathophysiology and the clinical components of the eye exam that are important in the evaluation of a patient with thyroid eye disease.

*Keywords:* thyroid eye disease, thyroid orbitopathy, thyroid-associated ophthalmopathy, Graves' disease, eyelid retraction, exophthalmos, strabismus

## 6.1 Introduction

Thyroid eye disease (TED) or thyroid-associated orbitopathy (TAO) is reported to affect 25 to 50% of patients with Graves' disease (GD) and up to 2% of patients with chronic autoimmune thyroiditis. Annual incidence is estimated to be 16 per 100,000 in women and 2.9 per 100,000 in men.[1,2] There is a bimodal age distribution with the highest incidence in the fifth and seventh decades. The major pathological features include expansion of orbital soft tissues and enlargement of extraocular muscles. These changes can lead to proptosis, exposure keratopathy, and restrictive strabismus with debilitating diplopia. In severe cases, crowding of the orbital apex can result in compression of the optic nerve with permanent vision loss if left untreated.[3] Currently available treatments for TED include medical therapy directed at treating hyperthyroidism and orbital inflammation, surgical therapy in the form of orbital decompression, eyelid surgery usually to recess the eyelids, strabismus surgery to realign the eyes, as well as radiation therapy as either radioactive iodine[4] or external beam orbital radiation. These treatments show variable efficacy over a wide spectrum of disease severity. This is at least in part due to our limited understanding of the pathophysiology behind TED. This chapter aims to provide a summary of the most current knowledge and evidence behind the pathogenesis of TED, clinical presentation, diagnostic studies, and treatment options.

## 6.2 Pathophysiology

Understanding the pathophysiology of TED begins with the mechanisms behind autoimmunity in GD. In GD, autoimmune response to the A-subunit of the thyroid-stimulating hormone receptor (TSHR), which is a G protein coupled receptor, results in autoantibodies known as thyroid-stimulating immunoglobulins (TSI).[5] TSI in circulation then bind the TSHR on the thyroid follicular cells, which then secrete thyroid hormone, leading to clinical hyperthyroidism. The cause or the trigger for the initiation of this autoimmune response, or loss of self-tolerance to TSHR, is unknown. There is, however, a close temporal correlation between onset of GD and TED, with the majority of patients developing eye symptoms within 18 months of autoimmune thyroid disease. This correlation is thought to suggest at least some overlapping common pathways underlying the two disease processes.[6]

Pathogenesis of TED can be understood as a complex interaction between autoimmunity, inflammation, cytokine response, and how these affect the downstream effector cells within the orbit leading to the clinical findings.[6]

### 6.2.1 Autoimmunity in Thyroid Eye Disease

As noted earlier, autoimmunity against TSHR is a fundamental component of GD. Given the temporal as well as many clinical correlations between TED and GD, autoimmunity against TSHR was assumed to play a role in TED. In fact, studies revealed that 98% of patients with TED have detectable TSHR autoantibodies.[7] With further improvement in sensitivity of modern assays for TSHR antibody detection, both TSI and second subtype TSHR binding inhibitory immunoglobulins (TBII) are detectable and highly correlated with clinical activity of TED.[8] Although TSHR was originally thought to be isolated to follicular cells within thyroid tissue, it has since been recovered in low levels in a variety of cell types, including orbital fibroblasts (OF). OF cultured from TED patients have higher levels of TSHR expression compared to controls, and those with active disease have higher levels of expression than those in inactive or chronic stage.[9] TSHR antibodies acting upon these upregulated TSHR within orbital tissue are thought to lead to downstream pathways as outlined below via the effector cells.[9]

Another potential autoantigen that has been implicated in TED is insulinlike growth factor 1 receptor (IGF-1R). IGF-1 R is a receptor tyrosine kinase with widespread expression and roles. Its expression is certainly not specific to GD, TED, or orbital tissues. It is, however, thought to form a functional complex with TSHR to propagate a synergistic response leading to changes in TED.[10] IGF-1 R has a threefold higher expression in OF from TED patients compared to controls, and induce hyaluronan (HA) synthesis.[11] However, the actual autoantibodies directed against IGF-1 R have been shown to be equivalent in TED and healthy controls,[10] and the exact binding activity of IGF-1 R antibodies on IGR-R1 on OF remains to be elucidated.

### 6.2.2 Effector Cells in Thyroid Eye Disease Orbit

The constellation of signs and symptoms of TED are attributable to volume expansion of extraocular muscles and orbital fat.

Examination of this orbital tissue reveals increased deposition of glycosaminoglycans (GAG) in the form of HA. HA is a high-molecular-weight, highly anionic and hydrophilic polysaccharide that is present within the connective tissue throughout the body. HA deposition within the endomysium of extraocular muscle fibers leads to extracellular, interstitial edema and subsequent extraocular muscle enlargement. In terms of orbital fat expansion, there is de novo adipogenesis triggered by signaling pathways linked to TSHR and IGF-1 R.

The main effector cell for both HA synthesis and adipogenesis carrying out the downstream signaling pathways for TSHR and IGF-1 R is thought to be the OF. Fibroblasts are ubiquitous connective tissue cells. In the orbit, two subpopulations of fibroblasts are thought to exist: thymocyte antigen 1 positive (Thy1 +) and Thy1-negative (Thy1–) OF. Thy1 + OF, when treated with transforming growth factor beta (TGF-β) differentiate into myofibroblasts with contractile properties, while Thy– OF differentiate into mature adipocytes when treated with peroxisome proliferator-activated receptor gamma (PPAR-γ) agonist.[12] Each of these subtypes are thought to be responsible for the heterogeneity in the presentation of TED, with some patients exhibiting enlargement of extraocular muscles predominantly versus proliferation of orbital fat.

The origin of these pluripotent OF is likely related to a population of progenitor cells known as fibrocytes, which are bone-marrow-derived cells expressing both fibroblastic and hematopoietic stem cell markers from monocyte lineage. They circulate in peripheral blood and are able to migrate to sites of injury, and in this case, orbital tissue in TED. In a similar manner to OF, fibrocytes are able to differentiate into myofibroblasts or adipocytes, express both TSHR and IGF-1 R, and secrete a similar set of inflammatory cytokines. Fibrocytes are found in higher levels in the peripheral circulation of TED patients compared to controls, and the concentration of TSHR-expressing fibrocytes in TED is similar to that of thyroid follicular cells.[13]

In response to both TSHR and IGF-1 R activation, HA synthesis and adipogenesis pathways are triggered in OF and fibrocytes. For HA synthesis interleukin-1 beta (IL-1β), TGF-β1, and platelet-derived growth factor (PDGF) have all been separately shown to be potent activators. PDGF also further increases expression of TSHR in OF, forming a type of positive feedback loop to potentiate its effect.[14] Interestingly, IL-1β-mediated stimulation of HA synthesis can be blocked by steroids[15] and PDGF-mediated response can be mitigated by a number of tyrosine kinase inhibitors, suggesting possible venues for targeted therapy in TED. Adipogenesis in OF is carried out by PPAR-γ signaling. There is an overexpression of PPAR-γ in the adipose tissue of active TED. Rosiglitazone, an anti-diabetic drug that is a PPAR-γ agonist, has also been shown to increase TSHR expression, further potentiating this pathway.[16] Both TSHR and IGF-1 R trigger differentiation of pre-adipocytic OF into mature adipocytes, leading to proliferation of orbital fat in TED.

### 6.2.3 Cellular Immunity and Role of Inflammation

Another component in the complex pathophysiology of TED is the role of cellular immunity and inflammation. In the active phase of TED, orbital inflammation is a key feature that manifests clinically as injection, chemosis, proptosis, lid edema, and pain, and is often acutely treated with steroids. Examination of enlarged extraocular muscles and orbital fat reveals extensive lymphocytic infiltration. While both T and B lymphocytes have been noted within the orbital tissue, CD4[+] T-cell population predominates. There is a reciprocal signaling between OF and lymphocytes in that activated OF secrete T-cell chemoattractants that recruit T cells to the orbit, which in turn further activate OF. Within extraocular muscles, Th1-type cytokine expression is seen with interferon gamma (IFN-γ), tumor necrosis factor alpha (TNFα), and IL-1β and IL-6. Within orbital fat, Th2-type profile with IL-4 and IL-10 is thought to be more common.[17] Th1 type is also more common in active phase of TED, while Th2 is seen in the chronic, stable phase.[18] Activated OF respond robustly to these cytokines, and in turn also secrete more to form a potentiating positive feedback loop. Overexpression of IL-1β, TNFα, IFN-γ, IL-6, IL-10, and IL-8 has been shown in orbital tissue in TED. IL-6 in particular is known to further increase the expression of TSHR, as well as B-cell activation. B lymphocytes in turn are responsible for the generation of the autoantibodies. Rituximab, a monoclonal antibody against B-cell antigen CD20, has shown promise in treatment of TED in recent studies.[19]

## 6.3 Clinical Presentation

The most salient clinical features of TED include unilateral or bilateral proptosis, eyelid retraction with "temporal flare," lid lag, lagophthalmos, and restrictive strabismus (▶ Fig. 6.1). The disease can be symmetric or vastly asymmetric. With regard to strabismus, the inferior rectus and medial rectus muscles are typically the most frequently affected muscles and can produce corresponding supraduction and abduction deficits. Decreased vision results from exposure keratopathy from a combination of features mentioned earlier, and in severe cases, compressive optic neuropathy. Additional signs and symptoms depending on the relative activity of the disease include eyelid erythema and edema, conjunctival injection (frequently over extraocular muscle insertions), and chemosis and caruncular edema. The acuity and activity of the disease can also be evaluated by assessing the resistance to retropulsion where the surgeon gently presses on the globes over closed eyelids and determines the

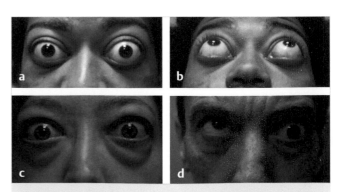

Fig. 6.1 (a) Exophthalmos. (b) Exophthalmos, Waters' view. (c) Upper eyelid retraction without exophthalmos. (d) Strabismus.

degree of resistance. When there is active inflammation, the resistance is generally higher than that of chronic fibrosis. According to an oft-cited cohort study, eyelid retraction is the most common feature of TED and is present in 90% of patients at some point during the clinical course. This was followed by proptosis, which was seen in 62%, restrictive extraocular motility (43%), and optic nerve dysfunction (6%). The most common subjective symptom was ocular pain, present in 30% of patients.[20]

TED is thought to have an active phase and a quiescent burnout phase, and this typical clinical course was described by Rundle in the so-called Rundle's curve.[21,22] Following the onset of active TED, Rundle's curve predicts a rapid escalation of signs of symptoms to reach maximum activity at 13 to 24 months.[23] The peak severity is delayed by a few months, before improving to reach a plateau level without ever resolving to the pre-TED level. The entire active phase generally lasts between 18 and 26 months.

As noted earlier, a distinction is made between clinical activity and clinical severity when describing the clinical status of TED. One classification system for grading clinical *severity* of TED is the NOSPECS (No physical signs or symptoms, Only signs, Soft tissue involvement, Proptosis, Extraocular muscle signs, Corneal involvement, and Sight loss) proposed by Werner in 1969.[24] This system, however, does not distinguish between the active and inactive phases of disease. The inflammatory *activity* of active TED is addressed by the clinical activity score (CAS) introduced by Mourits et al in 1989.[25] One point is assigned to each of the 10 items that comprise the CAS that describes pain, redness, edema, and impaired function (▶ Table 6.1). The sum of the points makes up the final activity score, regardless of the category. Since items 8 to 10 require comparison of values over two time points, only items 1 to 7 are used at the first visit. Scores greater than 3/7 at the first visit or 4/10 at subsequent visits are considered active inflammation.[23,26]

Classification systems combining clinical severity and activity have since been developed: the EUGOGO (European Group On Graves' Orbitopathy) system and the VISA (vision, inflammation, strabismus, and appearance) system.[27,28] The EUGOGO was established in 1999 and based on CAS system plus a set of

severity parameters, some of which are standard images to be compared to the patient's clinical findings.[27] Using these parameters, TED is classified as mild, moderate, severe, or sight-threatening. The VISA system was introduced in 2006 by Dolman and Rootman[28] and adopted by the International Thyroid Eye Disease Society (ITEDS). Sum of 1 point for vision, 10 points for inflammation, 6 points for strabismus, and 3 points for appearance make up the global severity grade out of 20 points.

# 6.4 Diagnostic Studies

In addition to the clinical examination with various scoring and classification systems outlined earlier, key diagnostic tests are used as adjuncts in evaluating a patient with TED. Some of the most relevant tests include orbital imaging, visual field test, and serology.

While orbital imaging is not required for the diagnosis of TED in the presence of typical clinical presentation with other supporting evidence, orbital imaging can provide invaluable information regarding the relative predominance of fat hypertrophy (type 1 orbitopathy) versus enlargement of extraocular muscles (type 2 orbitopathy), degree of apical crowding when assessing for risk of compressive optic neuropathy, and preoperative planning for orbital decompression. CT (computed tomography) is often the most common imaging modality given the combination of soft-tissue and bony anatomy details that can be obtained. More recent studies with magnetic resonance imaging (MRI) based volumetric measurements and objective assessment of disease activity with diffusion-weighted imaging have also demonstrated a role for MRI imaging.[29]

Evaluating for evidence of compressive optic neuropathy is an essential part of the clinical examination in TED. Compressive optic neuropathy is primarily a clinical diagnosis and good visual acuity, lack of a relative afferent pupillary defect, and lack of optic nerve swelling do not necessarily exclude its presence. Visual field defects, however, have been shown to be a sensitive screening measure for compressive optic neuropathy even in the absence of other signs and symptoms.[30,31,32] Both manual and automated perimetries have been used extensively for TED-associated compressive optic neuropathy. Inferior visual field defects are the most commonly seen pattern, which is thought to be related to the anatomy of the orbital apex where the location of the optic nerve within the lesser wing of the sphenoid in relation to the annulus of Zinn places the superior aspect of the optic nerve closest to the extraocular muscles, thereby making the superior portion most vulnerable to compression, resulting in an inferior visual field defect.

Finally, as discussed earlier, the thyroid function and antithyroid antibodies are closely related to the presumed pathogenesis of TED and are an essential part of determining disease activity and timing of surgical interventions. Both hyper- and hypothyroidism are to be avoided and TSH, T3, and free T4 levels are typically monitored in conjunction with the endocrinologist. Thyroid antibody levels do not need to be routinely monitored for the purposes of maintaining euthyroid state, but both TSI and TBII levels show positive correlation with CAS and prognosis of TED.[33,34] Thyroid antibody serologies are therefore a useful adjunct in both the diagnosis and management of TED.

**Table 6.1** Clinical activity score (CAS)

| Pain | 1 | Painful oppressive feeling on or behind the globe during the last 4 wk |
|---|---|---|
| | 2 | Pain with eye movement during the last 4 wk |
| Redness | 3 | Redness of the eyelids |
| | 4 | Conjunctival injection involving at least one quadrant |
| Edema | 5 | Edema of the eyelids |
| | 6 | Chemosis |
| | 7 | Edema of caruncle |
| | 8 | Increase in proptosis of ≥ 2 mm over 1–3 mo |
| Impaired function | 9 | Decrease in extraocular motility in any direction ≥ 5 degrees over 1–3 mo |
| | 10 | Decrease in best-corrected visual acuity of ≥ 1 line(s) on the Snellen chart over 1–3 mo |

Notes: 1 point is given for each item on clinical examination. The sum of all points represents the CAS for the patient, regardless of category.

# 6.5 Treatment

Treatment of TED consists of addressing the underlying thyroid dysfunction as well as the orbital inflammation and resultant functional deficits. First and foremost, the most important modifiable risk factor for TED is cigarette smoking, with an odds ratio of 7.7. Smokers have a higher risk of severe ophthalmopathy and there is a dose-dependent relationship, as well as temporal correlation and reversibility of its negative effects, making smoking cessation counseling an essential part of treatment of TED.[35]

For hyperthyroidism related to GD, currently available treatment options include antithyroid medications, thyroidectomy, and radioactive iodine (RAI) therapy. The preferred method of treatment by endocrinologists vary somewhat based on location: RAI is the most popular treatment modality in North America, while antithyroid medications are used much more frequently in Europe and abroad.[36] There is evidence for possible worsening of TED following RAI,[4,37] which can be prevented or blunted with systemic corticosteroids, while some advocate for thyroidectomy as a more definitive method to perhaps decrease the antigen load.

For TED in active phase, systemic steroids and orbital radiotherapy are the two main treatment options. Pulse IV (intravenous) methylprednisolone is generally thought to show the highest efficacy with increased tolerability while minimizing hepatotoxicity.[3] Orbital radiotherapy is particularly effective in cases with significant ocular dysmotility and compressive optic neuropathy, and is well tolerated when administered either with or without concurrent systemic steroids.[38]

Finally, surgical interventions for TED include orbital decompression, eyelid retraction repair, and strabismus surgery (to be discussed in greater detail throughout the book). Other than in cases of emergent orbital decompressions for progressive compressive optic neuropathy leading to vision loss, quiescence of disease activity for at least 6 months is recommended prior to pursuing surgery. Orbital decompression should be performed first, followed by eye muscle surgery, then eyelid retraction repair, due to the sequence of likely postoperative anatomic changes following each type of surgery.

# 6.6 Conclusion

TED is an entity that is difficult to understand and equally difficult to treat. Aside from the autoimmune etiology, there has been new light shed on the vasculogenesis in TED, which could be a potential target for treatment.[39] While steroids are a nonspecific treatment option for medical management, certain vascular growth factors could be locally targeted to decrease the inflammation, edema, and adipogenesis incited in TED. Currently, surgery is undertaken early on to relieve pressure in acute compressive optic neuropathy, or in the stable phase to improve the chronic clinical manifestations of the condition.

# References

[1] Wiersinga WM, Bartalena L. Epidemiology and prevention of Graves' ophthalmopathy. Thyroid. 2002; 12(10):855–860

[2] Wiersinga WM, Smit T, van der Gaag R, Koornneef L. Temporal relationship between onset of Graves' ophthalmopathy and onset of thyroidal Graves' disease. J Endocrinol Invest. 1988; 11(8):615–619

[3] Bahn RS. Graves' ophthalmopathy. N Engl J Med. 2010; 362(8):726–738

[4] Choi CJ, Gilbert AL, Lee NG. Radioactive iodine therapy and thyroid eye disease from an ophthalmologist's perspective. Int Ophthalmol Clin. 2015; 55 (4):63–72

[5] Wang Y, Smith TJ. Current concepts in the molecular pathogenesis of thyroid-associated ophthalmopathy. Invest Ophthalmol Vis Sci. 2014; 55(3):1735–1748

[6] Khong JJ, McNab AA, Ebeling PR, Craig JE, Selva D. Pathogenesis of thyroid eye disease: review and update on molecular mechanisms. Br J Ophthalmol. 2016; 100(1):142–150

[7] Ponto KA, Kanitz M, Olivo PD, Pitz S, Pfeiffer N, Kahaly GJ. Clinical relevance of thyroid-stimulating immunoglobulins in graves' ophthalmopathy. Ophthalmology. 2011; 118(11):2279–2285

[8] Gerding MN, van der Meer JW, Broenink M, Bakker O, Wiersinga WM, Prummel MF. Association of thyrotrophin receptor antibodies with the clinical features of Graves' ophthalmopathy. Clin Endocrinol (Oxf). 2000; 52 (3):267–271

[9] Wakelkamp IM, Bakker O, Baldeschi L, Wiersinga WM, Prummel MF. TSH-R expression and cytokine profile in orbital tissue of active vs. inactive Graves' ophthalmopathy patients. Clin Endocrinol (Oxf). 2003; 58(3):280–287

[10] Minich WB, Dehina N, Welsink T, et al. Autoantibodies to the IGF1 receptor in Graves' orbitopathy. J Clin Endocrinol Metab. 2013; 98(2):752–760

[11] Tsui S, Naik V, Hoa N, et al. Evidence for an association between thyroid-stimulating hormone and insulin-like growth factor 1 receptors: a tale of two antigens implicated in Graves' disease. J Immunol. 2008; 181(6):4397–4405

[12] Koumas L, Smith TJ, Feldon S, Blumberg N, Phipps RP. Thy-1 expression in human fibroblast subsets defines myofibroblastic or lipofibroblastic phenotypes. Am J Pathol. 2003; 163(4):1291–1300

[13] Gillespie EF, Papageorgiou KI, Fernando R, et al. Increased expression of TSH receptor by fibrocytes in thyroid-associated ophthalmopathy leads to chemokine production. J Clin Endocrinol Metab. 2012; 97(5):E740–E746

[14] Virakul S, van Steensel L, Dalm VA, Paridaens D, van Hagen PM, Dik WA. Platelet-derived growth factor: a key factor in the pathogenesis of graves' ophthalmopathy and potential target for treatment. Eur Thyroid J. 2014; 3 (4):217–226

[15] Kaback LA, Smith TJ. Expression of hyaluronan synthase messenger ribonucleic acids and their induction by interleukin-1beta in human orbital fibroblasts: potential insight into the molecular pathogenesis of thyroid-associated ophthalmopathy. J Clin Endocrinol Metab. 1999; 84(11):4079–4084

[16] Valyasevi RW, Harteneck DA, Dutton CM, Bahn RS. Stimulation of adipogenesis, peroxisome proliferator-activated receptor-gamma (PPARgamma), and thyrotropin receptor by PPARgamma agonist in human orbital preadipocyte fibroblasts. J Clin Endocrinol Metab. 2002; 87(5):2352–2358

[17] Hiromatsu Y, Yang D, Bednarczuk T, Miyake I, Nonaka K, Inoue Y. Cytokine profiles in eye muscle tissue and orbital fat tissue from patients with thyroid-associated ophthalmopathy. J Clin Endocrinol Metab. 2000; 85(3):1194–1199

[18] Aniszewski JP, Valyasevi RW, Bahn RS. Relationship between disease duration and predominant orbital T cell subset in Graves' ophthalmopathy. J Clin Endocrinol Metab. 2000; 85(2):776–780

[19] Salvi M, Vannucchi G, Currò N, et al. Efficacy of B-cell targeted therapy with rituximab in patients with active moderate to severe Graves' orbitopathy: a randomized controlled study. J Clin Endocrinol Metab. 2015; 100(2):422–431

[20] Bartley GB, Fatourechi V, Kadrmas EF, et al. Clinical features of Graves' ophthalmopathy in an incidence cohort. Am J Ophthalmol. 1996; 121(3): 284–290

[21] Rundle FF. Management of exophthalmos and related ocular changes in Graves' disease. Metabolism. 1957; 6(1):36–48

[22] Rundle FF, Wilson CW. Development and course of exophthalmos and ophthalmoplegia in Graves' disease with special reference to the effect of thyroidectomy. Clin Sci. 1945; 5(3–4):177–194

[23] Mourits MP, Koornneef L, Wiersinga WM, Prummel MF, Berghout A, van der Gaag R. Clinical criteria for the assessment of disease activity in Graves' ophthalmopathy: a novel approach. Br J Ophthalmol. 1989; 73(8):639–644

[24] Werner SC. Modification of the classification of the eye changes of Graves' disease: recommendations of the Ad Hoc Committee of the American Thyroid Association. J Clin Endocrinol Metab. 1977; 44(1):203–204

[25] Menconi F, Profilo MA, Leo M, et al. Spontaneous improvement of untreated mild Graves' ophthalmopathy: Rundle's curve revisited. Thyroid. 2014; 24(1): 60–66

[26] Barrio-Barrio J, Sabater AL, Bonet-Farriol E, Velázquez-Villoria Á, Galofré JC. Graves' ophthalmopathy: VISA versus EUGOGO classification, assessment, and management. J Ophthalmol. 2015; 2015:249125

[27] Wiersinga WM, Perros P, Kahaly GJ, et al. European Group on Graves' Orbitopathy (EUGOGO). Clinical assessment of patients with Graves' orbitopathy: the European Group On Graves' Orbitopathy recommendations to generalists, specialists and clinical researchers. Eur J Endocrinol. 2006; 155(3):387–389

[28] Dolman PJ, Rootman J. VISA classification for Graves orbitopathy. Ophthal Plast Reconstr Surg. 2006; 22(5):319–324

[29] Politi LS, Godi C, Cammarata G, et al. Magnetic resonance imaging with diffusion-weighted imaging in the evaluation of thyroid-associated orbitopathy: getting below the tip of the iceberg. Eur Radiol. 2014; 24(5):1118–1126

[30] Trobe JD, Glaser JS, Laflamme P. Dysthyroid optic neuropathy. Clinical profile and rationale for management. Arch Ophthalmol. 1978; 96(7):1199–1209

[31] Labonia AF, Carnovale-Scalzo G, Paola A, et al. Subclinical visual field alterations are commonly present in patients with Graves' orbitopathy and are mainly related to the clinical activity of the disease. Exp Clin Endocrinol Diabetes. 2008; 116(6):347–351

[32] Gasser P, Flammer J. Optic neuropathy of Graves' disease. A report of a perimetric follow-up. Ophthalmologica. 1986; 192(1):22–27

[33] Lantz M, Planck T, Asman P, Hallengren B. Increased TRAb and/or low anti-TPO titers at diagnosis of disease are associated with an increased risk of developing ophthalmopathy after onset. Exp Clin Endocrinol Diabetes. 2014; 122(2):113–117

[34] Eckstein AK, Plicht M, Lax H, et al. Thyrotropin receptor autoantibodies are independent risk factors for Graves' ophthalmopathy and help to predict severity and outcome of the disease. J Clin Endocrinol Metab. 2006; 91(9):3464–3470

[35] Prummel MF, Wiersinga WM. Smoking and risk of Graves' disease. JAMA. 1993; 269(4):479–482

[36] Burch HB, Burman KD, Cooper DSA. A 2011 survey of clinical practice patterns in the management of Graves' disease. J Clin Endocrinol Metab. 2012; 97(12):4549–4558

[37] Bartalena L, Marcocci C, Bogazzi F, et al. Relation between therapy for hyperthyroidism and the course of Graves' ophthalmopathy. N Engl J Med. 1998; 338(2):73–78

[38] Shams PN, Ma R, Pickles T, Rootman J, Dolman PJ. Reduced risk of compressive optic neuropathy using orbital radiotherapy in patients with active thyroid eye disease. Am J Ophthalmol. 2014; 157(6):1299–1305

[39] Wong LL, Lee NG, Amarnani D, et al. Orbital angiogenesis and lymphangiogenesis in thyroid eye disease: an analysis of vascular growth factors with clinical correlation. Ophthalmology. 2016; 123(9):2028–2036

# 7 Indications and Techniques for Orbital Decompression

*Benjamin S. Bleier and Suzanne K. Freitag*

**Abstract**

This chapter provides a detailed description of the surgical techniques for endoscopic decompression of the medial wall and floor of the orbit. Tips and pearls are included regarding prevention of diplopia and other complications. Lateral orbital wall decompression is also detailed, including the indications for its use alone or as an adjunct to medial wall decompression with the goals of maximizing proptosis reduction, minimizing diplopia and improving symmetry of the position of the globes.

*Keywords:* Orbital decompression, thyroid eye disease, endoscopic, medial wall, orbital floor, lateral wall, fat removal, bony strut

## 7.1 Indications for Orbital Decompression

Orbital decompression is performed in a variety of conditions and for various indications. The most common disease process leading to orbital decompression is thyroid eye disease. In this condition, the orbital fat and extraocular muscles enlarge due to inflammation. In severe cases, the enlarged muscles result in crowding at the orbital apex, which causes compression of the optic nerve as it passes through the orbital apex into the optic canal. Clinical signs of compressive optic neuropathy include decreased visual acuity, afferent papillary defect, and dyschromatopsia. Long-standing compressive optic neuropathy may result in optic nerve pallor and permanent visual loss. Further confirmation of optic neuropathy is done with automated visual field testing and orbital imaging (▶ Fig. 7.1). Computed tomography (CT) without contrast is adequate to assess the orbits in cases of thyroid orbitopathy. It is important to avoid unnecessary intravenous CT contrast in patients with thyroid eye disease, as there are reported cases of severe and immediate orbitopathy exacerbation following the administration of iodine-containing intravenous contrast.[1] Magnetic resonance imaging also nicely delineates the extraocular muscles and optic nerves. However, it is important to evaluate the bony orbital walls if orbital decompression is contemplated; hence, CT is the preferred method of imaging. Further, stereotactic image guidance systems are often employed in endoscopic orbital decompression and CT imaging is required for this.

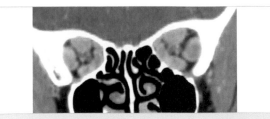

Fig. 7.1 Coronal CT (computed tomography) image through the orbital apices demonstrating significant enlargement of all extraocular muscles bilaterally due to thyroid orbitopathy resulting in crowding of apical structures including the optic nerves.

Other indications for orbital decompression surgery in patients with thyroid eye disease are to reduce proptosis causing corneal breakdown or severe cosmetic deformity. Exposure keratopathy is common in patients with thyroid eye disease because of the underlying autoimmune disorder, as well as proptosis and eyelid retraction resulting in increased ocular surface area exposed to the environment. If untreated, patients with severe exposure keratopathy may develop corneal ulceration or perforation resulting in visual loss. In addition, many patients with thyroid orbitopathy suffer psychosocially from their disfigurement.[2] Surgery to restore a more normal appearance is important.

Other conditions for which orbital decompression surgery may be indicated include orbital tumors or other space-occupying lesions such as vascular malformations that are causing compressive optic neuropathy, severe proptosis with exposure keratopathy, or extreme disfigurement. In these conditions, it is important to determine that opening the bony orbital walls is appropriate and will not lead to undesired tumor seeding of the spaces outside the orbit, as in the case of a malignancy.

## 7.2 Surgical Approaches to Orbital Decompression

Orbital decompression may be accomplished via bone removal from any of the orbital walls or from orbital fat removal with or without bony decompression.[3,4] Medial wall and floor decompression may be accomplished via a variety of external approaches, including transcutaneous, transconjunctival, and transcaruncular. However, the endoscopic approach has gained favor in recent years and this technique will be covered in detail below. Lateral wall decompression may be performed by removing bone from any location between the lateral orbital rim to the sphenoid trigone via a cutaneous incision. Orbital roof decompression has been reported in intractable cases.[5]

The decision of which wall or walls to decompress is based on surgeon preference and experience as well as a variety of variables including the presence or absence of diplopia, presence of compressive optic neuropathy, and the degree of proptosis. The risk of diplopia after orbital decompression is a significant factor in the decision to undergo this procedure.[6,7] Surgical techniques have been described to prevent diplopia, including preservation of the inferomedial strut of bone between the medial wall and floor of the orbit in cases where both walls are being removed for maximal decompression. This will be discussed in detail below.[8] A number of publications also advocate the utility of the balanced decompression to avoid diplopia, where the medial and lateral walls are decompressed in an effort to maintain globe centration in the orbit and prevent postoperative diplopia. Results are mixed, with postoperative diplopia ranging from 10 to 33%.[9,10,11,12] In cases of compressive optic neuropathy, it is thought that decompression of the medial orbital wall extending far posteriorly is the most effective method of relieving the compressive forces on the optic nerve in the orbital apex. This may be most safely and easily accomplished via an endoscopic endonasal approach.

Lateral wall decompression may be used alone or in combination with one or two other wall decompression. Its effectiveness in cases of compressive optic neuropathy has been debated. It may be safer and more effective in individuals with a larger bone mass in the sphenoid triangle.[13,14]

Many experts agree that there is no best method of orbital decompression and surgeons should utilize the techniques with which they are most comfortable and deliver the desired results. Ideally the approach should be tailored for each patient, since goals of surgery vary depending on indications.

## 7.3 Endoscopic Medial Orbital Wall and Floor Decompression

The endoscopic orbital decompression is an elegant method to decompress the medial and inferior orbit while eliminating disruption of normal external structures and preserving mucociliary function. The transantral approach to the medial wall and floor described by Walsh and Ogura[1,15] in 1957 has given way to modern endoscopic techniques first reported by Kennedy et al.[2,16] The extent of sinus dissection in preparation for decompression represents a balance in the need for preservation of physiologic sinus drainage pathways while limiting instrumentation of otherwise uninvolved structures within the sinonasal labyrinth. Each procedure is therefore tailored to the patient's site and degree of disease, anatomy, and presurgical vision status.

The endoscopic approach to decompress the medial orbital wall begins with a complete dissection of the adjacent sinus cavities. This entire dissection may be performed using a zero-degree endoscope. The uncinate process is first removed at its insertion on the maxillary line. Unlike traditional endoscopic sinus surgical approaches, the superior insertion of the uncinate is left in place in order to help protect the frontal recess from obstruction secondary to orbital fat prolapse. After removal of the uncinate, the maxillary may be visualized laterally and extended posteriorly and inferiorly. This should be performed even in cases where the orbital floor is not resected in order to avoid iatrogenic maxillary obstruction. Next the ethmoid bulla, basal lamella, and posterior ethmoid air cells are completely removed. It is critical to dissect these cells superiorly to the level of the skull base and laterally to the lamina in order to enable a maximal decompression. Residual posterior air cells, particularly those adjacent to the skull base, will tend to restrict the decompression and increase the potential for postoperative mucocele formation (▶ Fig. 7.2). In contradistinction, the inferior aspect of the agger nasi cell and superior rim of the ethmoid bulla may be left in place to further protect against obstruction of the frontal recess. Complete removal of the remainder of the ethmoid air cells will reveal the suture lines between the sphenoid and frontal bones and the lamina papyracea. Identification of these suture lines is critical as they represent the boundary of the medial bony decompression. Posteriorly, the sphenoid suture line may be identified as a focal thickening of the bone as it transitions from the thinner lamina. The decision to open the sphenoid sinus at this point will depend on the patient anatomy and surgical goals. If a maximal apical decompression is desired, it is often beneficial to partially resect the superior turbinate and widely open the sphenoid face to allow the orbital fat to prolapse posteriorly into the sphenoid

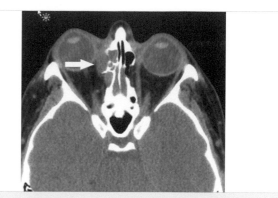

Fig. 7.2 Axial image of a postoperative mucocele in the right frontoethmoidal region (*white arrow*) resulting from inadequate resection of ethmoid partitions in a previous orbital decompression.

lumen. However, if the sphenoid is left intact, the superior turbinate will typically protect the sphenoid os from fat-related obstruction. Once the sinuses have been completely resected, the mucosa may be stripped from the lamina and lateral skull base to help prevent the risk of postoperative mucocele formation. The final consideration in the preparation of the medial decompression is whether or not to resect the middle turbinate. Resection carries risks of olfactory disruption, remnant lateralization with frontal obstruction, and postoperative epistaxis. Consequently, the middle turbinate should only be removed if its presence limits the decompression.

The next step is to completely remove the lamina papyracea, which, as noted, is bounded by the sphenoid, frontal, maxillary, and lacrimal bones (▶ Fig. 7.3). A wide osteotomy is critical as any residual bone will limit the degree of decompression. Once the bone has been removed, the periorbital fascial layer will be encountered. One may often be able to identify the medial rectus muscle and several venous structures through the periorbita. The surgeon should take note of these structures and attempt to avoid them while incising the periorbita. The extent of the periorbital incision should take into account the goals and adjunctive procedures being performed during the decompression. If a maximal decompression is desired, regardless of concerns for the induction of postoperative diplopia, then the medial periorbita may be stripped in its entirety. Conversely, a strip of periorbita may be left over the medial rectus muscle to function as a sling, which has been shown to limit diplopia rates.[3,17] Once the periorbita has been removed, the orbital fat may be feathered medially using blunt instrumentation and gentle tonic pressure on the globe in order to further lyse the periorbital fascial bands and enhance the degree of decompression (▶ Fig. 7.4).

Endoscopic decompression of the orbital floor requires a similar degree of adjacent sinus cavity resection as the medial approach. Though rarely performed, an isolated orbital floor decompression could be performed while preserving the basal lamella and posterior ethmoid air cells. Access to the orbital floor is facilitated by maximizing the vertical height of the maxillary antrostomy. Visualization may be further enhanced by using an angled endoscope. While the mucosa of the maxillary roof must be stripped to facilitate removal of the orbital floor, the mucosa may be preserved and re-draped over the exposed orbital fat at the conclusion of the procedure to facilitate remucosalization

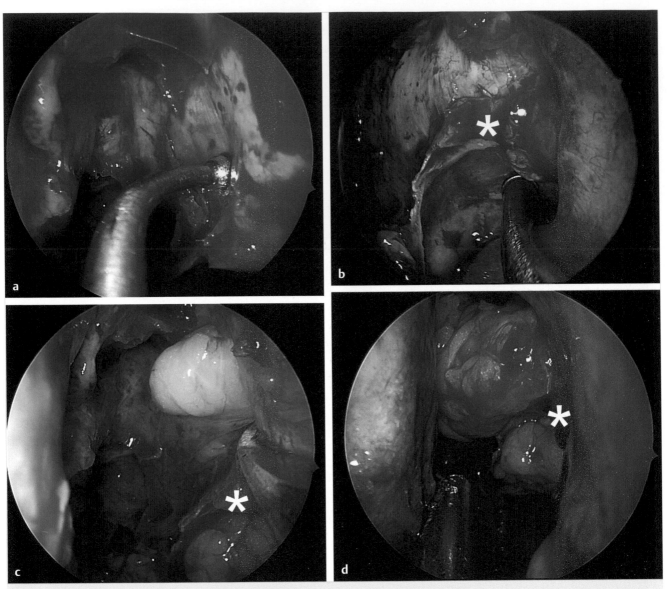

**Fig. 7.3** Endoscopic view of left medial and inferior decompression with preservation of the inferomedial bony strut (*asterisk*). **(a)** Removal of the lamina papyracea using a double-ball probe. **(b)** View of the medial and inferior periorbita following removal of the entire lamina and orbital floor to the level of the infraorbital nerve. Note the preservation of the inferomedial strut. **(c)** Incision of the periorbita from a posterior to anterior direction freeing the extraconal fat. **(d)** Postdecompression view of the extraconal fat after feathering of the fascial bands to maximize decompression. Note how the strut creates a retaining wall along the inferomedial orbit.

and expedite postoperative healing and reduce crusting. In patients whose goal is to achieve a maximal decompression, the entire floor may be easily removed by using a curette to down fracture the orbital strut. This fracture line will typically propagate to the level of the infraorbital canal, which represents the lateral limit of the endoscopic floor decompression.

As previously noted, in patients with no preoperative diplopia, the inferomedial bony strut may be preserved in order to limit globe prolapse and reduce the postoperative diplopia rate. This method was first described by Goldberg et al[18]via a transconjunctival approach and was later converted to an endoscopic technique by Wright et al[19] in 1999. In patients with preservation of the strut, no diplopia was reported; however, due to the

technical demands of the procedure, the strut could only be preserved in 71% of orbits. Our group subsequently developed a method of exclusively endoscopic orbital floor decompression using standard frontal sinus instrumentation, which allows for reliable preservation of the inferomedial strut in 100% of cases.[6,20] In this method, a 4-mm high-speed tapered 70-degree diamond burr (Medtronics, Jacksonville, FL, United States) is used to thin the bone from the lateral edge of the inferomedial strut to the medial border of the infraorbital canal under direct visualization using a 70-degree endoscope (▶ Fig. 7.5). A double-ball probe may then be used to down fracture the bone away from the periorbita taking care not to expose the orbital fat or inferior rectus muscle. The borders of the osteotomy may

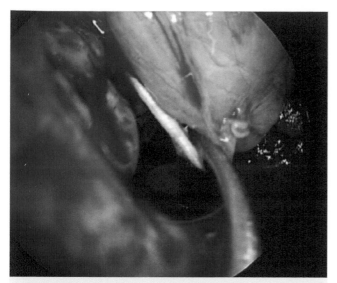

Fig. 7.4 Endoscopic view of the right medial orbit following periorbital resection. A probe can be seen lysing the residual fascial bands of the periorbital fat to maximize the degree of decompression.

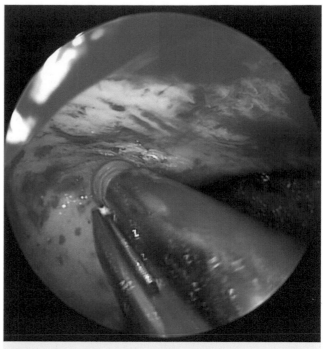

Fig. 7.5 Endoscopic view of the left orbital floor using a 70-degree endoscope. An angled drill can be seen thinning out the bone in preparation for controlled resection.

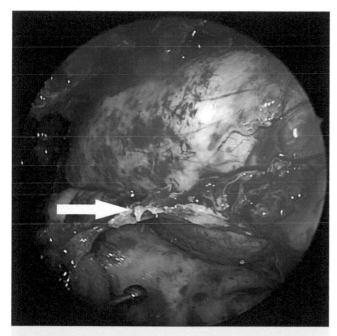

Fig. 7.6 Endoscopic view of left orbit following removal of the lamina and orbital floor with preservation of the inferomedial strut (*white arrow*).

## 7.4 Lateral Orbital Wall Decompression

The authors perform lateral wall decompression as an adjunct to medial wall and floor decompression in select patients. The decision to add lateral wall decompression is often made pre-operatively, but may be made intraoperatively, depending on the amount of decompression accomplished with the medial wall and floor. Indications for adjunctive lateral wall decompression include a desire for maximum decompression because of significant proptosis, to balance the medial decompression in a patient with no preoperative diplopia, or to increase the amount of decompression unilaterally for improved symmetry.

The lateral orbital wall decompression is begun after placement of a corneal protective shell and injection of local anesthetic with epinephrine for hemostasis. A variety of cutaneous incision locations provide access to the lateral orbit, including a lid crease incision extending laterally or a lateral canthotomy. We prefer a 2.5-cm-incision lateral canthotomy approach. Dissection is carried through the soft tissue overlying the lateral orbital rim, which is bared superiorly from the frontozygomatic suture down to the level of the zygomatic arch. The periosteum is incised vertically along the orbital rim, and a periosteal elevator is used in a subperiosteal plane to expose the bone inside the orbital rim (▶ Fig. 7.7). Care is taken to cauterize the zygomaticotemporal and zygomaticofacial neurovascular bundles as they are encountered. The periosteal elevation is carried posteriorly toward the orbital apex along the greater wing of the sphenoid, but stopping anterior to the infraorbital canal on the inferior aspect to avoid hemorrhage and damage to apical structures. Orbital access is easier if a wide area of periosteum

then be further expanded using a frontal sinus cobra through punch (Karl Storz, Tuttlingen, Germany) allowing for fine adjustments to the width of the remaining inferomedial strut (▶ Fig. 7.6). Once the osteotomy is complete, the periorbita may be incised allowing for decompression of the inferior periorbital fat into the maxillary sinus. In a review of 45 orbits decompressed using this technique, there was significant improvement in diplopia rates and with a mean proptosis reduction of 3.89 mm.[7,8]

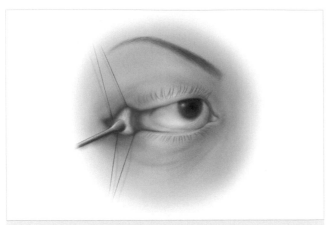

Fig. 7.7 Lateral orbitotomy for orbital decompression is performed via a lateral canthotomy incision. The lateral orbital rim has been exposed and a periosteal elevator is used in a subperiosteal plane to gain access to the lateral orbit.

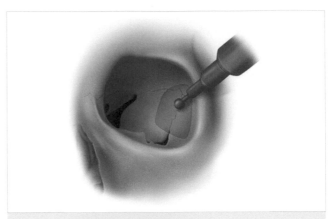

Fig. 7.8 Bone removal during lateral orbital decompression is performed using a drill with a cutting burr. A conservative bone removal as delineated in green shadow is often performed in our cases.

is elevated; hence, this is carried out superiorly to the level just below the zygomaticofrontal suture and inferiorly to the inferior-most aspect of the inferior orbital fissure. We have found that removal of the orbital rim is not usually necessary to access the orbit when this wide subperiosteal dissection is performed. Bone is then removed from the lateral orbit, beginning just inside the orbital rim and extending posteriorly to the trigone of the greater sphenoid wing. The vertical limits of bone removal are the superior and inferior orbital fissures. This may be performed with a variety of modalities, including drills or ultrasonic devices (▶ Fig. 7.8). We favor a high-speed drill with a 5-mm cutting burr because of its efficiency and availability. The amount of bone removal varies significantly among surgeons based on comfort level as well as patient anatomy, as there is variation in the amount of bone in the greater sphenoid wing trigone.[21] It is possible to safely drill to expose temporalis muscle laterally; however, consideration must be given to the risk of transmission of movement from the temporalis muscle to the orbital contents and globe during mastication if this defect is large.[22] Next, the periorbita is carefully opened with scissors just inferior to the lateral rectus muscle, starting at the orbital rim and extending posteriorly into the orbit. Orbital fat is encouraged to prolapse, and is most often removed for additional decompression. Several cubic centimeters ($cm^3$) can be removed safely from most orbits. The periosteum along the orbital rim is closed with 5–0 absorbable suture. The lateral commissure is repaired with an absorbable cerclage suture but is not reattached to the lateral orbital rim. The canthotomy incision is closed with cutaneous 6–0 absorbable suture.

# 7.5 Complications of Orbital Decompression Surgery

A variety of complications are possible after invasive orbital surgery, which include some that are inherent to most surgeries and others that are unique to this high-risk area. Special consideration must be given because of the anatomy of the orbit and its contents. The orbit is a fixed space surrounded by bony walls on all sides except anteriorly, and contains our most precious sensory organ, the eye, as well as the supporting vasculature and nervous system. Hence, the consequences of complications, which might be minor elsewhere, can be quite serious when they occur in the orbit.

General surgical complications may include infection, postoperative edema, and hemorrhage. Orbital infections can be devastating and precautions should be taken to avoid this risk. Intravenous antibiotics are given intraoperatively, and both topical and oral antibiotics should be prescribed postoperatively. Postoperative edema may worsen compressive optic neuropathy in these patients, and so intravenous corticosteroid should be given intraoperatively and oral corticosteroid should be prescribed postoperatively in a tapering fashion. Hemorrhage can be devastating because of the nature of the septated, fixed space in the orbit. Care must be taken to have patients stop anticoagulants for an appropriate period prior to surgery. Intraoperatively, hemostasis must be carefully maintained. Care in dissection and prevention of intraoperative hemorrhage is the optimal method. If bleeding does occur, use of electrocautery within the orbit is not advised, and other methods such as cold lavage are safer. Postoperatively, patients should have limited activity for 2 weeks and should not resume anticoagulant medications until several days after surgery. The eye should never be patched after orbital surgery. It is critical that patients are able to monitor their vision postoperatively and immediately report any changes. Retrobulbar hemorrhage can quickly result in permanent visual loss if unrecognized or untreated.

Complications that are unique to the orbit include loss of vision, elevated intraocular pressure, and diplopia. Visual loss can occur from physical damage to the globe or optic nerve from direct trauma, or thermal or electrical damage from cautery. Visual loss may also occur from elevated orbital pressure from hemorrhage or aggressive intraoperative retraction of orbital contents. Care must be taken to avoid the use of cautery in the orbit. Additionally, instruments should be removed from the orbit every few minutes to relieve pressure and allow perfusion of the globe and other orbital contents. Diplopia occurs when the two eyes are not aligned. In this setting, diplopia may result from restriction of extraocular motility, which may be a result of rectus muscle edema from retraction or manipulation.

Additionally, the neurovascular supply to the muscle may be damaged during retraction, as these vessels arise from the orbital apex and enter the intraconal side of the muscle approximately 1 cm from the apex.

When performing an endoscopic decompression, additional immediate complications may include high-flow arterial bleeding from sphenopalatine arterial branches, and much less commonly the internal carotid artery. A cerebrospinal fluid leak may also occur during the ethmoid and sphenoid dissection or when resecting the lamina papyracea off of the frontoethmoidal suture line. Finally, direct injury to the extraocular muscles may occur during the periorbital incision or when feathering the extraocular fat. This may be avoided by using a blunt probe or sickle knife during this portion of the procedure. Long-term complications may arise from postobstructive mucocele formation, which reinforces the importance of prophylactic sinusotomy and judicious mucosal stripping.

# References

[1] Fry EL, Fante RG. Acute orbital edema causing reversible blindness after the administration of intravenous contrast agent in a patient with thyroid eye disease. Ophthal Plast Reconstr Surg. 2008; 24(4):330–331

[2] Wickwar S, McBain H, Ezra DG, Hirani SP, Rose GE, Newman SP. The psychosocial and clinical outcomes of orbital decompression surgery for thyroid eye disease and predictors of change in quality of life. Ophthalmology. 2015; 122(12):2568–76.e1

[3] Kingdom TT, Davies BW, Durairaj VD. Orbital decompression for the management of thyroid eye disease: An analysis of outcomes and complications. Laryngoscope. 2015; 125(9):2034–2040

[4] Prat MC, Braunstein AL, Dagi Glass LR, Kazim M. Orbital fat decompression for thyroid eye disease: retrospective case review and criteria for optimal case selection. Ophthal Plast Reconstr Surg. 2015; 31(3):215–218

[5] Bingham CM, Harris MA, Vidor IA, et al. Transcranial orbital decompression for progressive compressive optic neuropathy after 3-wall decompression in severe graves' orbitopathy. Ophthal Plast Reconstr Surg. 2014; 30(3):215–218

[6] Mainville NP, Jordan DR. Effect of orbital decompression on diplopia in thyroid-related orbitopathy. Ophthal Plast Reconstr Surg. 2014; 30(2):137–140

[7] Wu CY, Niziol LM, Musch DC, Kahana A. Thyroid-related orbital decompression surgery: a multivariate analysis of risk factors and outcomes. Ophthal Plast Reconstr Surg. 2016

[8] Finn AP, Bleier B, Cestari DM, et al. A retrospective review of orbital decompression for thyroid orbitopathy with endoscopic preservation of the inferomedial orbital bone strut. Ophthal Plast Reconstr Surg. 2017; 33(5):334–339

[9] Alsuhaibani AH, Carter KD, Policeni B, Nerad JA. Orbital volume and eye position changes after balanced orbital decompression. Ophthal Plast Reconstr Surg. 2011; 27(3):158–163

[10] Takahashi Y, Kakizaki H, Shiraki K, Iwaki M. Improved ocular motility after balanced orbital decompression for dysthyroid orbitopathy. Can J Ophthalmol. 2008; 43(6):722–723

[11] Graham SM, Brown CL, Carter KD, Song A, Nerad JA. Medial and lateral orbital wall surgery for balanced decompression in thyroid eye disease. Laryngoscope. 2003; 113(7):1206–1209

[12] Kacker A, Kazim M, Murphy M, Trokel S, Close LG. "Balanced" orbital decompression for severe Graves' orbitopathy: technique with treatment algorithm. Otolaryngol Head Neck Surg. 2003; 128(2):228–235

[13] Mehta P, Durrani OM. Outcome of deep lateral wall rim-sparing orbital decompression in thyroid-associated orbitopathy: a new technique and results of a case series. Orbit. 2011; 30(6):265–268

[14] Goldberg RA, Perry JD, Hortaleza V, Tong JT. Strabismus after balanced medial plus lateral wall versus lateral wall only orbital decompression for dysthyroid orbitopathy. Ophthal Plast Reconstr Surg. 2000; 16(4):271–277

[15] Walsh TE, Ogura JH. Transantral orbital decompression for malignant exophthalmos. Laryngoscope. 1957; 67(6):544–568

[16] Kennedy DW, Goodstein ML, Miller NR, Zinreich SJ. Endoscopic transnasal orbital decompression. Arch Otolaryngol Head Neck Surg. 1990; 116(3):275–282

[17] Metson R, Samaha M. Reduction of diplopia following endoscopic orbital decompression: the orbital sling technique. Laryngoscope. 2002; 112(10):1753–1757

[18] Goldberg RA, Shorr N, Cohen MS. The medial orbital strut in the prevention of postdecompression dystopia in dysthyroid ophthalmopathy. Ophthal Plast Reconstr Surg. 1992; 8(1):32–34

[19] Wright ED, Davidson J, Codere F, Desrosiers M. Endoscopic orbital decompression with preservation of an inferomedial bony strut: minimization of postoperative diplopia. J Otolaryngol. 1999; 28(5):252–256

[20] Bleier BS, Lefebvre DR, Freitag SK. Endoscopic orbital floor decompression with preservation of the inferomedial strut. Int Forum Allergy Rhinol. 2014; 4(1):82–84

[21] Lefebvre DR, Yoon MK. CT-based measurements of the sphenoid trigone in different sex and race. Ophthal Plast Reconstr Surg. 2015; 31(2):155–158

[22] Fayers T, Barker LE, Verity DH, Rose GE. Oscillopsia after lateral wall orbital decompression. Ophthalmology. 2013; 120(9):1920–1923

# 8 Complications of Orbital Decompression and Management

*Jordan T. Glicksman, James N. Palmer, and Nithin D. Adappa*

**Abstract**
- Complications of endoscopic orbital decompression are rare, but can be life or vision threatening.
- Complications of orbital decompression may be irreversible, and therefore prevention is the best form of treatment.
- A solid grasp of patient anatomy, including risk factors for complications, is essential to prevent complications.
- Intraoperative complications include corneal abrasion, optic nerve injury, extraocular muscle injury, infraorbital nerve injury, nasolacrimal duct injury, arrhythmias, skull base injuries, and vascular injuries.
- Postoperative complications include diplopia, postsurgical sinus obstruction, subcutaneous emphysema, epistaxis, and inadequate decompression or asymmetry.
- A team approach with ophthalmology is critical for management of ocular complications.

*Keywords:* orbital decompression, complications, endoscopic, management, anatomy

## 8.1 Introduction

Since described by Kennedy et al[1] in 1990, endoscopic orbital decompression has largely replaced open decompressive procedures due to the decreased morbidity associated with an incisionless approach. While in most cases endoscopic orbital decompression is performed successfully, potential complications are important to consider, both by the surgeon and by the patient. While most complications of endoscopic decompression are minor and self-limiting, the complications of the procedure can lead to severe consequences, which can be life- or vision-threatening. The complications outlined in this chapter focus on those specific to the procedure, and not those related to a general anesthetic.

## 8.2 Patient Selection and Indications

Complications of orbital decompression can be broken down into intraoperative or postoperative complications.

### 8.2.1 Intraoperative Complications

The best method of treating complications is prevention. Therefore, it is critical for the surgeon to be aware of impending complications and for the surgeon to take steps to mitigate risk of them occurring. Intraoperative complications may include corneal abrasion, optic nerve injury, extraocular muscle injury, infraorbital nerve injury, nasolacrimal duct injury, bradycardia and asystole, skull base injuries/cerebrospinal fluid (CSF) leak, and vascular injuries (▶ Table 8.1).

## Corneal Abrasion

Corneal abrasion is typically prevented by the use of eye protection and lubrication during surgery. Corneal shields can be used to cover the eye, or the eyelids can be taped shut during the procedure. It is preferable not to place a tarsorrhaphy stitch for endoscopic sinus surgery, as this can make monitoring of the eye more challenging during the case. If a corneal abrasion occurs despite this, topical antibiotic ointments such as erythromycin or eye drops such as ciprofloxacin or ofloxacin may be prescribed. The ideal duration of treatment has not been studied, but it would be reasonable to continue treatment until the patient is symptom free for 24 hours. Topical anesthetic agents should be avoided as they can cause further trauma to the eye to go undetected by the patient. Evaluation by an ophthalmologist using slit-lamp biomicroscopy is recommended to ensure that corneal infection does not occur during the healing phase and that the corneal epithelial defect resolves completely.

## Optic Nerve Injury

Depending on the etiology of injury, this optic nerve injury may be suspected intraoperatively and confirmed postoperatively or may only be recognized postoperatively. In either case, an ophthalmology consultation is indicated, which should include a full examination and formal visual field testing. We would recommend discussing the use of steroids with the consulting ophthalmologist to address any potential swelling around the nerve.

A computed tomography (CT) scan may elucidate if swelling or a hematoma at the orbital apex is implicated, and could reveal a bony spicule impinging on the optic nerve. If the nerve is compressed by a bone fragment, then returning to the operating room for exploration and decompression would be indicated immediately.

A retrobulbar hematoma typically presents with bruising, pain, proptosis, mydriasis, chemosis, elevated intraocular pressure, and eventually visual loss (▶ Fig. 8.1). Typically color vision is impaired first as nerve fibers encoding color are located at the periphery of the nerve. To help prevent this complication, dissection should be performed meticulously and

**Table 8.1** Classification of complications

| Intraoperative complications | Postoperative complications |
|---|---|
| Corneal abrasion | Diplopia |
| Optic nerve injury | Sinus obstruction |
| Extraocular muscle injury | Subcutaneous emphysema |
| Infraorbital nerve injury | Epistaxis |
| Nasolacrimal duct injury | Inadequate decompression |
| Bradycardia and asystole | Asymmetry |
| Skull base injuries/cerebrospinal fluid leak | Retro-orbital hematoma |
| Major vascular injuries | |
| Retro-orbital hematoma | |

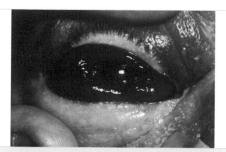

Fig. 8.1 Photograph of a patient with a retro-orbital hematoma secondary to anterior ethmoid artery injury. Chemosis, bruising, and mydriasis are demonstrated, which are all signs of this complication. A lateral canthotomy and cantholysis were required to decompress the orbit. (This image is provided courtesy of Dr. Raymond Sacks, MBBCH, FCS (SA) ORL, FRACS, MMed (ORL), University of Sydney, Sydney, Australia.)

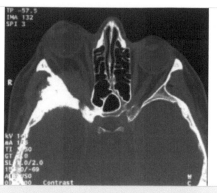

Fig. 8.2 Axial CT (computed tomography) scan image demonstrating retro-orbital hemorrhage. This case occurred secondary to trauma, but this complication can also occur following orbital decompression. (This image is provided courtesy of Dr. Raymond Sacks, MBBCH, FCS [SA] ORL, FRACS, MMed [ORL], University of Sydney, Sydney, Australia.)

vessels at risk of retracting into the orbit should be identified and coagulated prior to division, if division is required.

Ideally the signs and symptoms of a retrobulbar hematoma would be recognized clinically and would obviate the need for imaging (► Fig. 8.2). In the case of a hematoma following endoscopic orbital decompression, these signs may be masked by the decompressive nature of the procedure. If the orbit has not been decompressed to the orbital apex, then emergent decompression may be warranted given the small window before vision loss. Adjunctive medical therapy such as mannitol or acetazolamide could also be considered. If packing was placed intraoperatively, it should be removed to decrease pressure on the orbital contents.

## Extraocular Muscle Injury

The medial rectus muscle is at risk whenever the periorbita is violated. Whereas in most endoscopic sinus procedures it is undesirable to penetrate the lamina papyracea, removal of this structure is required for endoscopic orbital decompression. Care should be taken when dividing the periorbita to avoid penetrating the orbital contents deeply and lacerating the extraocular muscles. Although a variety of incisions have been described, the key point is the incisions through periorbita should be done in a controlled fashion and any form of debrider should never be used to resect periorbita. Injury to the medial rectus will result in diplopia and may require future strabismus surgery. Unfortunately, diplopia may persist in some fields of gaze even after successful strabismus surgery and therefore prevention is the best treatment.

## Infraorbital Nerve Injury

The infraorbital canal is the lateral limit of orbital floor decompression. It is important to recognize the position of the nerve prior to decompressing the orbital floor. If bleeding occurs in the vicinity of the nerve, care should be taken in achieving hemostasis to avoid thermal injury. Damage to the infraorbital nerve results in midfacial numbness and/or paresthesia. Ference et al[2] demonstrated the nerve traverses within the

maxillary sinus in 8% of patients without an infraorbital ethmoid air cell and in 28% of patients in whom this variation exists. Care must be taken to avoid infraorbital nerve injury, as it is often irreversible. Management is typically conservative.

## Nasolacrimal Duct Injury

The nasolacrimal duct is vulnerable to injury when a maxillary antrostomy is carried too far anteriorly. In general, angled scopes are recommended to identify the true maxillary antrostomy and removal of the entire uncinate process. An angled view also allows visualization of the harder lacrimal bone that protects the nasolacrimal duct. If image guidance is available, navigation can demonstrate the border of the nasolacrimal duct. In most cases, even if an injury occurs, patients are typically asymptomatic. If complications occur, it typically is in the form of epiphora and a dacryocystorhinostomy can be performed to correct this issue.

## Bradycardia and Asystole

Bradycardia and asystole are possible complications of ocular manipulation due to the oculocardiac reflex. This reflex is mediated by the ophthalmic branch of the trigeminal nerve. The afferent pathway involves the ciliary ganglion, gasserian ganglion, and trigeminal sensory nucleus. Vagal efferents lead to parasympathetic stimulation of the heart, which can result in bradycardia and asystole.

Factors known to perpetuate this reflex include hypercarbia, hypoxemia, light anesthesia, young age, and strength and duration of the stimulus.[3] It is important to ensure the anesthesiologist you are working with is aware of this potential complication and potential exacerbating factors to minimize the risk. Communication with the anesthesiologist during the case is probably the most important aspect of care to prevent or minimize these issues. Should a patient develop bradycardia or asystole, medical management such as atropine can be administered. Persistent or recurrent bradycardia or periods of asystole may warrant external pacing and aborting the case.

## Skull Base Injuries/Cerebrospinal Fluid Leak

Skull base injuries are rarely encountered during endoscopic sinus surgical procedures. Preoperative CT imaging allows the surgeon to identify risk factors for skull base injury, such as a low-lying cribriform plate. If recognized intraoperatively, a variety of patching materials (e.g., mucosa, fascia, fat, or commercially available dural analogs) can be used to repair the leak.

It is important to recognize that an injury to the brain or its vasculature can occur when the skull base is violated. Postoperative imaging and serial clinical examination can lead to the diagnosis, and if present would warrant neurosurgical consultation (▶ Fig. 8.3).

## Vascular Injury

Major vascular injuries are possible during orbital decompression surgery. It is important to consider the anatomy of the anterior/posterior ethmoid arteries when reviewing the preoperative imaging.

An anterior ethmoid artery that is situated below the skull base in a mesentery is particularly vulnerable to injury. This can result in epistaxis, or if the artery retracts laterally into the orbit, a retrobulbar hematoma. Depending on how far along the case has progressed, consideration of a lateral canthotomy and inferior cantholysis as well as an intraoperative ophthalmology consult would be warranted. Definitive treatment involves completing the orbital decompression. Fortunately, the posterior ethmoid artery is usually found within the skull base and is therefore less likely to be at risk of injury.

The internal carotid artery is vulnerable in cases with a dehiscence in the lateral sphenoid wall. Additionally, an Onodi cell may predispose a patient to carotid injury. It is critically important not to twist any horizontal septations between the sphenoid and Onodi cell. The septation may attach to the bone overlying the internal carotid, and torsion of the septation may lead to carotid injury with resulting catastrophic bleeding and stroke.

In the event of internal carotid injury, every effort must be made to control the bleeding immediately. The anesthetist should be notified once this complication is suspected. The patient will almost certainly require a transfusion of blood products.

Large bore intravenous lines must be established, and crystalloid products should be administered while awaiting blood transfusion. Most importantly, the area of injury should be

tightly packed to tamponade the bleeding. Large bore suction should be used to facilitate visualization. If a second surgeon is available, then a four-handed, two-surgeon technique is preferable. Valentine and Wormald[4] describe the use of a 10 × 10 mm patch of muscle harvested from the sternocleidomastoid muscle to help facilitate hemostasis. Muscle from the tongue may be more readily available and could be used as an alternative. The patient would require urgent transfer to an interventional radiology suite for consideration of balloon occlusion or possibly stent insertion.

## 8.2.2 Postoperative Complications

Postoperative complications include diplopia, sinus obstruction, subcutaneous emphysema, epistaxis, and inadequate decompression or asymmetry (▶ Table 8.1). Retro-orbital hematoma can also present as an early complication.

### Diplopia

Patients with preoperative diplopia must be aware that surgery may not correct their double vision. Postoperative diplopia in patients with this morbidity preoperatively would not be considered a surgical complication.

The incidence of new-onset postoperative diplopia has been variable in the literature and may affect up to one-third of patients undergoing orbital decompression. It is thought to result from altered vectors of the extraocular muscles, and consultation with an ophthalmologist specializing in strabismus surgery is indicated. This topic is covered in detail in Chapter 11.

### Sinus Obstruction

If the orbital contents are decompressed too far anteriorly, the protruding contents may obstruct the frontal sinus. Decompression should therefore not extend into the frontal recess. Should this occur, a CT scan and MRI (magnetic resonance imaging) would be helpful in planning subsequent management (▶ Fig. 8.4). Medial positioning of extraocular muscles may

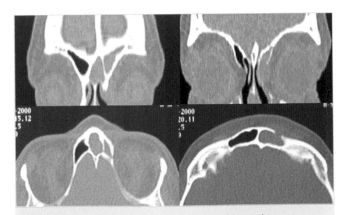

Fig. 8.4 CT (computed tomography) scan (top: coronal images; bottom: axial images) demonstrating a left frontal mucocele. This occurred secondary to frontal sinus obstruction from fat protruding into the frontal recess. This necessitated a frontal sinusotomy for drainage. (These images are provided courtesy of Dr. Raymond Sacks, MBBCH, FCS (SA) ORL, FRACS, MMed (ORL), University of Sydney, Sydney, Australia.)

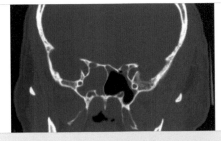

Fig. 8.3 Coronal CT (computed tomography) scan image demonstrating a left-sided injury to the skull base at planum sphenoidale from aggressive manipulation during an orbital decompression. (This image is provided courtesy of courtesy of Dr. Raymond Sacks, MBBCH, FCS [SA] ORL, FRACS, MMed [ORL], University of Sydney, Sydney, Australia.)

prohibit debulking of orbital fat. Reconstruction of the medial orbital wall may be considered, or alternatively surgery to improve the patency of the frontal sinus may be pursued (e.g., a Draf III procedure).

The maxillary sinus can become obstructed if an inadequate maxillary antrostomy is performed. A large antrostomy provides improved access and visualization when performing surgery and also will help prevent this complication.

### Subcutaneous Emphysema

Subcutaneous emphysema may result from bag mask ventilation following extubation, or if the patient exerts positive pressure into the nose (e.g., coughing or sneezing). For this reason, bag mask ventilation should be avoided postoperatively if possible. Fortunately, this is a self-limiting complication that usually resolves within 1 to 2 weeks.

### Epistaxis

Epistaxis following sinus surgery, including orbital decompression, is typically minor. To help reduce the risk of postoperative bleeding, it is important to ensure hemostasis at the end of the case. When postoperative epistaxis is encountered, topical decongestants, cautery, and/or packing may be useful. In the case of major bleeding, control should be achieved in a monitored setting, ideally in the operating room. Bleeding from branches of the anterior ethmoid artery or sphenopalatine artery is typically addressed with ligation. Embolization by an interventional radiologist can be considered if a sphenopalatine artery bleed is suspected. Epistaxis secondary to an anterior or posterior ethmoid artery bleed typically requires a surgical ligation.

### Inadequate Decompression and Asymmetry

The average endoscopic medial orbital decompression leads to a 3.5-mm reduction in proptosis.[5] In cases where this is an inadequate result, the addition of an open decompressive procedure may enhance the effect by an additional 2 mm.[6] Orbital floor and lateral wall decompression are also commonly performed to increase the amount of decompression where indicated. Patients should be aware that there may not be perfect symmetry following the procedure.

## 8.3 Diagnostic Workup

Generally, diagnostic workup is not indicated following uncomplicated endoscopic orbital decompression surgery. Ophthalmic examination including visual acuity, color vision, extraocular motility and intraocular pressure should be checked upon the patient awakening in the recovery area and should be monitored during the course of hospital admission, or the following day if the patient is discharged on the day of surgery.

Most complications are minor and do not require investigations. However, when a serious complication is suspected, an appropriate diagnostic workup should be performed.

In patients with suspected optic nerve injury, severe corneal abrasion, or any other suspected ocular complication, the ophthalmologic team should be closely involved.

In the unlikely event of a skull base injury and CSF leak, CT imaging would be appropriate, as would consideration of beta-2 transferrin testing. Intrathecal injection of fluorescein is commonly used to help localize small CSF leaks, although its use is off-label.

## 8.4 Surgical Anatomy

A solid grasp of surgical anatomy is required for a safe endoscopic orbital decompression. Critical structures at risk of injury include the extraocular muscles, anterior and posterior ethmoid arteries, optic and infraorbital nerves, skull base, and nasolacrimal duct.

The medial rectus muscle is the most at-risk muscle when performing orbital surgery and the inferior rectus muscle can be injured as well. In patients with Graves' ophthalmopathy, these muscles are usually thickened and inflamed and sit adjacent to the periorbita. Care must be taken not to injure these muscles when incising the periorbita.

As in routine endoscopic sinus surgery, it is important to recognize the anatomy of the ethmoid arteries and in particular the anterior ethmoid artery. If located in a mesentery below the skull base, the anterior ethmoid injury may be particularly vulnerable. If injured, it may retract into the orbit and result in a retrobulbar hematoma.

The nasolacrimal apparatus includes the superior and inferior lacrimal puncta and canaliculi, the common canaliculus, the lacrimal sac, and nasolacrimal duct. Hasner's valve is at the distal end of the nasolacrimal duct as it enters the inferior meatus. The nasolacrimal duct travels through the lacrimal bone, maxilla, and inferior turbinate, anterior to the maxillary sinus. If a maxillary antrostomy is carried too far anteriorly, the duct can be injured and scarring may lead to obstruction and epiphora.

The optic nerve courses along the superior aspect of the lateral sphenoid wall before entering the orbit through the optic foramen. In patients with an Onodi cell, the nerve may be intimately related to the horizontal septation of the cell or even contained within the air cell. It is important to recognize these anatomical variants to prevent injury to the nerve.

The infraorbital nerve runs along the roof of the maxillary sinus. It marks the lateral extent of the inferior orbital decompression. It is particularly vulnerable to injury when contained within the maxillary sinus lumen. This variation is more frequently seen in patients with an infraorbital air cell.

The lateral lamella of the ethmoid bone is the thinnest component of the anterior skull base and is therefore at the greatest risk of penetration. The skull base naturally slopes inferiorly from anterior to posterior. A steeper slope of the skull base has been demonstrated to be a risk factor for skull base injury and CSF leak.[7] Similarly, a deep skull base increases the risk of CSF leak.[8] In the Keros classification system, the depth of the lateral lamella is measured relative to the fovea ethmoidalis (1–3 mm is type I, 4–7 mm is type II, and > 7 mm is type III). Patients with a skull base that has a higher Keros classification are therefore at greater risk of injury to the base of skull.

## 8.5 Postoperative Care

Postoperative care for patients with complications of endoscopic orbital decompression depends on the nature and severity of the complication. Management of the complications presented in this chapter has already been described. At many centers, patients undergoing orbital decompression are routinely admitted overnight for monitoring. Patients with major injuries such as vascular injury, skull base injury, or arrhythmias will require care in an intensive care setting. Minor complications such as subcutaneous emphysema can be observed in a less acute setting.

## 8.6 Outcomes

Fortunately, the complications of orbital decompression are rare, in particular those which are severe. Publications examining orbital decompression surgery are limited to case series of less than 200 patients, which makes it difficult to capture the infrequent and severe complications. There is a bias in peer-reviewed articles toward under-reporting complications. Investigators who have low complication rates and less severe complications are more likely to publish their results than those with higher complication rates. Therefore, it is difficult to accurately estimate the incidence of complications following endoscopic orbital decompression.

A systematic review, published by Leong et al in 2009, pooled 11 studies with a total of 613 endoscopically decompressed orbits, performed without adjunctive open procedures. The pooled complication rate was 5.2%. In a more recent series of 115 orbits in 73 patients, Yao et al[9] reported a complication rate of 6.9%, none of which were severe. In a series of 114 orbits in 77 patients, Kingdom et al[10] reported a complication rate of 2.6% (including 1 patient with permanent V2 numbness and another with bilateral corneal abrasions that resolved within 24 hours).

## References

[1] Kennedy DW, Goodstein ML, Miller NR, Zinreich SJ. Endoscopic transnasal orbital decompression. Arch Otolaryngol Head Neck Surg. 1990; 116(3):275–282

[2] Ference EH, Smith SS, Conley D, Chandra RK. Surgical anatomy and variations of the infraorbital nerve. Laryngoscope. 2015; 125(6):1296–1300

[3] Lang S, Lanigan DT, van der Wal M. Trigeminocardiac reflexes: maxillary and mandibular variants of the oculocardiac reflex. Can J Anaesth. 1991; 38(6): 757–760

[4] Valentine R, Wormald PJ. Controlling the surgical field during a large endoscopic vascular injury. Laryngoscope. 2011; 121(3):562–566

[5] Leong SC, Karkos PD, Macewen CJ, White PS. A systematic review of outcomes following surgical decompression for dysthyroid orbitopathy. Laryngoscope. 2009; 119(6):1106–1115

[6] Metson R, Dallow RL, Shore JW. Endoscopic orbital decompression. Laryngoscope. 1994; 104(8, Pt 1):950–957

[7] Heaton CM, Goldberg AN, Pletcher SD, Glastonbury CM. Sinus anatomy associated with inadvertent cerebrospinal fluid leak during functional endoscopic sinus surgery. Laryngoscope. 2012; 122(7):1446–1449

[8] Ramakrishnan VR, Suh JD, Kennedy DW. Ethmoid skull-base height: a clinically relevant method of evaluation. Int Forum Allergy Rhinol. 2011; 1 (5):396–400

[9] Yao WC, Sedaghat AR, Yadav P, Fay A, Metson R. Orbital decompression in the endoscopic age: the modified inferomedial orbital strut. Otolaryngol Head Neck Surg. 2016; 154(5):963–969

[10] Kingdom TT, Davies BW, Durairaj VD. Orbital decompression for the management of thyroid eye disease: an analysis of outcomes and complications. Laryngoscope. 2015; 125(9):2034–2040

# 9 Strabismus and Eyelid Surgery in Thyroid Eye Disease

*Bo Young Chun, Suzanne K. Freitag, and Dean M. Cestari*

## Abstract

This chapter provides an overview of the medical and surgical management of the problems commonly encountered by thyroid eye disease patients with strabismus. Restrictive strabismus can be disabling for patients, and having an understanding of the various surgical and nonsurgical options for treatment is important. Placement of prism in spectacles or injection of botulinum toxin into extraocular muscles may temporize or obviate the need for strabismus surgery. Eyelid retraction results in keratopathy, discomfort, disfigurement, and rarely corneal perforation and visual loss. This chapter discusses the gamut of treatment options from ocular lubrication to placement of fillers or botulinum toxin. A highly effective surgical technique for upper and lower eyelid recession is described.

*Keywords:* thyroid eye disease, strabismus, eyelid surgery, eyelid retraction, blepharoplasty, tarsorrhaphy, extraocular muscle, prism, eyelid recession, spacer graft

## 9.1 Introduction

Thyroid eye disease (TED) may affect a variety of orbital and adnexal structures. Patients with mild disease often have upper and/or lower eyelid retraction. Eyelids may also be affected by edema in the acute phase of the disease, and by steatoblepharon in the acute or chronic stage as a result of the characteristic orbital fat hypertrophy in thyroid orbitopathy. Patients with more severe disease may develop diplopia from inflammation of the extraocular muscles, resulting in restrictive myopathy. A variety of conservative measures are helpful to manage these problems during the active stage of disease, and will be discussed in this chapter. In addition, corrective surgery may be performed; however, the timing and order of these surgeries is critical in order to maximize patient outcomes. When surgeries are performed during the active stage of disease, the outcomes are less likely to be stable over time. If orbital decompression is planned to reduce proptosis, this should be performed as the first rehabilitative surgery, as this procedure can affect extraocular muscle function. Orbital decompression is discussed in detail in Chapter 7. Next, if strabismus surgery is planned, it should be performed prior to eyelid surgery, as recession of vertical extraocular muscles may result in additional eyelid retraction. Finally, eyelid surgery may be undertaken if indicated.

## 9.2 Management of Strabismus Associated with Thyroid Eye Disease

### 9.2.1 Etiology

Enlargement of the extraocular muscles with sparing of their tendons is a common feature of TED that often results in an incomitant strabismus with binocular diplopia.[1,2] In the initial acute phase of TED, there is lymphocytic infiltration and interstitial edema of the extraocular muscles with deposition of glycosaminoglycans and hyaluronic acid as well as adipogenesis.[3,4] Extraocular muscle inflammation stimulates fibroblast activity resulting in mucopolysaccharide and collagen formation. Later the inflammation subsides, often leaving chronic fibrotic change, which results in limitation of extraocular motility and diplopia in patients with TED.[4]

### 9.2.2 Typical Patterns of Strabismus in Thyroid Eye Disease

Mild periorbital edema in association with limitation of elevation of one eye may be the first symptom of strabismus due to TED. Impaired ductions are observed in nearly 80% of TED patients and binocular diplopia is the initial presentation in 15 to 20% of TED patients.[5,6,7] Clinically, the inferior rectus muscle is most commonly affected (60–80%), followed by the medial rectus muscle (42–44%) and then the superior rectus muscle, although any extraocular muscle can be affected in TED.[4,6,8,9] It is not known why some muscles are more commonly affected than others. The inferior rectus muscle is the bulkiest and most tonically active extraocular muscle and it may be that the degree of muscle activity and hence the blood supply is a factor.[4] Magnetic resonance imaging (MRI) of the orbits is useful in assessment of disease activity and in showing muscle involvement and optic nerve compression.[4] Finally, the diagnosis of strabismus due to TED can be confirmed by forced duction testing, which reveals restriction of passive movements of the eyeball.

Enlargement and tightening of an extraocular muscle with relative sparing of its antagonist muscle causes the eye to deviate toward the affected muscle.[10] Symptoms of diplopia in the primary position may not be present if the angle of deviation is small and falls within the patient's fusional range, which decreases with time.[10] Sparing of the contralateral yoke muscle may cause a significant imbalance that often results in an esotropia when the medial rectus muscle is involved or a hypotropia from the inferior rectus muscle. Strabismus due to TED is usually incomitant, meaning that the angle of deviation changes depending on the direction of gaze.[4,10]

Patients with TED may have isolated horizontal or vertical strabismus, but many patients have a combination of the two depending on the extent of muscle involvement. The most commonly seen vertical deviation is a hypotropia, unilateral or bilateral, that results from a tight inferior rectus muscle. These patients often have concomitant excyclotorsion since the inferior rectus muscle's secondary action is to excyclotort the globe. Esotropia is by far the most common horizontal deviation in TED due to tightening of the medial rectus muscle and relative sparing of the lateral rectus muscle, its antagonist. Since the lateral rectus muscles are rarely involved, exotropia is almost never seen in TED.

## 9.2.3 Nonsurgical Management of Strabismus Associated with Thyroid Eye Disease

### Prism

Prisms bend light and can be used to move images onto the fovea of the deviated eye so that disparate images can be fused. Prisms can be grounded into spectacle lenses (▶ Fig. 9.1) or a Fresnel prism can be applied on top of a spherocylindrical lens (▶ Fig. 9.2). A Fresnel prism is a type of compact lens originally developed by French physicist Augustin-Jean Fresnel for lighthouses. The Fresnel principle states that prismatic power can be achieved by employing a concentric set of prismatic rings and in this way a Fresnel prism can be made much thinner than a comparable conventional prism. In most cases, the cost of Fresnel prisms is much lower than ground-in prisms and they are particularly effective in comitant, small-angle strabismus or for the temporary elimination of small-angle diplopia in primary position while TED patients are waiting for strabismus surgery.

Fresnel prisms, however, have some major disadvantages. They often cause degradation of visual acuity in the distance compared with traditional ground-in prisms, especially when using a prism greater than 12 prism diopters.[11] They cause increased optical aberrations, loss of contrast, and light scatter that can be intolerable to many patients, and these symptoms typically worsen when using Fresnel prisms of increasing strength. Furthermore, many patients do not like the cosmetic appearance of the lens because the grooves of the Fresnel lens are visible. Overall, Fresnel prisms can be used in select patients and in one study, only 8% of subjects continued using them once satisfactory treatment of diplopia was achieved.[12]

A more permanent prism option is the ground-in prism, in which the prism is incorporated into the spectacle lens. However, these lenses tend to be thick and relatively heavy, often causing similar optical aberrations as Fresnel prisms. Many optical shops will not grind more than a total of 6 to 10 prism diopters, making this option only good for small-angle, comitant deviations. Since the strabismus associated with TED is usually incomitant, prisms often do not work well because they create a zone of binocular vision that is too small to provide improvement in functionality.[9,10] Further, patients with TED often have variation and worsening of their strabismus, making a permanent prism a poor option, as it cannot be frequently and inexpensively changed.

### Botulinum Toxin Injection

Botulinum toxin is a lethal toxin produced by the bacterium *Clostridium botulinum*. It acts at the presynaptic terminal of the neuromuscular junction to decrease the release of acetylcholine, thereby blocking neuromuscular transmission to cause flaccid muscular paralysis for 3 to 4 months. The toxin begins to work within 1 to 3 days and has its maximum effect in 7 to 10 days.

Injection of botulinum toxin to treat strabismus, reported in 1981, is considered to be its first ever use for therapeutic purposes. A small amount of toxin is injected into the tight muscle in order to weaken its primary action. For example, in a TED patient with esotropia due to an enlarged and tight medial rectus muscle, toxin is injected into the medial rectus.

In the initial phase of TED, patients can experience discomfort with eye movements that results from restriction of ductions. They will often assume a compensatory head turn to put the eyes in a position of least deviation in order to prevent diplopia.[10,13] At this stage, botulinum toxin injection into the affected extraocular muscle can produce temporary alignment in primary position and eliminate an abnormal head turn. Several studies have demonstrated that botulinum toxin injections can improve the ocular misalignment in patients with TED resulting in improved ocular ductions and resolution of diplopia, thus avoiding the need for strabismus surgery in some cases.[13,14,15,16] The best candidates for botulinum toxin injection are patients with esotropia, relatively small-angle horizontal and vertical deviations, and those with smaller degrees of exclotorsion.[16] In addition, prisms can be effective at eliminating a small residual angle of deviation following botulinum toxin injection.

A disadvantage of using botulinum toxin for strabismus is that the effect of the toxin cannot be accurately titrated and the resulting effect is unpredictable. Thus, injections can improve the angle of deviation but may not completely eliminate the diplopia. Additionally, TED patients with strabismus often wait many months prior to being a surgical candidate in order to ensure that their misalignment is stable. Since botulinum toxin has an effect for 3 to 4 months, the monitoring period begins after the toxin has worn off, thus delaying definitive surgical treatment by many months.

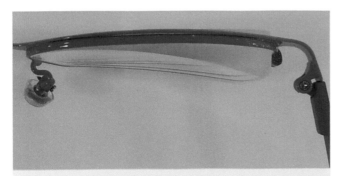

**Fig. 9.1** Prisms ground into spectacle lenses.

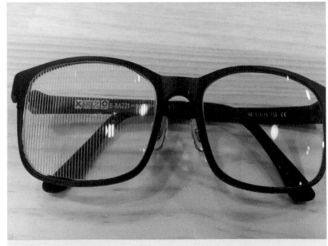

**Fig. 9.2** A Fresnel prism applied on top of a spectacle lens.

## 9.2.4 Indications for Surgical Intervention

Strabismus surgery is indicated in a patient with TED who has binocular diplopia in primary position or an abnormal head position that is adopted to minimize or eliminate diplopia. Once it is determined that there is an indication to perform surgery, the surgeon must decide on the correct timing for surgery, as it should not be carried out until the inflammatory phase has become inactive, thyroid function has normalized, and orbital decompression has been performed, if indicated.[4] Since the inflammatory phase typically lasts 12 to 18 months, it is important to document the approximate start date of the eye symptoms. Prior to performing surgery, the surgeon must make sure that strabismus measurements are stable over a period of 4 to 6 months.[4,9,10] Patients who have a prolonged clinical disease course and who are experiencing debilitating diplopia are often eager to have surgery as soon as possible and it is important to properly manage patient expectations. The surgeon should explain that despite careful surgical planning, up to 30% of patients will develop clinically significant changes in their deviation after 6 months of stable measurements.[4,17] As mentioned earlier, if orbital decompression is planned, it should occur prior to any strabismus surgery because eye misalignment will worsen in about 20% and improve in 25 to 36% of patients due to shifting of orbital contents.[18] Eyelid surgery should be delayed until after strabismus surgery because operating on the inferior rectus or superior rectus muscles may result in eyelid retraction given the proximity of the eyelid retractor muscles to the vertical rectus muscles.

## 9.2.5 Surgical Management of Strabismus Associated with Thyroid Eye Disease

### Surgical Goal

Surgical goals and realistic expectations should be defined and discussed with the patient prior to surgery. Surgery of restrictive strabismus, particularly in TED, is challenging, because a full field of binocular single vision in patients with TED is difficult to obtain due to the incomitant characteristics of the strabismus.[10,19] Therefore, the goal of strabismus surgery in TED patients should be to create a zone of binocular single vision that is as large as possible.[18,19,20,21] The practical goal should be to achieve a zone of binocular single vision in primary position at distance and near, in addition to the reading position with or without the aid of prisms.[4,9,10] It is important to make the patient understand the possibility of residual deviation and new diplopia in certain gaze directions requiring a new head turn or maneuver, and the possibility of having multiple surgeries.[10] There are many possible surgical methods to accomplish this goal including recessions of the affected extraocular muscles with or without adjustable sutures, Faden procedures, or interposition of spacers to lengthen the involved muscle.[19,21,22,23,24]

### Recessions of the Affected Extraocular Muscles with or without Adjustable Sutures

The affected extraocular muscles in patients with TED are usually tight and fibrotic. Standard surgical treatment for strabismus associated with TED is recession of the tight muscles. Resection is rarely carried out, and gaining access to the muscles can be difficult.[4] Surgery is performed under general anesthesia and an experienced assistant is recommended. A Fison retractor is helpful to expose tight muscles. When the muscle is extremely tight, it may be necessary to disinsert it using a scalpel while protecting the globe with the strabismus hook. A forced duction test should be performed in order to grade the tightness of all the muscles. The position of the muscle insertion should be measured prior to and after disinsertion.[4,10] The insertion of a very tight muscle may move up to 2 mm anteriorly after disinsertion of the muscle, and the muscle could be under-recessed if this is not recognized during surgery.[4,10]

Surgical results in strabismus associated with TED can be highly unpredictable, due to the intrinsic changes to the extraocular muscles, which may lead to variable responses to standard dose surgery, with reoperation rates reported between 17 and 45%.[25,26,27,28] The adjustable suture technique is effective in improving outcomes, as it allows more precise alignment of the eyes in the immediate postoperative period.[29] However, there is some controversy over using adjustable sutures when recessing the inferior rectus muscle. Several authors have reported late overcorrection of preoperative hypotropia using adjustable sutures in strabismus associated with TED.[25,29,30] Kerr found that nonabsorbable sutures provided an advantage in reducing late overcorrections.[31] In addition, several authors suggest targeting the postoperative deviation angle to undercorrect preoperative hypotropia in order to prevent a late overcorrection.[4,29] The aim should be to achieve binocular single vision in about 10 degrees of downgaze. This facilitates reading and walking down steps while requiring only a minimal chin-up head position for distance vision.[4,29] In addition, semi-adjustable suture techniques have been proposed to prevent late overcorrection due to muscle slippage, including in patients with TED.[32] An alternative method is to recess the inferior rectus muscle with a fixed suture while recessing the contralateral superior rectus with an adjustable suture.[4]

Recession of an inferior rectus muscle in patients with TED results in between 3 and 4 prism diopters of effect per millimeter of recession.[4,29] Large recession of an inferior rectus muscle results in limitation of depression.[10] With very large recession of the inferior rectus, the superior oblique increases its action of downgaze. Considering that the inferior rectus is an adductor and the superior oblique is an abductor, the eye abducts in downgaze, resulting in an A-pattern with incyclotorsion and diplopia occurring after a very large recession of the inferior rectus.[4,10] To prevent this phenomenon, the inferior rectus should be moved in a nasal direction by half an insertion width during surgery in order to reduce the A-pattern.[4,10] When there is no excyclotorsion in the presence of a tight inferior rectus muscle, a tight superior oblique muscle should be considered and if present, the superior oblique muscle will be

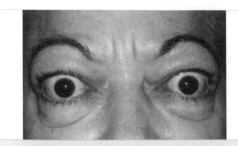

**Fig. 9.3** External photograph of patient with thyroid eye disease demonstrating retraction of bilateral upper and lower eyelids.

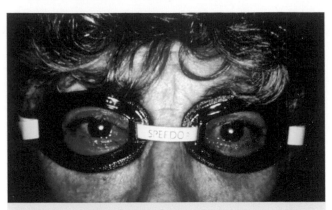

**Fig. 9.4** External photograph of patient with exposure keratopathy due to thyroid eye disease. She elects to wear swimming goggles when she goes outdoors to protect the eyes and maintain a moist ocular surface. Notice the conjunctival injection medially and inferolaterally and the presence of a glistening coat of lubricating ointment on the ocular surface and eyelashes.

tight during the traction test after disinsertion of the interior rectus muscle and should be recessed as well[4,10,33,34]

Large muscle recessions may need to be accompanied by additional conjunctival recession to avoid postoperative restriction through conjunctival tethering. To prevent this, the forced duction test should be performed not only prior to surgery, but also after conjunctival suturing.[10] In addition, close attention should be paid when dissecting Tenon's capsule, particularly around the inferior rectus muscle, because the possibility of a slipped muscle after large recession is somewhat high, partly due to its short arc of contact with the globe and the presence of Tenon's capsule, which may predispose to nonadhesion to the sclera.[4,10]

In summary, strabismus surgery, particularly with the adjustable suture technique, can be highly effective in patients with strabismus due to TED. Correcting restrictive strabismus caused by TED is challenging, because routine surgical dosing tables do not seem to be as effective in cases of strabismus due to TED.[21] The adjustable suture technique is effective in improving outcomes, as it allows more precise alignment of the eyes in the immediate postoperative period[21,29] However, the adjustable technique cannot prevent late overcorrection after inferior rectus recession in patients with strabismus due to TED. Therefore, some authors suggest that adjustment of these patients to undercorrection of at least 2 prism diopters to compensate for postoperative overcorrection after inferior rectus recession.[29] Most patients are very grateful to have their most disabling problem related to TED resolved or improved as much as possible.

# 9.3 Management of Eyelid Malposition Associated with Thyroid Eye Disease

## 9.3.1 Eyelid Retraction

Eyelid retraction is the most common sign of TED and is found in 70% of upper eyelids and 20% of lower eyelids of patients recently diagnosed with TED.[35] Studies suggest that the levator palpebrae superioris muscle is the most commonly involved extraocular muscle in thyroid orbitopathy.[36,37] The exact mechanism of upper eyelid retraction is poorly understood, but is thought to be the result of levator inflammation acutely, which is followed later by fibrosis. Müller's muscle has also been implicated in upper eyelid retraction as a result of sympathetic

stimulation during the acute phase of TED and by enlargement and fibrosis in the chronic phase.[38] Lower eyelid retraction has been postulated to be a result of either proptosis or lamellar shortening from retractor muscle inflammation and fibrosis. Studies measuring inferior fornix depth and analyzing postsurgical decompression data have suggested that proptosis is likely the primary cause of lower eyelid retraction.[39,40]

Eyelid retraction may result in symptoms related to dryness such as pain, foreign body sensation, and epiphora, and contact lenses may become intolerable. Other autoimmune mechanisms directly affecting the ocular surface have also been implicated as a cause of these symptoms.[41] Eyelid retraction is often cosmetically troublesome to patients, resulting in poor self-esteem, depression, and avoidance of social situations (▶ Fig. 9.3).[42]

First-line therapy for eyelid retraction is conservative, nonsurgical management involving improvement of ocular surface lubrication. Placement of fluorescein ophthalmic solution on the corneas and viewing with a cobalt blue filtered light via slit-lamp biomicroscopy is useful in assessing corneal dryness and pathology. Preservative-free artificial teardrops, gels, and ointments should be used frequently and routinely throughout the day. Many patients with eyelid retraction have poor eyelid closure (lagophthalmos), and it is important in these cases to tape the eyelids closed at night, being careful to avoid tape abrading the corneas, or wear a moisture chamber device or goggles (▶ Fig. 9.4). However, some patients will remain uncomfortable despite this therapy and will have more significant ocular surface issues requiring more aggressive management.

## 9.3.2 Minimally Invasive Treatment of Upper Eyelid Retraction

Several minimally invasive methods of improving upper eyelid retraction may be considered, including the injection of botulinum toxin, hyaluronic acid gel filler, or corticosteroid into the involved muscles. Injection of botulinum toxin into the levator muscle just above the superior tarsus may be performed either transcutaneously or transconjunctivally. Botulinum toxin works by binding to presynaptic nerve terminals and blocking the release of acetylcholine. This provides 3 to 4 months of improvement in eyelid retraction and may be useful during either the active or chronic stage of disease. The disadvantages of this procedure are the inability to precisely titrate the effect, which may result in undesired ptosis or diplopia because of inadvertent spread of toxin to extraocular muscles.[43,44,45,46,47,48]

Hyaluronic acid (HA) gels are commonly used today as cosmetic fillers. Their efficacy is temporary, lasting about 3 to 6 months, and there are ever-expanding uses for these products. Injection of approximately 0.5 mL of HA filler above the tarsus in the plane of the levator muscle will result in lowering of a retracted upper eyelid.[49] The effect may be slightly more controllable than with botulinum toxin injection, although ultrasonic imaging has demonstrated that there is migration of the gel around the area of injection. A disadvantage of both botulinum toxin and HA filler is the high cost of the product and difficulty with obtaining insurance coverage. Also, both botulinum toxin and HA filler have a temporary effect and will likely need to be repeated during the course of the disease. This indication is off-label use of both of these products.

Injection of corticosteroid, such as triamcinolone, has been reported to be effective in the treatment of upper eyelid retraction, and several studies have touted its efficacy when injected into the subconjunctival space at the superior aspect of the tarsus during the acute phase of the disease. Injections are performed at regular intervals several weeks apart until the desired eyelid height is reached. Several injections are usually required and this procedure is not thought to be effective in the chronic, fibrotic stage of disease.[50,51,52] Injection of particulate material such as steroid in the periorbital area poses a risk for elevated intraocular pressure as well as sight-threatening embolic intraocular events.

## 9.3.3 Surgical Management of Upper Eyelid Retraction

The mainstay of surgical treatment of upper eyelid retraction is recession of the levator palpebrae superioris or Müller's muscle or both via either an internal transconjunctival or an external transcutaneous approach. Multiple descriptions of variations on these procedures date back to the 1980s.[53,54,55] There are advantages and disadvantages to both approaches. Both approaches allow for disinsertion and recession of the levator aponeurosis and Müller's muscle in a graded fashion. Internal transconjunctival surgery has the advantage of leaving no cutaneous scar; however, there is less ability to place sutures to control contour or fix overcorrection. External surgery may result in a longer recovery period because of the cutaneous incision; however, there is the potential for finer control intraoperatively by placement of sutures to adjust lid contour and height. The external full-thickness blepharotomy described by Elner et al has been a mainstay procedure for many surgeons. The eyelid is incised at the crease and dissection is carried in a graded fashion at the superior border of the tarsus through the levator aponeurosis, Müller's muscle, and conjunctiva until the desired eyelid lowering is achieved (▶ Fig. 9.5).[56] An additional advantage of the external approach is the option to perform concurrent blepharoplasty with fat debulking via the same incision.

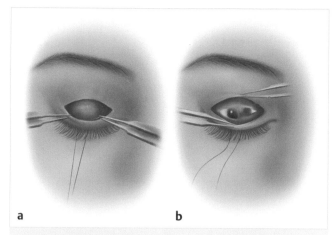

**Fig. 9.5** Repair of upper eyelid retraction via full-thickness blepharotomy. (**a**) The skin is incised along the eyelid crease and dissection is performed in a graded fashion through the levator aponeurosis, Müllers' muscle, and conjunctiva until the lid is lowered to the desired height. (**b**) A small band of conjunctiva may be left in place in order to preserve the eyelid contour.

These procedures, whether performed internally or externally, are often fraught with frustration, as the lid has a tendency to shift position during the postoperative weeks to months. Success rates have been reported as high as 86.5%,[57] while reoperation rates are reported from 8 to 23%.[58] The lid usually creeps upward over time, but in some cases may fall; hence, slight overcorrection at the time of surgery may be desirable. Also, timing surgery when eyelid position and thyroid serology levels have been stable for many months may result in a more stable postsurgical result. Several authors have reported variations on traditional upper eyelid recession techniques, in an effort to improve predictability of postsurgical eyelid height, including use of adjustable sutures,[59,60] transposition of the lateral horn of the levator,[61] use of spacer grafts including reflected orbital septum,[62] and preservation of a strut of conjunctiva and retractors in the medial aspect of the lid.[63]

## 9.3.4 Surgical Management of Lower Eyelid Retraction

Repair of lower eyelid retraction in TED can be equally challenging, as the negative vector anatomy, with the eye more prominent than the cheek, creates a need for the lid to be moved not only upward, but also outward to cover the inferior globe (▶ Fig. 9.6). Surgical correction of proptosis with orbital decompression is often helpful in reducing lower eyelid retraction.[64] If this is not desired or feasible, then surgery may be directed toward the lower eyelid. The basic principle is to release the lower eyelid retractor muscles to allow the lid to move upward. However, given the natural tendency of wound healing and the effect of gravity, the lid is at risk of returning to its presurgical position. An effective method of preventing this involves placement of a graft between the inferior tarsal border and the disinserted retractor muscles on the conjunctival side of the eyelid. A number of materials have been proposed, dating back to the 1980s, including polytetrafluoroethylene (PTFE), Mersilene

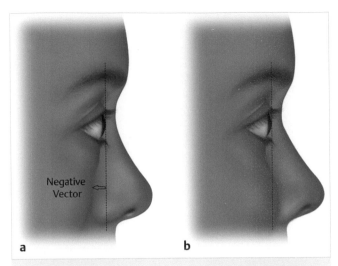

**Fig. 9.6** "Negative vector" anatomy. **(a)** In negative vector midface anatomy, the globe is more prominent than the cheek. This can result in challenges when attempting to surgically elevate the lower eyelid, as the desired vector of eyelid movement is not only upward, but also upward and anterior to cover the globe. **(b)** Comparison with a normal midface to globe anatomy where the cheek is more prominent than the eye.

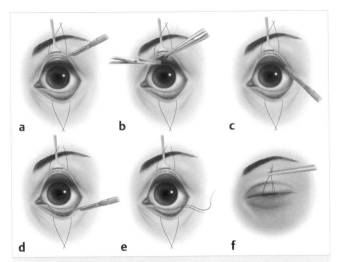

**Fig. 9.7** Surgical technique for simultaneous repair of upper and lower eyelid retraction. **(a)** After placement of silk traction sutures, the upper eyelid is everted and an incision is made through the full thickness of the tarsus 4 to 5 mm above the inferior margin of the tarsus. **(b)** The tarsus with attached conjunctiva is harvested above this incision line to be used as the lower eyelid posterior spacer graft. **(c)** In a graded fashion, the levator and Müller's muscle are incised via the upper lid tarsus donor site in order to recess the upper eyelid. **(d)** An incision is made in the lower eyelid through conjunctiva and lower eyelid retractors at the base of the tarsus along the length of the eyelid to create a recipient bed for the spacer graft. **(e)** The tarsal graft is placed into the recipient bed in the lower lid with the conjunctival side against the globe. It is sutured into position with 6–0 plain gut running suture. **(f)** The silk traction sutures in the upper and lower eyelids are tied together as a temporary tarsorrhaphy.

mesh, donor sclera, hard palate mucosa, donor tarsus, ear or nasal cartilage, porous polyethylene, synthetic bioengineered tarsus, autologous dermis, porcine acellular dermal matrix, and autologous tarsus.[65,66,67,68,69,70,71,72,73,74] Some of these donor and synthetic materials have been noted to cause chronic inflammation and result in fibrous capsule formation, extrusion, and other complications. Most of the donor grafts melt over time, resulting in recurrence of eyelid retraction.[75] Therefore, the ideal posterior spacer graft is composed of autologous tissue. Cartilage and hard palate grafts are options, but may not be comfortable because of stiffness or production of secretions that are not native to the ocular surface. Autologous tarsus is a fantastic graft choice for this indication, as it is flexible and comfortable against the globe, and will not shrink over time, providing lasting structural support to the lower eyelid.

## 9.3.5 Surgical Technique for Simultaneous Repair of Upper and Lower Eyelid Retraction

A highly effective technique for repair of ipsilateral upper and lower eyelid retraction is a simultaneous procedure incorporating internal upper eyelid recession and placement of an autologous tarsus posterior spacer graft into the lower eyelid. It is quick and easy to perform, provides a durable result, and is minimally invasive, requiring no cutaneous incisions (▶ Fig. 9.7). The procedure begins with injection of local anesthetic into the upper and lower eyelids and placement of a corneal protective cover. A 4–0 silk traction suture is placed in the margin of the upper and lower eyelids centrally. The upper eyelid is everted and a caliper is used to make a curvilinear mark 4 mm above the inferior tarsal border along the length of the tarsus. The tarsus is incised with a no. 15 blade and the tarsus

and conjunctiva is harvested from above this incision, taking care to dissect the levator muscle attachments from the anterior surface of the tarsus. This is the maximum amount of tarsus that can be safely harvested in order to protect the upper eyelid from horizontal tarsal kink, and less can be used as dictated by severity of lower eyelid retraction. The free tarsoconjunctival graft is placed in saline-soaked gauze until later in the procedure. Next, the upper lid is recessed via the donor site. A Desmarres retractor is used to evert the upper eyelid and Westcott scissors are used to make sequential incisions in the levator aponeurosis and Müller's muscle in a graded fashion along the horizontal length of the eyelid. The lid is reverted back to normal position and the corneal protective cover is removed to assess the eyelid height. This graded recession is repeated until the upper lid is at the desired height and contour. Next, the lower lid is everted using the traction suture and a blade or sharp Westcott scissors are used to incise the conjunctiva and retractors at the inferior tarsal border. The retractors are recessed and a recipient bed is created for the tarsoconjunctival graft. The graft is sutured into position using a running 6–0 plain gut suture. Care is taken to bury the knot to avoid corneal abrasion. The traction sutures in the lid margins are left in place at the end of the procedure and are tied together in a square knot as a temporary tarsorrhaphy. Ophthalmic antibiotic ointment and a patch are placed over the eye for 3 to 5 days (▶ Fig. 9.8).

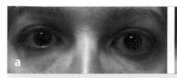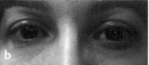

**Fig. 9.8 (a)** Preoperative external photograph of a woman with thyroid eye disease with retraction of the left upper and lower eyelids and mild retraction of the right upper eyelid. **(b)** Postoperative external photograph of the same woman status post internal recession of both upper eyelids and internal recession of the left lower eyelid with placement of a posterior spacer tarsus graft harvested from the left upper eyelid.

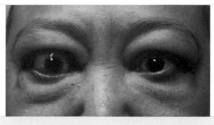

**Fig. 9.9** Lateral tarsorrhaphy. This external photograph demonstrates a left permanent lateral tarsorrhaphy that has been placed in this patient with acute thyroid eye disease resulting in eyelid retraction with severe corneal exposure and ulceration.

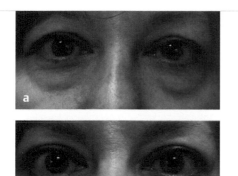

**Fig. 9.10 (a)** Preoperative external photograph of a woman with thyroid eye disease with steatoblepharon of both lower eyelids. **(b)** Postoperative photograph of the same patient after transconjunctival bilateral lower blepharoplasty with debulking of fat pads. Although she has mild eyelid retraction, she is pleased with the cosmetic outcome.

## 9.4 Permanent Lateral Tarsorrhaphy for Eyelid Retraction Repair

Creation of a small permanent lateral tarsorrhaphy can be quite effective in decreasing the exposed ocular surface area in patients with proptosis and eyelid retraction. This procedure can easily be performed in an office or bedside setting with a small injection of local anesthetic. The anterior and posterior lamellae of the eyelid are split along the gray line with a no. 11 blade and polyglycolic acid suture is used to oppose the raw tarsal edges. Then the skin edges are closed with the same suture (▶ Fig. 9.9). Lateral tarsorrhaphy is not as aesthetically desirable as posterior spacer graft recession surgery, but can be very effective in select patients.

## 9.5 Upper and Lower Blepharoplasties in Thyroid Eye Disease

Upper and lower blepharoplasties are often requested by patients suffering from TED because of orbital and eyelid fat

hypertrophy and prolapse resulting in undesirable cosmesis. These procedures can be safely performed in patients with TED, keeping in mind several considerations. Patients should be in the stable phase of disease prior to undertaking this procedure, as fat prolapse may recur if there is active inflammation. Upper lid blepharoplasty should involve conservative skin removal, since excess skin excision can result in postoperative lagophthalmos, which can be particularly problematic in patients who have proptosis and keratopathy at baseline. Preaponeurotic and nasal fat pads can be debulked for improved eyelid appearance. Brow/retro-orbicularis oculi fat (ROOF) should not be debulked, as this can result in a dimpled skin texture and drooping of the deflated brows. Consideration can be given to injection of hypertrophic ROOF fat with corticosteroid, which after one or several treatments may result in a decrease in fat volume. Lower blepharoplasty should be performed cautiously with attention to preventing increased eyelid retraction. External lower blepharoplasty with skin excision can significantly worsen lid retraction in these patients. An internal approach with careful fat removal is likely safer in this regard (▶ Fig. 9.10); however, excessive fat removal even from an internal approach may result in eyelid deflation and retraction.

## References

[1] Yeatts RP. Quality of life in patients with Graves ophthalmopathy. Trans Am Ophthalmol Soc. 2005; 103:368–411
[2] Coulter I, Frewin S, Krassas GE, Perros P. Psychological implications of Graves' orbitopathy. Eur J Endocrinol. 2007; 157(2):127–131
[3] Eckstein AK, Johnson KT, Thanos M, Esser J, Ludgate M. Current insights into the pathogenesis of Graves' orbitopathy. Horm Metab Res. 2009; 41(6):456–464
[4] Harrad R. Management of strabismus in thyroid eye disease. Eye (Lond). 2015; 29(2):234–237
[5] Asman P. Ophthalmological evaluation in thyroid-associated ophthalmopathy. Acta Ophthalmol Scand. 2003; 81(5):437–448
[6] de Waard R, Koornneef L, Verbeeten B, Jr. Motility disturbances in Graves' ophthalmopathy. Doc Ophthalmol. 1983; 56(1–2):41–47
[7] Kendler DL, Lippa J, Rootman J. The initial clinical characteristics of Graves' orbitopathy vary with age and sex. Arch Ophthalmol. 1993; 111(2):197–201
[8] Dyer JA. The oculorotary muscles in Graves' disease. Trans Am Ophthalmol Soc. 1976; 74:425–456
[9] Nardi M. Squint surgery in TED: hints and fints, or why Graves' patients are difficult patients. Orbit. 2009; 28(4):245–250
[10] Al Qahtani ES, Rootman J, Kersey J, Godoy F, Lyons CJ. Clinical pearls and management recommendations for strabismus due to thyroid orbitopathy. Middle East Afr J Ophthalmol. 2015; 22(3):307–311
[11] Véronneau-Troutman S. Fresnel prisms and their effects on visual acuity and binocularity. Trans Am Ophthalmol Soc. 1978; 76:610–653

[12] Tamhankar MA, Ying GS, Volpe NJ. Effectiveness of prisms in the management of diplopia in patients due to diverse etiologies. J Pediatr Ophthalmol Strabismus. 2012; 49(4):222–228

[13] Lyons CJ, Vickers SF, Lee JP. Botulinum toxin therapy in dysthyroid strabismus. Eye (Lond). 1990; 4(Pt 4):538–542

[14] Kikkawa DO, Cruz RC, Jr, Christian WK, et al. Botulinum A toxin injection for restrictive myopathy of thyroid-related orbitopathy: effects on intraocular pressure. Am J Ophthalmol. 2003; 135(4):427–431

[15] Scott AB. Botulinum toxin injection into extraocular muscles as an alternative to strabismus surgery. Ophthalmology. 1980; 87(10):1044–1049

[16] Akbari MR, Ameri A, Keshtkar Jaafari AR, Mirmohammadsadeghi A. Botulinum toxin injection for restrictive myopathy of thyroid-associated orbitopathy: success rate and predictive factors. J AAPOS. 2016; 20(2):126–130.e1

[17] Lee YH, Oh SY, Hwang JM. Is 6 months of stable angle of strabismus enough to perform surgery in patients with strabismus related to thyroid ophthalmopathy? Br J Ophthalmol. 2010; 94(7):955–956

[18] Finn AP, Bleier B, Cestari DM, et al. A retrospective review of orbital decompression for thyroid orbitopathy with endoscopic preservation of the inferomedial orbital bone strut. Ophthal Plast Reconstr Surg. 2017; 33(5):334–33

[19] Jellema HM, Braaksma-Besselink Y, Limpens J, von Arx G, Wiersinga WM, Mourits MP. Proposal of success criteria for strabismus surgery in patients with Graves' orbitopathy based on a systematic literature review. Acta Ophthalmol. 2015; 93(7):601–609

[20] Dagi LR, Elliott AT, Roper-Hall G, Cruz OA. Thyroid eye disease: honing your skills to improve outcomes. J AAPOS. 2010; 14(5):425–431

[21] Volpe NJ, Mirza-George N, Binenbaum G. Surgical management of vertical ocular misalignment in thyroid eye disease using an adjustable suture technique. J AAPOS. 2012; 16(6):518–522

[22] Yoo SH, Pineles SL, Goldberg RA, Velez FG. Rectus muscle resection in Graves' ophthalmopathy. J AAPOS. 2013; 17(1):9–15

[23] Schittkowski M, Fichter N, Guthoff R. Strabismus surgery in Grave's disease: dose-effect relationships and functional results. Klin Monatsbl Augenheilkd. 2004; 221(11):941–947

[24] Esser J, Schittkowski M, Eckstein A. Graves' orbitopathy: inferior rectus tendon elongation for large vertical squint angles that cannot be corrected by simple muscle recession. Klin Monatsbl Augenheilkd. 2011; 228(10):880–886

[25] Scott WE, Thalacker JA. Diagnosis and treatment of thyroid myopathy. Ophthalmology. 1981; 88(6):493–498

[26] Nguyen VT, Park DJJ, Levin L, Feldon SE. Correction of restricted extraocular muscle motility in surgical management of strabismus in graves' ophthalmology. Ophthalmology. 2002; 109(2):384–388

[27] Prendiville P, Chopra M, Gauderman WJ, Feldon SE. The role of restricted motility in determining outcomes for vertical strabismus surgery in Graves' ophthalmology. Ophthalmology. 2000; 107(3):545–549

[28] Evans D, Kennerdell JS. Extraocular muscle surgery for dysthyroid myopathy. Am J Ophthalmol. 1983; 95(6):767–771

[29] Peragallo JH, Velez FG, Demer JL, Pineles SL. Postoperative drift in patients with thyroid ophthalmopathy undergoing unilateral inferior rectus muscle recession. Strabismus. 2013; 21(1):23–28

[30] Sprunger DT, Helveston EM. Progressive overcorrection after inferior rectus recession. J Pediatr Ophthalmol Strabismus. 1993; 30(3):145–148

[31] Kerr NC. The role of thyroid eye disease and other factors in the overcorrection of hypotropia following unilateral adjustable suture recession of the inferior rectus (an American Ophthalmological Society thesis). Trans Am Ophthalmol Soc. 2011; 109:168–200

[32] Kushner BJ. An evaluation of the semiadjustable suture strabismus surgical procedure. J AAPOS. 2004; 8(5):481–487

[33] Thacker NM, Velez FG, Demer JL, Rosenbaum AL. Superior oblique muscle involvement in thyroid ophthalmopathy. J AAPOS. 2005; 9(2):174–178

[34] Holmes JM, Hatt SR, Bradley EA. Identifying masked superior oblique involvement in thyroid eye disease to avoid postoperative A-pattern exotropia and intorsion. J AAPOS. 2012; 16(3):280–285

[35] Bartley GB, Fatourechi V, Kadrmas EF, et al. Chronology of Graves' ophthalmopathy in an incidence cohort. Am J Ophthalmol. 1996; 121(4):426–434

[36] Davies MJ, Dolman PJ. Levator muscle enlargement in thyroid eye disease-related upper eyelid retraction. Ophthal Plast Reconstr Surg. 2017; 33(1):35–39

[37] Ohnishi T, Noguchi S, Murakami N, et al. Levator palpebrae superioris muscle: MR evaluation of enlargement as a cause of upper eyelid retraction in Graves disease. Radiology. 1993; 188(1):115–118

[38] Cockerham KP, Hidayat AA, Brown HG, Cockerham GC, Graner SR. Clinicopathologic evaluation of the Mueller muscle in thyroid-associated orbitopathy. Ophthal Plast Reconstr Surg. 2002; 18(1):11–17

[39] Rootman DB, Golan S, Pavlovich P, Rootman J. Postoperative changes in strabismus, ductions, exophthalmometry, and eyelid retraction after orbital decompression for thyroid orbitopathy. Ophthal Plast Reconstr Surg. 2017; 33(4):289–293

[40] Rajabi MT, Jafari H, Mazloumi M, et al. Lower lid retraction in thyroid orbitopathy: lamellar shortening or proptosis? Int Ophthalmol. 2014; 34(4):801–804

[41] Versura P, Campos EC. The ocular surface in thyroid diseases. Curr Opin Allergy Clin Immunol. 2010; 10(5):486–492

[42] Wickwar S, McBain H, Ezra DG, Hirani SP, Rose GE, Newman SP. The psychosocial and clinical outcomes of orbital decompression surgery for thyroid eye disease and predictors of change in quality of life. Ophthalmology. 2015; 122(12):2568–76.e1

[43] Biglan AW. Control of eyelid retraction associated with Graves' disease with botulinum A toxin. Ophthalmic Surg. 1994; 25(3):186–188

[44] Uddin JM, Davies PD. Treatment of upper eyelid retraction associated with thyroid eye disease with subconjunctival botulinum toxin injection. Ophthalmology. 2002; 109(6):1183–1187

[45] Shih MJ, Liao SL, Lu HY. A single transcutaneous injection with Botox for dysthyroid lid retraction. Eye (Lond). 2004; 18(5):466–469

[46] Morgenstern KE, Evanchan J, Foster JA, et al. Botulinum toxin type a for dysthyroid upper eyelid retraction. Ophthal Plast Reconstr Surg. 2004; 20(3):181–185

[47] Costa PG, Saraiva FP, Pereira IC, Monteiro ML, Matayoshi S. Comparative study of Botox injection treatment for upper eyelid retraction with 6-month follow-up in patients with thyroid eye disease in the congestive or fibrotic stage. Eye (Lond). 2009; 23(4):767–773

[48] Salour H, Bagheri B, Aletaha M, et al. Transcutaneous dysport injection for treatment of upper eyelid retraction associated with thyroid eye disease. Orbit. 2010; 29(2):114–118

[49] Kohn JC, Rootman DB, Liu W, Goh AS, Hwang CJ, Goldberg RA. Hyaluronic acid gel injection for upper eyelid retraction in thyroid eye disease: functional and dynamic high-resolution ultrasound evaluation. Ophthal Plast Reconstr Surg. 2014; 30(5):400–404

[50] Lee JM, Lee H, Park M, Baek S. Subconjunctival injection of triamcinolone for the treatment of upper lid retraction associated with thyroid eye disease. J Craniofac Surg. 2012; 23(6):1755–1758

[51] Lee SJ, Rim TH, Jang SY, et al. Treatment of upper eyelid retraction related to thyroid-associated ophthalmopathy using subconjunctival triamcinolone injections. Graefes Arch Clin Exp Ophthalmol. 2013; 251(1):261–270

[52] Chee E, Chee SP. Subconjunctival injection of triamcinolone in the treatment of lid retraction of patients with thyroid eye disease: a case series. Eye (Lond). 2008; 22(2):311–315

[53] Putterman AM, Fett DR. Müller's muscle in the treatment of upper eyelid retraction: a 12-year study. Ophthalmic Surg. 1986; 17(6):361–367

[54] Small RG. Surgery for upper eyelid retraction, three techniques. Trans Am Ophthalmol Soc. 1995; 93:353–365, discussion 365–369

[55] Ben Simon GJ, Mansury AM, Schwarcz RM, Modjtahedi S, McCann JD, Goldberg RA. Transconjunctival Müller muscle recession with levator disinsertion for correction of eyelid retraction associated with thyroid-related orbitopathy. Am J Ophthalmol. 2005; 140(1):94–99

[56] Elner VM, Hassan AS, Frueh BR. Graded full-thickness anterior blepharotomy for upper eyelid retraction. Arch Ophthalmol. 2004; 122(1):55–60

[57] Shortt AJ, Bhogal M, Rose GE, Shah-Desai S. Stability of eyelid height after graded anterior-approach lid lowering for dysthyroid upper lid retraction. Orbit. 2011; 30(6):280–288

[58] Golan S, Rootman DB, Goldberg RA. The success rate of TED upper eyelid retraction reoperations. Orbit. 2016; 35(6):335–338

[59] Ueland HO, Uchermann A, Rødahl E. Levator recession with adjustable sutures for correction of upper eyelid retraction in thyroid eye disease. Acta Ophthalmol. 2014; 92(8):793–797

[60] Tucker SM, Collin R. Repair of upper eyelid retraction: a comparison between adjustable and non-adjustable sutures. Br J Ophthalmol. 1995; 79(7):658–660

[61] Ceisler EJ, Bilyk JR, Rubin PA, Burks WR, Shore JW. Results of Müllerotomy and levator aponeurosis transposition for the correction of upper eyelid retraction in Graves disease. Ophthalmology. 1995; 102(3):483–492

[62] Watanabe A, Shams PN, Katori N, Kinoshita S, Selva D. Turn-over orbital septal flap and levator recession for upper-eyelid retraction secondary to thyroid eye disease. Eye (Lond). 2013; 27(10):1174–1179

[63] Nimitwongsakul A, Zoumalan CI, Kazim M. Modified full-thickness blepharotomy for treatment of thyroid eye disease. Ophthal Plast Reconstr Surg. 2013; 29(1):44–47

[64] Cho RI, Elner VM, Nelson CC, Frueh BR. The effect of orbital decompression surgery on lid retraction in thyroid eye disease. Ophthal Plast Reconstr Surg. 2011; 27(6):436–438

[65] Olver JM, Rose GE, Khaw PT, Collin JR. Correction of lower eyelid retraction in thyroid eye disease: a randomised controlled trial of retractor tenotomy with adjuvant antimetabolite versus scleral graft. Br J Ophthalmol. 1998; 82(2): 174–180

[66] Ribeiro SF, Shekhovtsova M, Duarte AF, Velasco Cruz AA. Graves lower eyelid retraction. Ophthal Plast Reconstr Surg. 2016; 32(3):161–169

[67] Dailey RA, Marx DP, Ahn ES. Porcine dermal collagen in lower eyelid retraction repair. Ophthal Plast Reconstr Surg. 2015; 31(3):233–241

[68] Oestreicher JH, Pang NK, Liao W. Treatment of lower eyelid retraction by retractor release and posterior lamellar grafting: an analysis of 659 eyelids in 400 patients. Ophthal Plast Reconstr Surg. 2008; 24(3):207–212

[69] Feldman KA, Putterman AM, Farber MD. Surgical treatment of thyroid-related lower eyelid retraction: a modified approach. Ophthal Plast Reconstr Surg. 1992; 8(4):278–286

[70] Cohen MS, Shorr N. Eyelid reconstruction with hard palate mucosa grafts. Ophthal Plast Reconstr Surg. 1992; 8(3):183–195

[71] Mourits MP, Koornneef L. Lid lengthening by sclera interposition for eyelid retraction in Graves' ophthalmopathy. Br J Ophthalmol. 1991; 75(6):344–347

[72] Karesh JW, Fabrega MA, Rodrigues MM, Glaros DS. Polytetrafluoroethylene as an interpositional graft material for the correction of lower eyelid retraction. Ophthalmology. 1989; 96(4):419–423

[73] Downes RN, Jordan K. The surgical management of dysthyroid related eyelid retraction using Mersilene mesh. Eye (Lond). 1989; 3(Pt 4):385–390

[74] Gardner TA, Kennerdell JS, Buerger GF. Treatment of dysthyroid lower lid retraction with autogenous tarsus transplants. Ophthal Plast Reconstr Surg. 1992; 8(1):26–31

[75] Sullivan SA, Dailey RA. Graft contraction: a comparison of acellular dermis versus hard palate mucosa in lower eyelid surgery. Ophthal Plast Reconstr Surg. 2003; 19(1):14–24

# 10 Orbital Trauma Management, Reconstruction, and External Approaches to the Orbit

*Daniel R. Lefebvre*

**Abstract**

Orbital trauma and reconstruction involves careful evaluation and management of critical soft-tissue structures and complex bony anatomy. The consequences of incorrect or unsafe management can include disfiguring cosmesis, pain, intracranial injury, double vision, and even blindness. When the bony orbit is accessed via endonasal endoscopic surgery, an orbital "fracture" is essentially created as the access route into the orbit. In many cases, formal reconstruction may not be necessary, but as access window size increases, the potential need for reconstruction increases. This chapter reviews the concepts and basis for orbital reconstruction in the setting of traumatic orbital blowout fractures to serve as a basis for consideration of reconstruction in the setting of endonasal endoscopic orbital surgery.

*Keywords:* orbital trauma, orbital blowout fracture, white-eyed blowout fracture, orbital reconstruction, orbital compartment syndrome, canthotomy/cantholysis

## 10.1 Introduction

While the orbit itself occupies a proportionally small fraction of volume of the whole human body (30-mL average total volume), it is densely packed with complex and vital anatomy—namely, the eye, optic nerve with its dural sheath contiguous with the intracranial space, ocular motor nerves and muscles, various sensory nerves, arteries (from the carotid siphon), and veins (draining to the cavernous sinus). The orbital shape is cone-like, but actually much more complex than a simple cone. The orbital walls are a combination of concavities and convexities and angulations, foramina, and fissures, and these are all important to the status of the eye in terms of its position and alignment, which have both cosmetic and functional implications. Nonetheless, the orbit can sustain a moderate amount of traumatic disruption and can heal functionally and cosmetically quite well without surgical reconstruction.[1] Despite this, when surgical reconstruction of the orbit is indicated, it must be done safely and accurately to restore the normal orbital anatomy; otherwise, the surgery itself may be responsible for a host of functional and cosmetic adverse outcomes such as enophthalmos, strabismus, eyelid retraction, and even blindness.

The orbital surgeon most frequently encounters disruption of the orbital walls in the setting of trauma. Indirect orbital "blowout" fractures involve the orbital floor, medial orbital wall, or both, and generally occur from a blunt force applied to the eye area, such as a punch by a fist or a hit from a baseball, without disruption of the orbital rim. The disruption of the internal orbital wall can range from essentially nondisplaced with very little anatomical consequence to the orbit and nondisplaced but with entrapment of orbital tissue (a so-called trapdoor fracture) to moderately displaced with herniation of orbital contents possibly causing a measureable change in orbital volume and function and large fractures with significant change to the orbital volume and function.

In endonasal endo-orbital surgery, the orbit is accessed via the medial orbital wall, orbital floor, and sometimes both. Depending on the size of the bony window created, reconstruction may be appropriate; the precise indications for reconstruction in this setting are still being elucidated. In general, the larger the orbital disruption, the more likely a reconstruction would be appropriate. In a review of 23 cases of endonasal removal of orbital cavernous hemangiomas, lesions that were intraconal in location more commonly required a binaural approach with an associated larger bone window to the orbit compared to extraconal lesions, with intraconal lesions accounting for all cases (6 out of 16) in which the orbit was reconstructed.[2] The purpose of this chapter is to review the evaluation and management of orbital disruption vis-à-vis orbital blowout fractures, which can then serve as a basis for the evaluation and implementation of orbital reconstruction in association with endonasal orbital procedures. The surgical approaches described can also be used for enhanced access during combined endoscopic/external orbital surgery.

## 10.2 Diagnostic Workup for the Orbital Blowout Fracture Patient

In cases in which there is an isolated orbital blowout fracture (i.e., the orbital rims are intact), the leading theory for the mechanism of injury is that the eye itself has been retropulsed into the orbit by blunt force trauma and as a result the hydrostatic pressure within the orbit has increased substantially to a threshold point at which the orbital wall (usually the floor and less commonly the medial wall) "blows out" into the adjacent paranasal sinus to relieve this pressure.[3] It has been presumed that this fracture serves as a safety-valve mechanism to relieve the pressure on the eye before the eyeball itself ruptures, and indeed it is rare in practice to see an open globe injury in association with a pure orbital blowout fracture resulting from blunt trauma. Eye injuries do occur in association with approximately one-third of orbital blowout fractures and can include corneal abrasion, traumatic iritis, microhyphema and hyphema (blood in the anterior chamber of the eye), traumatic iris tears/mydriasis, commotio retinae (bruising of the retina), retinal tear or detachment, traumatic optic neuropathy, orbital hemorrhage, and orbital emphysema.[4] Soft-tissue injuries may also occur, such as a laceration of the lacrimal canaliculus of the eyelid that may occur from a lateral shear force applied to the lid during blunt trauma. If an extraocular muscle is entrapped (or even tethered by adjacent orbital tissue) within the fracture site, the oculocardiac reflex may occur, which can lead to potentially life-threatening bradycardia and even asystole.[5] Thus, all orbital trauma patients should have a full trauma assessment including evaluation for other injuries and monitoring of vital signs. Because identification of the associated ocular injuries referenced above requires specialized equipment and techniques, a full eye examination with an ophthalmologist is advisable, who should perform slit-lamp biomicroscopy and dilated fundus examination. Visual acuity can be measured one eye at a time with a vision checking card by anyone in the health care team, along with assessment of pupils (looking for direct and consensual responses as well as assessing for an afferent pupillary defect), and gross assessment of ocular motility by having the patient follow the examiner's finger in a wide circle. Any significant dysmotility could be a clue to an underlying orbital fracture. Other signs suggesting an orbital fracture would be frank misalignment of the eye such as strabismus or hypoglobus, relative enophthalmos (although this is often masked by the associated orbital edema in the acute setting), or hypesthesia of the cheek or lip. A laceration medial to the lacrimal punctum should raise suspicion for a canalicular laceration. A periorbital laceration with fat present within the wound indicates the orbital septum and orbit proper have been violated, and one should consider the possibility of intraorbital injury (muscle, nerve, globe) or a retained intraorbital foreign body.

If the orbit is quite tense and firm such that the lids are not able to be readily opened and the globe is under obvious pressure, there is an orbital compartment syndrome. This is an emergency and requires timely release of the orbital pressure, which is usually accomplished via a lateral canthotomy and inferior cantholysis in an effort to avoid central retinal artery occlusion or optic nerve ischemia, which can be catastrophic after 60 to 90 minutes. This technique will be described later in this chapter as part of the swinging eyelid transconjunctival approach.

If the eye is deformed or soft or there is any other concern for an open globe injury, the area should be protected with a shield so that no further manipulations are applied to the globe until evaluation by an ophthalmologist.

Imaging is indicated when there is concern for an orbital fracture or foreign body as described earlier. This should be computed tomography (CT) of the facial bones/orbits with coronal and sagittal reconstructions. Plain X-ray films of the orbit are not sensitive enough to detect many orbital fractures and not detailed enough for surgical reconstruction planning. A CT scan with only axial images is an incomplete study for the purpose of evaluating orbital trauma, as it is nearly impossible to assess the orbital floor on axial view—at a minimum, a coronal reconstruction must be obtained. Soft-tissue and bone windows should both be evaluated directly by the surgeon. The soft-tissue window can show blood in the orbit, tissue edema, and the status of the globe and extraocular muscles. The bone window

enables proper assessment of the thin orbital walls (particularly the floor and medial wall, which are so thin that nondisplaced fractures are often not visible on soft-tissue windows). The images must be directly viewed by the evaluating surgeon; one cannot simply rely on reading the report for the scan. It is regrettably too common an occurrence that a CT scan is read as "normal" when in fact a fracture or other abnormality exists.[6] Unfortunately, it tends to be trapdoor fractures that are underrecognized most frequently because of their nondisplaced configuration; these tend to occur in children and require urgent surgical repair.[7]

## 10.2.1 Indications for and Timing of Surgical Repair of Orbital Blowout Fractures

Like many conditions in medicine, and in oculoplastic and orbital surgery in particular, there are few hard rules regarding orbital fracture management. One exception though is the "white-eyed" blowout fracture, or "trapdoor" fracture, most commonly seen in pediatric patients. This is a fracture in which the orbital floor (less commonly the medial orbital wall) is fractured and minimally displaced, actually springing back into near normal anatomical alignment but unfortunately entrapping soft tissue (such as orbital fat or a rectus muscle) within the fracture itself. These fractures externally appear to have minimal edema and ecchymosis, and the eye itself is often "white and quiet"[8] (▶ Fig. 10.1). Most striking is the severe limitation of movement of the globe—often an inability to supraduct in floor fractures, or to abduct in medial wall fractures. Some cases can be associated with the oculocardiac reflex, in which bradycardia and nausea may develop during attempted ductions. These fractures can be missed by radiologists or surgeons not familiar with this fracture pattern (▶ Fig. 10.2). Nonetheless, it is essential to *not* miss such a fracture, because treatment involves urgent (same-day) surgical treatment. Delayed treatment of a trapdoor fracture exposes the patient to the risk of permanent injury to the rectus muscle entrapped within the fracture, which can undergo contracture from ischemia and lead to permanent strabismus and muscle dysfunction that is difficult to correct.

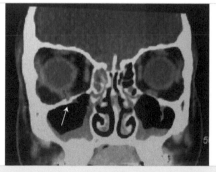

Fig. 10.2 A coronal reconstruction of maxillofacial CT (computed tomography), soft-tissue window. This scan was read by a radiologist as "no fracture identified." A clue to the fracture is the soft-tissue abnormality between the right inferior rectus muscle and right orbital floor–this is the soft tissue entrapped by the trapdoor fracture and is what tethers the eye and limits supraduction.

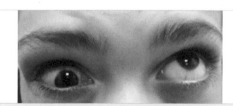

Fig. 10.1 A "white-eyed" or "trapdoor" blowout fracture of the right orbital floor in a 12-year-old boy who was struck by a baseball. The right eye exhibits severe limitation of supraduction, but otherwise there are minimal external signs of trauma.

A review article by Burnstine in 2002 collated data to offer evidence-based recommendations concerning the indications and timing for orbital fracture repair.[9] Repairing a white-eyed blowout fracture within 24 to 48 hours is supported by level A1 evidence. The other indications and timing recommendations for fracture repair are not as strong, and rely on the addition of clinical judgment. A floor fracture associated with diplopia within 30 degrees of primary gaze from limited supraduction or infraduction that persists beyond a week should be repaired ideally within 7 to 14 days, with newer data suggesting repair within 7 days having better long-term results.[10] Fractures that have a disproportionate amount of soft-tissue disruption compared to the fracture size (e.g., a minimally depressed floor fracture but with a significant "teardrop" deformity of the inferior rectus muscle) may also benefit from earlier repair.[11] Enophthalmos at presentation is generally always associated with a large fracture or combined floor and medial wall fracture, and the enophthalmos can be expected to only worsen as edema subsides; thus, such a fracture should be considered for repair. Any fracture of 50% or greater of the surface of the orbital floor or combined floor and medial wall should be considered for surgical repair because of the high likelihood of developing problematic enophthalmos. The normal discrepancy of exophthalmometry measurements between the two eyes in normal individuals is up to 2 mm.[12] Thus, the development of latent enophthalmos of 2 mm or greater may be an indication for surgical repair if cosmetically unacceptable to the patient. Even after repair, however, some enophthalmos can persist from internal soft-tissue scarring, imperfect reconstruction, or orbital fat atrophy following trauma and surgery.[13] Still, delayed repair of a fracture in a patient who has manifested latent enophthalmos can have good success and should not be discounted.[14]

## 10.2.2 Implant Materials for Orbital Reconstruction

A variety of implant materials have been employed for orbital fracture reconstruction, including autologous tissue (e.g., nasal septum cartilage, calvarial bone graft) and alloplastic materials (such as nylon foil, porous polyethylene sheeting, and titanium mesh). The author uses almost exclusively alloplastic implants because of their ease of use, lack of donor site morbidity, and safety and effectiveness.

One implant material that is thin, flexible, and inexpensive is nylon foil. This is a clear sheet with physical characteristics similar to X-ray film, and is available in a variety of thicknesses. The author most commonly uses 0.4-mm sheets for small isolated orbital floor or medial wall fractures with excellent surrounding bony support. It can also be used as a "wraparound" implant for combined floor and medial wall fractures, particularly when the inferomedial orbital strut is intact.[15] The material is smooth and this is viewed as a positive attribute in terms of not adhering to orbital tissues such as rectus muscles, but this can also make the implant prone to shifting. Thus, a single microscrew is often placed anteriorly to stabilize the implant and prevent migration.[16] Smooth implants, while being nonadherent, do carry a risk of encapsulation and subsequent hematic cyst formation.[17]

Porous polyethylene is flexible and malleable while retaining some rigidity, and as a result of being porous undergoes fibrovascular ingrowth into the implant itself, which serves to stabilize the implant and in theory avoid infection and encapsulation. These implants are available in variable thicknesses, including 0.45, 0.85, 1, and 1.5 mm. They are also available with an optional smooth "barrier" surface to prevent fibrovascular ingrowth on one or both surfaces. Porous polyethylene is "sticky" and adheres to the orbital soft tissues (fat, periosteum) and is generally resistant to shifting. The author most commonly employs nonbarrier porous polyethylene sheets for medium-sized blowout fractures with good surrounding bony support. There have been reported cases of latent implant inflammation.[18] Barrier sheets are susceptible to capsular formation and hemorrhage similar to any other smooth implant.[19] For larger fractures, porous polyethylene sheets can be cantilevered from the orbital rim with a titanium miniplate; composite implants of porous polyethylene with an inner layer of titanium (for rigidity and enhanced malleability) are also available. Beware, though, that porous polyethylene, being flexible, can bow as the orbit swells postoperatively, or could be drawn down to a depressed bone plate during the fibrovascular in growth phase. This could have the effect of creating a concave orbital floor configuration (as opposed to convex) and can lead to latent enophthalmos or diplopia (▶ Fig. 10.3).

Titanium alloy is an inert and lightweight nonferrous metal with appropriate rigidity for implant reconstruction. Because of its ability to hold shape, manufacturers have been able to fabricate preformed orbital implants that are based on an averaging of CT scan data of many patients to create implants that replicate the natural shape of the orbit. These implants span the orbital floor to the medial orbital wall, and maintain the natural

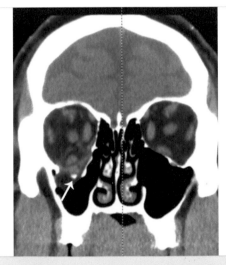

Fig. 10.3 A maxillofacial CT (computed tomography; soft tissue, coronal reconstruction) scan obtained at postoperative month 3 in a patient with persistent vertical diplopia in down gaze following orbital fracture repair with a porous polyethylene sheet. The scan shows a very large fracture spanned by the porous polyethylene sheet with some soft tissue below the implant. The very large size of the fracture (essentially the whole floor with very little residual bony support) may have been better reconstructed with a rigid implant to avoid "bowing" into the maxillary sinus.

convexity of the orbital floor medially and the natural angle from the floor to medial wall transition by the inferomedial orbital strut. They are available in left or right configurations, small and large sizes, and are fenestrated to allow drainage of blood and fluid out of the orbit into the adjacent paranasal sinus. The author prefers these implants for reconstruction in large fractures where there is little of the floor left, floor fractures with disruption of the inferomedial orbital strut, and combined floor and medial wall fractures, especially if there is disruption of the inferomedial orbital strut. Once the implant is cut to size (if needed) and the shape fine-tuned (if needed), it is placed and fixated to the internal inferior orbital rim laterally with a single microscrew. Screws can also be placed on the anterior face of the inferior orbital rim with screw points that fold over the rim; however, efforts should be made to avoid this as the screws and implant could be palpable or could contribute to scarring and lower lid retraction postoperatively. Because the implant is fenestrated, secondary removal if necessary can be difficult as the orbital soft tissues will be strongly adherent to the implant. Care must be taken to ensure tissue or muscle is not herniated around the implant and that bare extraocular muscle is not in contact with the implant or a restrictive strabismus could result. There have been reports of "orbital adherence syndrome" in which the orbital tissues/extraocular muscles/eyelid become tightly scarred to the titanium implant and are very difficult to remedy.[20] And while the rigidity of the implant is on balance a strength and reason for its use, one must be careful when cantilevering the implant that the rise posteriorly is not too high, or else an optic nerve compression or direct nerve injury could result, with catastrophic consequences. Unlike nylon foil or porous polyethylene, which will generally "mold" to the native surrounding orbital shape, the titanium implant will not do this and thus correct position and angulation *must* be ensured intraoperatively, and rechecked carefully after screw fixation.

While preformed implants reconstruct the orbital shape quite well, custom-made patient-specific implants are available. These are created by the manufacturer based on individual patient CT imaging data with the goal of reconstructing an orbit to closely match the contralateral normal orbit. These implants can be made from titanium or alloplastic material. Cost and production lead time limit their use in most primary fracture repair settings, but this type of implant can be valuable in difficult secondary reconstructions.

## 10.3 Surgical Techniques

### 10.3.1 Transconjunctival Approach to the Orbital Floor

A variety of approaches exist to access the orbital floor, including transcutaneous incisions below the lashes, transcutaneous incision over the orbital rim directly, and transconjunctival incision, often performed with a lateral canthotomy and inferior cantholysis (i.e., the "swinging eyelid" approach).[21] There has been a movement away from transcutaneous approaches to the orbit, as these can be associated with visible scarring and cicatricial ectropion of the eyelid. The author most commonly employs the swinging-eyelid approach to the floor; however, in

children with small trapdoor fractures in whom wide exposure is not as critical, the floor is often accessed without disturbing the lateral canthus.

The patient is supine on the operating table and under general anesthesia. The lateral canthus and lower eyelid are injected with local anesthetic (2% lidocaine with epinephrine 1:100,000 mixed 1:1 with 0.75% bupivacaine with the addition of hyaluronidase). The patient is administered 10 mg of intravenous dexamethasone if not medically contraindicated and 1 to 2 g of intravenous cefazolin (or other antibiotic if allergic). After prepping and draping in the usual sterile fashion a corneal scleral protecting shield is placed over the operative eye. Prior to placing the shield, forced duction testing can be performed in which the conjunctiva of the eye is carefully grasped with toothed forceps near the limbus (where conjunctiva is fused with Tenon's fascia) and the eye is rotated up and down and side to side to assess for any restriction of movement. A curved Stevens tenotomy scissors is then used to perform a lateral canthotomy (cutting full thickness across the lateral eyelid commissure within a horizontal lateral canthal rhytid for approximately 0.5 to 1 cm toward the lateral orbital rim) and inferior cantholysis (turning the scissors to point toward the patient's feet and cutting the firm tissues of the inferior crus of the lateral canthal band and orbital septal attachments to "release" the eyelid). The closed scissors are then placed through the lateral canthal incision and directed medially in the preseptal/postorbicularis plane across the lower lid until the tips reach alignment with the most medial eyelashes, and the scissors are opened to perform a blunt preseptal dissection. The scissors are then backed out laterally and opened such that one tine of the scissors remains in the preseptal plane and the other tine is over conjunctiva. The scissors are then used to cut the fused layers of conjunctiva, lower lid retractors, and orbital septum from the inferior border of the tarsal plate across the eyelid proceeding lateral to medial, taking care not to disrupt the lacrimal canaliculus medially. This yields an efficient preseptal exposure and avoids any thermal injury to the conjunctival and orbital septum from the use of monopolar cautery. Hemostasis is obtained with careful use of bipolar cautery if needed. A 4–0 silk traction suture is placed through the cut end of the conjunctiva and lower lid retractors and clamped superiorly to the head drape, while a Desmarres retractor holds the eyelid inferiorly. A malleable retractor is used to hold the orbital soft tissues down to isolate the inferior orbital rim. The overlying soft tissues can then be cut with a no. 15 blade or at this point with a monopolar cautery device. Care is taken to ensure that the cheek and lid skin is not rolled up superiorly and overlying the rim by the assistant applying downward traction on the cheek skin. The periosteum of the orbital rim is then elevated with a Freer periosteal elevator and the orbital fracture is revealed. Careful subperiosteal dissection is performed around the fracture site medially and laterally, and then the herniated tissues are elevated back into the orbit using a hand-over-hand technique between the Freer elevator and malleable retractor. Sometimes a skeletonized infraorbital nerve/neurovascular bundle is encountered, and this must carefully be separated from the overlying orbital soft tissues. Medially, care is taken to not disrupt the origin of the inferior oblique extraocular muscle, which originates near the entrance to the nasolacrimal duct. The dissection proceeds to the posterior extent of the fracture

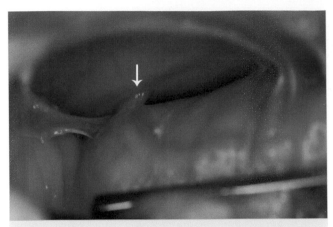

**Fig. 10.4** Surgeon's view of the right orbital floor in a cadaver dissection showing the orbital perforating neurovascular bundle exiting the mid-infraorbital canal and entering the orbital soft tissues.

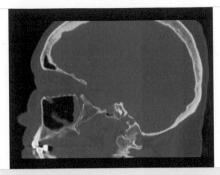

**Fig. 10.5** A postoperative maxillofacial CT (computed tomography) scan, bone window, sagittal reconstruction, demonstrating appropriate placement of a titanium orbital implant reconstruction of the orbital floor. The implant maintains the appropriate contour of the floor, rising posteriorly to the "posterior ledge" of the maxilla.

so that all orbital soft tissues are returned to the orbit and the fracture is entirely exposed. Free fragments of bone are carefully removed during dissection so that they do not become lost in the orbital fat and intraconal space, from which pain, globe, or nerve injury or vision loss could result. There is a perforating neurovascular bundle from the center of the orbital floor from the infraorbital canal into the orbit[22] (► Fig. 10.4). If this is intact, it should be identified, cauterized, and lysed so that it is not inadvertently lacerated, which could lead to hemorrhage. Sometimes the floor fracture extends all the way posteriorly to the palatine bone. There are essentially no critical structures along the orbital floor to prevent full dissection and release of the fracture all the way posteriorly; however, pauses should be taken every few minutes to avoid sustained retraction on the orbital soft tissues, which puts stress on the globe and optic nerve. Once the fracture is entirely exposed and all soft tissues have been elevated back into the orbit, the fracture site is covered with an implant. In small fractures or trapdoor fractures in which the bony defect is small, the author prefers a 0.45-mm porous polyethylene sheet or a 0.4-mm nylon sheet. The porous polyethylene is generally not fixated, while the nylon sheet is fixated anteriorly with a single 4-mm self-drilling microscrew. For medium-sized fractures, the author prefers 0.85- or 1.0-mm porous polyethylene sheets, usually fashioned in a "guitar-pick" shape to span the fracture circumferentially. For very large fracture, the author prefers preformed titanium orbital implants that are fixated anteriorly with one or two 4-mm self-drilling microscrews on the inner surface of the orbital rim. These implants are cut down to size as needed and then carefully positioned taking great care to ensure there is no herniation of orbital soft tissue around the edges of the implant and that the implant is directly on bone in the subperiosteal space. The implant should be resting on the posterior-most bone behind the fracture site, called the posterior ledge, which is often the palatine bone in such large fractures. This ensures that the trajectory of the floor is maintained (which is a rising trajectory proceeding posteriorly; see ► Fig. 10.5). Forced duction testing is then performed to ensure the eye is freely mobile, confirming that there is no tissue entrapment. It is very rare for the author to suture the periosteum or orbicularis muscle, but instead a

"sutureless" technique is employed.[23] When a lateral canthotomy/cantholysis has been performed, this is repaired with a double-armed 5–0 Polyglactin suture placed intratarsally from the cut edge of the tarsus to the firm tissue of the lateral canthal band in horizontal mattress fashion. The lateral canthal angle is reformed with a 7–0 Polyglactin sutured cerclage placed gray line to gray line from the upper to lower eyelid, with the knot placed within the lateral wound. A 6–0 fast gut suture is used to close the conjunctiva of the lower eyelid with two simple interrupted sutures (one at the medial third and one at the lateral third), taking care to take very small purchase of conjunctiva only. The skin of the lateral canthus is then closed with 6–0 fast gut simple interrupted sutures. The protecting shield is removed from the eye, the patient is undraped, and the skin is cleansed, followed by the application of erythromycin ophthalmic ointment to the operative eye. The patient is then awoken from anesthesia and extubated and taken to the recovery room and observed for any bleeding (► Fig. 10.6, composite).

## 10.3.2 Retrocaruncular Transconjunctival Approach to the Medial Orbital Wall

A skin incision (e.g., Lynch-type incision) can be avoided in accessing the medial orbit by employing a retrocaruncular approach.[24,25] This is a transconjunctival incision placed between the caruncle and the plica semilunaris, and affords excellent exposure to the medial orbit with essentially no morbidity and excellent cosmesis when performed properly.

The patient is prepared as previously described for orbital surgery.

To allow exposure of the caruncle and plica semilunaris, either the assistant or a self-retaining eyelid speculum is used to hold the eyelids in the open position. The caruncle is grasped with a toothed Bishop forceps and elevated anteriorly. Blunt-tipped Westcott scissors are used to cut through the conjunctiva immediately between the caruncle and plica semilunaris. It is import for the scissors to be oriented toward the midline of the face and away from the globe. Additionally, the scissors

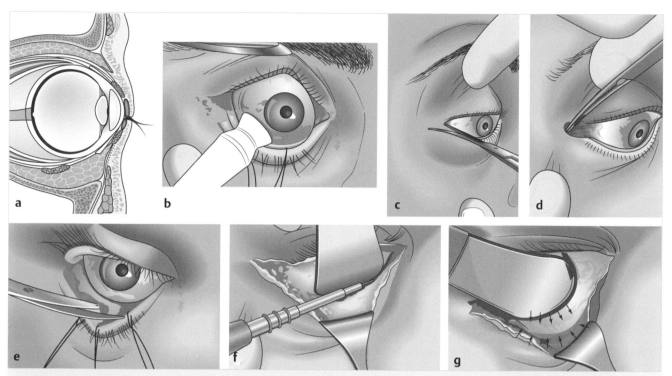

**Fig. 10.6** **(a,b)** The swinging eyelid transconjunctival approach to the orbital floor. **(c,d)** Lateral canthotomy and inferior cantholysis. **(e)** The preseptal dissection and release of the conjunctiva from the inferior tarsal border is performed with the Stevens tenotomy scissors. **(f)** Periosteum along inferior orbital rim incised with monopolar cautery device. **(g)** Subperiosteal exposure of the orbital floor. (Adapted from Ellis E, III. Surgical approaches to the orbit in primary and secondary reconstruction. Facial Plast Surg 2014;30(5):537–544.)

should be oriented posteriorly at approximately a 45-degree angle so that the common canaliculus of the lacrimal drainage system is not inadvertently cut. Once this initial incision is created, it can be carefully extended superiorly and inferiorly with the Westcott scissors, taking care to avoid injury to the globe and extraocular muscles. Closed curved Stevens tenotomy scissors are then placed through the incision and advanced to "palpate" the posterior lacrimal crest. The scissors are then opened to bluntly dissect and then orbital Sewell or small malleable retractors are placed to maintain exposure. The periosteum overlying the posterior lacrimal crest can be incised with a crescent blade or a Colorado needle-tipped monopolar cautery device. A subperiosteal dissection can then commence. The superior zone of dissection is along the frontoethmoidal suture line, and care must be taken not to lacerate the anterior ethmoid neurovascular bundle. If this structure is encountered and it impedes, the dissection bipolar cautery is applied and the bundle may be carefully lysed. Inferiorly, the dissection is along the inferomedial orbital strut. Care is taken not to create iatrogenic fracture of these fragile bones. Once the fracture in the lamina papyracea is isolated, the herniated orbital soft tissues are carefully elevated back into the orbit using the Freer elevator and small malleable retractor. Unlike the orbital floor, in which there are essentially no critical structures along the floor posteriorly, the medial orbital wall leads directly to the optic canal and optic nerve as one proceeds posteriorly. Frequent rest periods to release tissue retraction and gentle manipulations are key to avoiding injury to the optic nerve. Taking note of the depth of dissection (the medial orbital wall is approximately

40 mm in length on average) and the presence of the posterior ethmoid neurovascular bundle (which is on average 6 mm anterior to the optic canal) can help maintain situational awareness during dissection. Note that up to a third of patients may have an accessory ethmoidal neurovascular bundle (middle ethmoidal artery) between the anterior and posterior foramina; thus, this is not an absolutely reliable landmark.[26] Stereotactic image guidance can be a helpful adjunct if available.

Once the soft tissues are reduced out of the fracture, the fracture may be covered with an implant of the surgeon's choice. The author typically uses a 0.4-mm nylon foil or a 0.85-mm porous polyethylene sheet. The implant is cut to an oval shape and placed such that it rests on intact bone circumferentially, while the orbital soft tissues are held back with a malleable retractor. If there is very good security of the implant over intact bone, fixation is generally not necessary; however, if the implant has only slight overlap on bone or if there is some movement of the implant during forced duction testing, the implant can be fixated with a single 4-mm microscrew placed through the anterior inferior edge of the implant into the region of the posterior lacrimal crest. Note that significant movement of the implant during forced duction testing should prompt the surgeon to explore for soft tissue that has not been properly released from the fracture or that has herniated around the implant—this must be rectified to avoid postoperative restrictive strabismus or even severe injury to the muscle if it itself is entrapped by the implant.

Once the implant is secure and forced duction testing is satisfactory, the soft tissues by the caruncle are returned to their

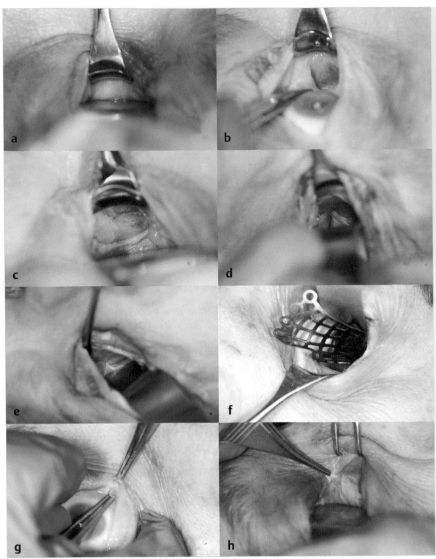

**Fig. 10.7** Retrocaruncular approach to the medial orbital wall. **(a)** The caruncle and plica semilunaris are retracted in preparation for conjunctival incision with the Westcott scissors. **(b)** A Desmarres retractor is pulled medially, while a curved Stevens tenotomy scissor is used to bluntly dissect through soft tissue to the posterior lacrimal crest. **(c)** The periosteum at the posterior lacrimal crest has been incised and elevated and the lamina papyracea is now exposed. **(d)** The anterior ethmoidal neurovascular bundle is exposed, and may be cauterized and divided. **(e)** The lamina papyracea of the medial orbital is now well-visualized. **(f)** After the fracture is reduced, an implant is placed along the medial orbital wall. **(g,h)** The conjuctival incision by the caruncle may be left open or may be lightly secured with a suture such as 6-0 gut or 7-0 polyglactin. (Used with permission from Shen Yun-Dun, Paskowitz Daniel, Merbs Shannath, Grant Michael, Retrocaruncular *Approach for the Repair of Medial Orbital Wall Fractures*. New York, NY: Thieme; 2015: 100-104.)

normal anatomical position. Suturing is not mandatory. If there is a tendency noted for some soft tissue to protrude by the caruncle, a 6–0 fast gut simple interrupted may be placed from the posterior aspect of the caruncle to the conjunctiva. The protecting shield is removed from the eye, the patient is undraped, and the skin is cleansed, followed by the application of erythromycin ophthalmic ointment to the operative eye. The patient is then awoken from anesthesia and extubated and taken to the recovery room and observed for any bleeding (► Fig. 10.7).

## 10.3.3 Combined Floor and Medial Wall Fracture

When both the floor and medial wall of the orbit are disrupted, there exists a greater potential for enophthalmos and potential ocular dysmotility to develop. The decision-making process and surgical approach employed can become more complicated. In general, the same concepts as applied for isolated floor or medial wall fractures apply to combined fractures in terms of deciding on whom to operate. Very small fractures with

minimal displacement and minimal change to the overall orbital volume likely do not mandate repair and may be observed. Some fractures with apparently minimal displacement in terms of magnitude may still require repair if the total size of the fracture is large, that is, the small displacement is multiplied by the surface area of the fracture and leads to significant orbital volume expansion and enophthalmos. Large fractures, which most often manifest by early enophthalmos, require repair. A not uncommon scenario is a combined fracture in which the orbital floor is of moderate to large size and the medial wall fracture is small or very minimally displaced. If very minimally displaced and/or if the area of size is small (e.g., a single ethmoid air cell), then it may be acceptable to repair only the floor and leave the medial wall untreated. On the other hand, it is a mistake to not repair a medial wall fracture in the setting of combined floor and medial wall disruption if the displacement or size is significant—this will lead to postoperative enophthalmos even if the floor is perfectly reconstructed.

Another consideration in combined fractures is the status of the inferomedial orbital strut. This structure represents an important buttress for the orbit, and is the point of inflection

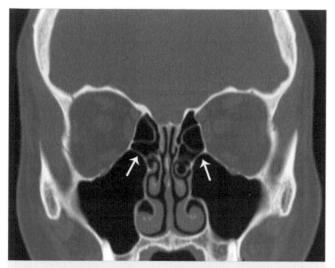

Fig. 10.8 Maxillofacial CT (computed tomography) scan, bone window, and coronal reconstruction. The inferomedial orbital strut (*arrows*) serves as a buttress for the orbit, and is an important surgical and structural landmark in orbital reconstruction.

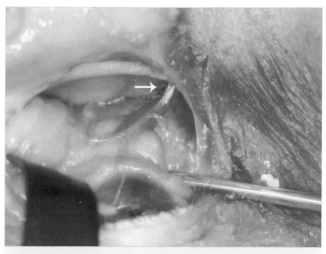

Fig. 10.9 Surgeon's view of left orbit, cadaver dissection, showing origin of the inferior oblique muscle by the internal and medial aspects of the inferior orbital rim.

between the orbital floor and the medial orbital wall (▶ Fig. 10.8). When this structure is disrupted, one can be sure the orbital volume has been significantly expanded—the strut is generally strong and disruption requires significant traumatic force. When the strut is intact, the surgeon has the benefit of an anatomical landmark that preserves the natural contour of the patient's orbit and also serves as a structural support point for an implant. When it is disrupted, it tends to be displaced inferomedially. In this situation, the surgeon does not have a clear reference point for the transition from floor to medial wall or for the rise of the orbital floor proceeding posteriorly (except for the palatine bone most posteriorly). In this situation, an implant could be placed too medially and too flat, leading to inadequate orbital reconstruction and postoperative enophthalmos. Recognition of this is extremely important during surgery, and the surgeon in such cases should rely on the palatine bone posteriorly to serve as a posterior "ledge" in order to obtain the correct rise of the floor, and the origin of the inferior oblique muscle as a point near the transition from floor to medial wall.

The inferior oblique muscle originates just lateral to the bony nasolacrimal duct entrance, immediately behind the inferior orbital rim medially (▶ Fig. 10.9). Thus, it is situated between the orbital floor and medial orbital wall. During surgery, care must be taken to avoid injury to this structure, as problematic torsional diplopia that is difficult to cure can result.[27]

## 10.3.4 Surgical Approach for Combined Floor/Medial Wall Fractures of the Orbit

The author begins combined fracture repair with the swinging-eyelid approach via the lower lid as described earlier. A judicious lateral canthal release and incision of the periosteum high up the lateral orbital rim can afford excellent exposure of the orbital floor with exposure up onto the medial orbital wall. In many cases, this is adequate to allow a safe and complete repair of the combined floor and medial wall fracture. Once the floor

component has been isolated and soft tissue released from the maxillary sinus, the subperiosteal dissection proceeds medially and superiorly from the inferomedial orbital strut up to the lamina papyracea and the medial fracture is isolated from below and then anteriorly and posteriorly, and the soft tissues are elevated from the ethmoid sinus proceeding superiorly and posteriorly. Care is taken to observe rest periods from retraction in the orbit, and to dissect with a "light touch" medially to avoid further fracture of the lamina papyracea or penetration into the skull base superiorly. If the soft tissues are not able to be easily elevated or the orbit is "tight" and access to the medial wall is limited from the floor, the author will then make a separate incision to the medial orbit via a retrocaruncular incision as described earlier. This then allows further exposure of the medial fracture, in particular direct exposure to the superior aspect of the fracture and allows the dissection vector to be applied in a safer downward manner away from the skull base.

When a retrocaruncular and swinging eyelid approaches are employed together, there is excellent access into the orbit; however, the inferior oblique muscle stands in the way of unencumbered 180-degree access. It is best to work around the inferior oblique muscle if possible, but not at the expense of repeatedly traumatizing it via direct manipulations over the course of an operation. If the surgeon must have full 180-degree access, the conjunctival incision of the lower lid and retrocaruncular area may be connected carefully with Westcott scissors and the inferior oblique muscle may be released. Historically, it was purported that the inferior oblique muscle could simply be "stripped" away from bone along with periosteum and then allowed to heal back into position secondarily. The author has not found this to be reliable and prefers to mark the muscle at its origin with double-armed 6–0 Polyglactin suture prior to sharply releasing the muscle at its origin below this suture. Then at the conclusion of reconstruction, the preplaced suture is sewn to the tendinous stump origin on the internal inferior orbital rim in a horizontal mattress fashion to ensure the muscle is secured in the correct anatomical location.

## 10.3.5 Implant Placement for Combined Floor/Medial Wall Fractures

The implant types most commonly used by the author for combined floor/medial wall fractures include nylon foil and preformed titanium plates for the orbital floor and wall. In some cases, it may be appropriate to use two separate implants: one for the floor and one for the medial wall. This would generally be performed in the setting of a retrocaruncular incision combined with a swinging-eyelid approach, not connected, and with an intact intrinsic optical signal. More commonly, a single implant is used to cover both the medial wall and floor fractures.

When the inferomedial orbital strut is intact, a nylon foil sheet can be used to "wrap around" the medial wall and floor, resting on the strut at the transition point for support and contour orientation as described earlier. The sheet is cut to an ellipsoid shape that will span the fracture anteroposteriorly along its minor axis and reach from the level of the frontoethmoidal suture to the lateral aspect of the orbital floor along its major axis. A 4–0 silk suture can be passed through one end of the major axis, and then with the fracture fully exposed using malleable retractors, the implant is placed via the lower lid/ floor area and the suture grasped through the retrocaruncular/ medial wall area with a curved hemostat and "pulled" into position. The suture is then released and removed. Care is taken to ensure that the implant covers the fractured areas entirely and that no soft tissues (particularly the superior oblique muscle or medial rectus muscle by the superior aspect of the medial fracture) have herniated around the implant.

When the inferomedial orbital strut is disrupted, or in cumulatively large fractures, the author prefers to use a preformed titanium orbital floor and wall implant (▶ Fig. 10.10). Placement of the implant is accomplished by placing first the superomedial aspect of the implant into the orbit via the lower eyelid approach, while all soft tissues are held back with malleable retractors. Large fractures requiring a large implant benefit from release of the inferior oblique muscle (with subsequent reattachment as previously described) to allow safe and accurate implant placement. Once the implant is in place, it is con-

firmed to be in correct alignment in relation to the frontoethmoidal suture superiorly, the palatine bone posteriorly, and the angle of the lateral aspect of the implant floor to the angle of the inferior orbital fissure. The implant should not be so medial or anterior as to impinge on the nasolacrimal duct. In cases in which the anatomy is distorted, stereotactic image guidance can be used to confirm position in an attempt to mirror the uninjured orbit. The implant should be recessed from the inferior orbital rim, that is, no hardware should be palpable transcutaneously. Care is taken to ensure no soft tissue has herniated around the implant. The implant is then secured with a 4-mm self-drilling microscrew on the internal aspect of the inferior orbital rim laterally. Forced duction testing confirms freedom of eye movement and the wounds are closed as previously discussed.

## 10.3.6 Access to the Orbital Roof via Upper Eyelid Crease Incision

Orbital roof fractures, when repair is warranted, are generally treated in conjunction with neurosurgery as there is usually other cranial trauma and manipulations of the orbital roof that carry a risk of cerebrospinal fluid leak or other intracranial iatrogenic injury. Access to the orbital roof is more commonly indicated in the setting of draining an abscess or accessing a mass involving the frontal and/or ethmoid sinuses. When wide exposure of the roof is required, a coronal flap is appropriate, as this allows release of the supraorbital neurovascular bundle from its notch or foramen and allows unrestricted access to the orbital roof, particularly medially. To avoid a coronal flap, an eyelid crease incision can be used to reach the orbital roof with great access to all but the most anteromedial aspect.[28]

The upper eyelid crease is marked preoperatively. The patient is prepared for orbital surgery as described previously. A 4–0 silk traction suture is placed centrally above the upper lid eyelashes and this is used to hold the eyelid on downward traction by carefully clamping to the drape. A no. 15 blade is used to incise the skin of the upper eyelid within the marking of the crease. The depth of incision is just through skin to orbicularis muscle, but not deeper in order to avoid injury to the levator palpebrae superioris aponeurosis. Curved Stevens tenotomy scissors are then used to cut through the orbicularis muscle with the scissors oriented parallel to the eyelid surface with the goal of entering the preseptal plane superiorly. Blunt and sharp dissections are performed superiorly in the preseptal plane up to a level overlying the superior orbital rim. A Desmarres retractor is used to retract the skin and soft tissue superiorly. Hemostasis is obtained with careful use of bipolar cautery. The supraorbital notch is palpated and dissection is maintained lateral to this landmark to avoid injury to the supraorbital neurovascular bundle. A malleable retractor is used to hold back the orbital soft tissues below the superior orbital rim, and the soft tissue and periosteum over the rim are then incised with a Colorado needle–tipped monopolar cautery device from just lateral to the supraorbital notch proceeding laterally to the lateral orbital rim. This incision can be carried along the rim to the level of the lateral canthus. A Freer periosteal elevator is then used to elevate the arcus marginalis periosteum and the subperiosteal space of the orbital roof is entered. The

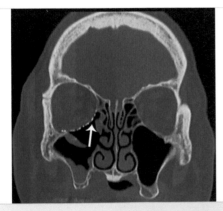

Fig. 10.10 Combined floor and medial wall fracture of the right orbit with disruption of the inferomedial orbital strut. A preformed titanium orbital floor and wall implant has been placed to reconstitute the natural orbital contour and provide stability in the absence of the strut (*arrow*).

periosteum of the roof will then generally elevate quite readily centrally. Dissection is performed deep to the supraorbital notch and the frontoethmoidal suture line can be approached in this way. Laterally, the periosteum will elevate readily as well. The zygomaticotemporal neurovascular bundle may be encountered. Generally, this is left intact, but may be cauterized with bipolar cautery and lysed if necessary. Small defects in the orbital roof do not require direct reconstruction. In some cases, the author will place a cellulose film over a small roof defect to prevent orbital soft-tissue herniation during early phases of healing while the periosteum is reconstituting. Larger defects may benefit from placement of a 0.4-mm nylon foil sheet or a 0.45-mm porous polyethylene sheet. Note that when very large areas of the orbital roof are removed (as in a transcranial orbitotomy), reconstruction may require titanium or porous polyethylene–titanium composite implants to prevent cerebral herniation into the orbit. At the conclusion of surgery, the retractors and traction sutures are removed and the eyelid crease incision is closed with interrupted 6–0 fast gut suture. When an abscess has been evacuated, the author will place a drain in the superior subperiosteal space exiting from a lateral sub-brow stab incision.

## 10.4 Postoperative Care

In general, an eye patch is not placed following orbital surgery, as this could potentially mask a developing hemorrhage. An exception to this is in cases in which there may have been above-average bleeding and/or the patient is expected to have a difficult exit from general anesthesia (e.g., a smoker who is expected to cough, etc.)—in these cases, a standard pressure patch of two eye pads placed over the closed eyelid and affixed with tape under tension may be placed in an effort to apply pressure to the orbit and maintain hemostasis during the extubation process and immediate postoperative period. This patch *must* be removed promptly in the recovery area so that the orbit may be observed for any subsequent signs of active bleeding.

The patient should have vision assessed once awake enough to cooperate. This can be as simple as ensuring the patient is capable of counting the examiner's fingers and of reporting normal brightness sense. The vision is often quite blurry because of ointment and intraocular pressure change (usually decreased) immediately after surgery. Many patients feel lights are bright immediately postoperatively, which is usually due to the blurring, ocular irritation from intraoperative manipulations, and sometimes a dilated pupil (which can be normal, especially when epinephrine-containing local anesthetic is used). Inability to count fingers or the report of "dim" or "dark" vision should prompt concern for optic nerve insult. It is important to understand the details of a pupil examination. A unilaterally dilated pupil does *not* indicate injury to the optic nerve. More likely the pupil is pharmacologically dilated from local anesthetic contacting the eye, from sustained pressure in the orbit during surgery, or from traumatic mydriasis sustained in the original injury (which would be present preoperatively). Neuroanatomically, the pupils are innervated to constrict together. Normally, when a light is shone to an eye, that pupil will constrict (the direct response). The pupil of the other eye

should also constrict (the consensual response). This forms the basis for assessing optic nerve function via pupil testing. Thus, if light is shone to the right eye only, both pupils should constrict. In the swinging flashing test, the light is alternated between the two eyes. The pupils of each eye should remain constricted to the light. If one pupil is pharmacologically dilated, the test can still be performed, because the undilated pupil should remain reactive regardless of which eye is receiving the light. If the pupil of the right eye dilates once the light is moved to the left eye, this would indicate a problem with the left afferent system (such as an optic neuropathy) and would be called an *afferent pupillary defect*. Thus, even if one pupil is completely unreactive (e.g., from atropine eyedrops used to treat traumatic iritis), the status of the afferent visual system can be assessed by observing the status of the normal (other) pupil in response to light applied to each eye separately—the reactive pupil should react both directly and consensually. If an afferent pupillary defect is present, one should search for a cause such as hemorrhage, implant malposition, or direct nerve injury. Any suspicion for hemorrhage or implant impingement on the optic nerve should lead to immediate return to the operating room for exploration.

Most isolated blowout fractures in the author's practice are not kept overnight postoperatively unless there was above-average bleeding intraoperatively, there was a delayed hemorrhage requiring take-back to the operating room, or if the patient lives a great distance from the hospital. Patients are instructed to avoid any bending, straining, or heavy lifting for 1 week postoperatively. Erythromycin ophthalmic ointment or equivalent is applied twice daily to the operative eye for 1 week. The author does not routinely prescribe postoperative systemic antibiotics. Cool compresses are applied every hour for 10 minutes while awake for the first 48 hours postoperatively. The patient is instructed to avoid any nose blowing or drinking through a straw for 4 weeks following surgery. In general, postoperative examination is performed at 1 week, 1 month, and 3 months.

## 10.5 Complications

### 10.5.1 Hemorrhage and Orbital Compartment Syndrome

A hemorrhage can occur anytime during surgery or in the recovery area immediately postoperatively or even days after surgery. A significant hemorrhage, in which the orbit becomes firm and the eyelids tense, is an emergency. The diagnosis is made on clinical examination alone in which the orbit is tensely firm to palpation, there is exophthalmos, and usually the eyelids are difficult or impossible to manually open. Sometimes pain may be quite severe and well out of the normal postoperative pain expectation. Any loss of vision or the presence of an afferent pupillary defect, if able to be assessed, is an ominous sign that the eye and optic nerve are under significant insult and the risk of permanent vision loss is a time-sensitive reality—retinal death can occur within 60 to 90 minutes of ischemia. There is no role for imaging in the acute setting as this would only delay treatment. Likewise, in the acute setting, there is no role for medical therapy such as intraocular pressure-lowering eyedrops or systemic acetazolamide. If the bleeding is in the recovery area of the operating suite, any accessible sutures should be released, and a lateral canthotomy and inferior cantholysis should be performed to release the orbital pressure and to potentially allow egress of blood. The patient should urgently be returned to the operating room and placed under general anesthesia and the orbit explored to identify the source of bleeding and control it with bipolar cautery. In most cases, once this is accomplished, the wound may be reclosed. The author prefers to admit the patient for overnight observation and to maintain bed rest and blood pressure control. Any bleeding diathesis (such as thrombocytopenia or coagulation problem) should be remedied. If the bleeding is particularly difficult to control, particularly in the absence of a reasonable cause such as severe postoperative rise in blood pressure, etc., a hematology evaluation can be considered to rule out a previously undiagnosed bleeding tendency, such as von Willebrand's disease.

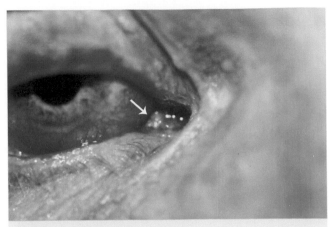

**Fig. 10.11** External photograph of a patient referred for chronic eye discharge, lower eyelid retraction, and strabismus, showing a transconjunctival exposure of a porous polyethylene implant (*arrow*) placed some years earlier for repair of an orbital fracture.

### 10.5.2 Canalicular Laceration

Iatrogenic canalicular laceration can occur during orbital fracture repair surgery from overaggressive lower eyelid retraction or from direct cutting during dissection. A canalicular laceration is suspected in the setting of any laceration medial to the lacrimal punctum. This can be confirmed via passage of a Bowman lacrimal probe through the punctum and canaliculus. A canalicular laceration must be repaired with direct re-anastomosis over a silicone stent such as a self-retaining monocanalicular stent or Crawford-type nasolacrimal stent. If the operating surgeon is not familiar with canalicular laceration repair or the required stenting material is not available, it is acceptable to perform a superficial closure of the lid and have the patient treated by a surgeon with canalicular repair experience within 24 to 48 hours—following this time, the chance for a successful canalicular repair is greatly reduced, with the potential consequence of permanent tearing.

### 10.5.3 Incorrect Implant Position

An implant protruding anteriorly over the orbital rim may lead to orbital septal scarring and subsequent cicatricial eyelid retraction, which is extremely difficult to repair. Medially, if the implant is anteriorly displaced, it may become exposed through the conjunctiva, as the conjunctiva is not as strong as skin and is more prone to breakdown and implant exposure, which can lead to infection and conjunctival scarring and strabismus (▶ Fig. 10.11). An implant placed extremely posteriorly on the floor may apply pressure to the infraorbital nerve exiting the foramen rotundum, leading to persistent hypesthesia and/or chronic pain. Medially, an implant placed too posteriorly will abut the optic foramen, and could potentially apply pressure to the optic nerve, leading to vision loss ranging from a visual field defect to blindness. If the inferomedial orbital strut is displaced, it is possible to place the implant too medially, which leads to an inadequate orbital reconstruction and can cause enophthalmos and strabismus/diplopia. In the sagittal plane, an implant along the floor should rise posteriorly, with the target of resting on the palatine bone. Most cases of poor implant positioning here involve the implant being placed too "flat" without any

rise posteriorly. This leads to inadequate orbital reconstruction and postoperative enophthalmos. A potentially worse scenario is when the implant rise is too great, which is most likely to happen when the floor implant has been cantilevered from the inferior orbital rim. If the rise angle is too severe, significant pressure, and even sharp injury, to the inferior rectus muscle, globe, or optic nerve can occur with catastrophic consequences. A patient with significantly decreased or complete loss of vision in the postoperative recovery area should be taken back to the operating room and have the implant removed—obtaining imaging in this case could lead to delay and potentially contribute to permanent loss of vision.

### 10.5.4 Diplopia and Strabismus

It is normal for patients to have altered ocular motility postoperatively in relation to edema and shifting of the rectus muscles from a herniated position to the normal anatomical position. Patients can be reassured that this diplopia can be expected to correct itself over days to weeks. What is not normal in the immediate postoperative period is severe limitation of movement. If the limitation of movement is severe and global and the orbit is tense, an orbital compartment syndrome may be developing. If the movement is generally full except for one direction (e.g., there is zero adduction), there may be a restrictive or paralytic problem. Forced duction testing can be performed and if significant restriction is present, one should be concerned for tissue entrapment around the implant. This should be fixed expediently. If the eye moves freely, and there are no signs or concerns for significant malposition, the patient may be observed for improvement of function over days to a week. If the eye remains unrestricted but with limited movements, imaging can be considered (either MRI [magnetic resonance imaging] or CT orbits with contrast) to evaluate the extraocular muscles for edema or injury. Some patients will experience persistent double vision despite timely repair and excellent orbital reconstruction without any overt extraocular muscle pathology. Such patients should be referred to an ophthalmologist specializing in the evaluation and treatment of strabismus, who may treat the patient with prism in spectacles and/or strabismus surgery.

## 10.5.5 Eyelid Retraction

The development of cicatricial lower eyelid retraction can be quite serious to the patient, as it is unsightly and uncomfortable. The eye becomes exposed and dry, leading to redness and tearing. In the most severe forms, the cornea can become so dry as to become infected and even perforate. Once the scarring process of eyelid scarring begins, it is extremely challenging to halt. Some patients may go on to require multiple surgeries including removal of hardware and placement of tissue grafts. The best approach here is prevention. In the author's referral practice, this complication seems to occur most frequently when the transconjunctival dissection has not been performed precisely (e.g., evidence of cutting *through* the tarsus, or notation in the operative report of an unexpected full-thickness eyelid laceration acquired during dissection requiring repair). Additionally, these cases seem to involve an overzealous closure of the conjunctival wound, with multiple different sutures used to close periosteum, septum or orbicularis, and conjunctiva. If the retraction is mild, massage and anti-inflammatory treatments (such as injection of 5-FU [5-fluorouracil] and triamcinolone into the middle lamella of the eyelid) are instituted. In more severe cases, secondary reconstruction may be necessary. The author prefers to wait at least approximately 6 months if possible to allow the postoperative inflammation to subside. Historically, hard palate grafting was used as a middle and posterior lamella spacer graft. A modern technique with less donor site morbidity is the use of nasal mucosal graft, such as from the inferior turbinate or nasal septum. Allografts, such as processed cadaver dermis, may also be used.

# 10.6 Conclusion

The orbit is a complicated and critical area that is both resilient to trauma and disruption while simultaneously being delicate and sensitive to manipulation. The concepts of orbital fracture management have evolved to a generally reliable approach for evaluation and treatment, which can in turn serve as a basis for orbital reconstruction considerations related to endonasal endoscopic orbital surgery.

# References

[1] Putterman AM. Management of blow out fractures of the orbital floor. III. The conservative approach. Surv Ophthalmol. 1991; 35(4):292–298

[2] Bleier BS, Castelnuovo P, Battaglia P, et al. Endoscopic endonasal orbital cavernous hemangioma resection: global experience in techniques and outcomes. Int Forum Allergy Rhinol. 2016; 6(2):156–161

[3] Gilliland GD, Gilliland G, Fincher T, Harrington J, Gilliland JM. Assessment of biomechanics of orbital fracture: a study in goats and implications for oculoplastic surgery in humans. Am J Ophthalmol. 2005; 140(5):868–876

[4] Kreidl KO, Kim DY, Mansour SE. Prevalence of significant intraocular sequelae in blunt orbital trauma. Am J Emerg Med. 2003; 21(7):525–528

[5] Kim BB, Qaqish C, Frangos J, Caccamese JF, Jr. Oculocardiac reflex induced by an orbital floor fracture: report of a case and review of the literature. J Oral Maxillofac Surg. 2012; 70(11):2614–2619

[6] Chen T, Gu S, Han W, Zhang Q. The CT characteristics of orbital blowout fracture and its medicolegal expertise. J Forensic Leg Med. 2009; 16(1):1–4

[7] Parbhu KC, Galler KE, Li C, Mawn LA. Underestimation of soft tissue entrapment by computed tomography in orbital floor fractures in the pediatric population. Ophthalmology. 2008; 115(9):1620–1625

[8] Jordan DR, Allen LH, White J, Harvey J, Pashby R, Esmaeli B. Intervention within days for some orbital floor fractures: the white-eyed blowout. Ophthal Plast Reconstr Surg. 1998; 14(6):379–390

[9] Burnstine MA. Clinical recommendations for repair of isolated orbital floor fractures: an evidence-based analysis. Ophthalmology. 2002; 109(7):1207–1210, discussion 1210–1211, quiz 1212–1213

[10] Matteini C, Renzi G, Becelli R, Belli E, Iannetti G. Surgical timing in orbital fracture treatment: experience with 108 consecutive cases. J Craniofac Surg. 2004; 15(1):145–150

[11] Harris GJ, Garcia GH, Logani SC, Murphy ML. Correlation of preoperative computed tomography and postoperative ocular motility in orbital blowout fractures. Ophthal Plast Reconstr Surg. 2000; 16(3):179–187

[12] Migliori ME, Gladstone GJ. Determination of the normal range of exophthalmometric values for black and white adults. Am J Ophthalmol. 1984; 98(4):438–442

[13] Clauser L, Galiè M, Pagliaro F, Tieghi R. Posttraumatic enophthalmos: etiology, principles of reconstruction, and correction. J Craniofac Surg. 2008; 19(2):351–359

[14] Scawn RL, Lim LH, Whipple KM, et al. Outcomes of orbital blow-out fracture repair performed beyond 6 weeks after injury. Ophthal Plast Reconstr Surg. 2016; 32(4):296–301

[15] Nunery WR, Tao JP, Johl S. Nylon foil "wraparound" repair of combined orbital floor and medial wall fractures. Ophthal Plast Reconstr Surg. 2008; 24(4):271–275

[16] Park DJ, Garibaldi DC, Iliff NT, Grant MP, Merbs SL. Smooth nylon foil (SupraFOIL) orbital implants in orbital fractures: a case series of 181 patients. Ophthal Plast Reconstr Surg. 2008; 24(4):266–270

[17] Chao DL, Ko MJ, Johnson TE. Hematic cyst around orbital floor implant masquerading as choroidal mass. JAMA Ophthalmol. 2015; 133(3):e143534

[18] Aryasit O, Ng DS, Goh AS, Woo KI, Kim YD. Delayed onset porous polyethylene implant-related inflammation after orbital blowout fracture repair: four case reports. BMC Ophthalmol. 2016; 16:94

[19] Mihora LD, Holck DE. Hematic cyst in a barrier-covered porous polyethylene/titanium mesh orbital floor implant. Ophthal Plast Reconstr Surg. 2011; 27(5):e117–e118

[20] Lee HB, Nunery WR. Orbital adherence syndrome secondary to titanium implant material. Ophthal Plast Reconstr Surg. 2009; 25(1):33–36

[21] Bonawitz S, Crawley W, Shores JT, Manson PN. Modified transconjunctival approach to the lower eyelid: technical details for predictable results. Craniomaxillofac Trauma Reconstr. 2016; 9(1):29–34

[22] Patel AV, Rashid A, Jakobiec FA, Lefebvre DR, Yoon MK. Orbital branch of the infraorbital artery: further characterization of an important surgical landmark. Orbit. 2015; 34(4):212–215

[23] Lane KA, Bilyk JR, Taub D, Pribitkin EA. "Sutureless" repair of orbital floor and rim fractures. Ophthalmology. 2009; 116(1):135–138.e2

[24] Shorr N, Baylis HI, Goldberg RA, Perry JD. Transcaruncular approach to the medial orbit and orbital apex. Ophthalmology. 2000; 107(8):1459–1463

[25] Shen YD, Paskowitz D, Merbs SL, Grant MP. Retrocaruncular approach for the repair of medial orbital wall fractures: an anatomical and clinical study. Craniomaxillofac Trauma Reconstr. 2015; 8(2):100–104

[26] Mason E, Solares CA, Carrau RL, Figueroa R. Computed tomographic exploration of the middle ethmoidal artery. J Neurol Surg B Skull Base. 2015; 76(5):372–378

[27] Tiedemann LM, Lefebvre DR, Wan MJ, Dagi LR. Iatrogenic inferior oblique palsy: intentional disinsertion during transcaruncular approach to orbital fracture repair. J AAPOS. 2014; 18(5):511–514

[28] Szabo KA, Cheshier SH, Kalani MY, Kim JW, Guzman R. Supraorbital approach for repair of open anterior skull base fracture. J Neurosurg Pediatr. 2008; 2(6):420–423

# 11 Optic Nerve Decompression

*Adam P. Campbell and Ralph B. Metson*

**Abstract**

The endoscopic endonasal approach for decompression of the optic nerve may be used in the treatment of patients with optic neuropathy due to either traumatic or nontraumatic etiologies. The combination of endoscopic instrumentation and image-guidance technology provides the surgeon with excellent visualization and anatomic localization along the entire course of the optic canal for safe and effective nerve decompression.

*Keywords:* optic neuropathy, optic nerve decompression

## 11.1 Introduction

Endoscopic optic nerve decompression is a natural extension of the technique of endoscopic orbital decompression first described in the 1990s.[1,2,3] In patients with visual loss caused by compressive optic neuropathy, removal of bone from the optic canal to relieve pressure along the nerve sheath can be a vision-saving procedure.[3]

## 11.2 Patient Selection and Indications

Optic neuropathy is generally divided into two broad categories: traumatic and nontraumatic. The most common indication for optic nerve decompression historically has been traumatic optic neuropathy.

The role of optic nerve decompression for traumatic optic neuropathy is controversial and early studies suggest that neither corticosteroids nor surgical optic nerve decompression offers benefit over observation.[4] In order to answer this question, a randomized controlled trial named the International Optic Nerve Trauma Study (IONTS) was created but struggled with patient recruitment. The protocol was changed to a nonrandomized study of 127 patients and found no benefit of corticosteroids or surgical decompression. The final study recommendations were that patients with visual loss from trauma to the optic nerve should be first treated with high-dose systemic steroids rather than surgical decompression but that treatment should be individualized for each patient.[5] Multiple retrospective studies subsequent to the IONTS have suggested improvement in visual acuity with optic nerve decompression following failure of visual improvement with steroids.[6,7,8]

For patients with nontraumatic optic neuropathy, however, optic nerve decompression may prevent further deterioration of the optic nerve or even reverse the visual loss that has already occurred. Neuropathy with vision loss is most likely due to direct neuronal compression leading to a conduction block and resultant demyelination. Therefore, many patients experience rapid recovery following pressure release and continued recovery as the nerve continues to remyelinate.[9] The most common indications for such decompression are the following:
- Fibro-osseous lesions (e.g., fibrous dysplasia involving the optic canal).
- Neoplasms (e.g., meningioma of the skull base).
- Non-neoplastic masses (e.g., lymphangioma along the lateral sphenoid sinus).
- Inflammatory conditions (e.g., Graves' disease or orbital pseudotumor).

For most patients with optic neuropathy from Graves' disease, decompression of the orbital apex without formal optic canal decompression is sufficient to address the pathology. Some ophthalmologists, however, feel that patients with severe optic neuropathy from Graves' disease unresponsive to high-dose steroids should undergo optic nerve decompression at the time of orbital decompression.

## 11.3 Diagnostic Workup

In traumatic optic neuropathy, patients are often involved in high-speed or multisystem trauma and should first be evaluated by a trauma team. A computed tomography (CT) scan should be performed to evaluate for orbital, orbital apex, or skull base injuries. In nontraumatic optic neuropathy, most patients initially present with complaints of blurred or hazy vision with a normal funduscopic exam. Prior to optic nerve decompression, a complete ophthalmologic examination should be performed within 1 week prior to surgery. Often this examination may reveal visual field defects, change in color vision (dyschromatopsia), afferent pupillary defect, or even optic disc pallor in advanced disease. A magnetic resonance imaging (MRI) with and without contrast may be obtained to radiographically evaluate the optic nerve. Once optic nerve compression has been diagnosed, systemic corticosteroids may provide some relief while awaiting surgical intervention.

## 11.4 Surgical Anatomy

The optic nerve may be divided into three segments: intraorbital, intracanalicular, and intracranial. Optic nerve decompression aims to relieve compressive forces within the intracanalicular portion of the nerve. The canal of the optic nerve is formed by the two struts of the lesser wing of the sphenoid and carries both the optic nerve and the ophthalmic artery.

## 11.5 Surgical Technique

The patient is placed in a supine position on the operating table. The eyes are draped in the surgical field and protected with scleral shields. Lidocaine (1%) with epinephrine (1:100,000) is injected along the lateral nasal wall, middle turbinate, and posterior nasal septum.

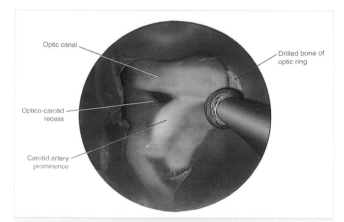

**Fig. 11.1** Endoscopic view of the left nasal cavity following wide sphenoidotomy. The posterior lamina papyracea has been resected to reveal underlying periorbita, which is contiguous with the optic nerve sheath. A diamond burr is used to thin bone along the optic canal. (Reproduced with permission of Metson R. Optic nerve decompression. In: Kennedy D, Myers E, eds. Masters Techniques in Otolaryngology: Head and Neck Surgery. Rhinology. 1st ed. New York, NY: Wolters Kluwer; 2016.)

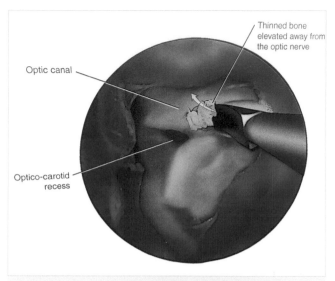

**Fig. 11.2** Thinned bone along the medial surface of the optic canal is elevated from the underlying nerve with a microcurette. (Reproduced with permission of Metson R. Optic nerve decompression. In: Kennedy D, Myers E, eds. Masters Techniques in Otolaryngology: Head and Neck Surgery. Rhinology. 1st ed. New York, NY: Wolters Kluwer; 2016.)

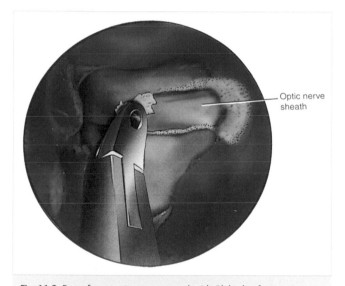

**Fig. 11.3** Bony fragments are removed with Blakesley forceps to expose the underlying optic nerve sheath. (Reproduced with permission of Metson R. Optic nerve decompression. In: Kennedy D, Myers E, eds. Masters Techniques in Otolaryngology: Head and Neck Surgery. Rhinology. 1st ed. New York, NY: Wolters Kluwer; 2016.)

If necessary for adequate surgical exposure, the surgeon should perform a septoplasty or resect the middle turbinate at the beginning of the procedure. A sphenoethmoidectomy is then performed in the standard fashion. The sphenoid face is opened widely, and the prominence of the bony optic nerve canal is identified as it courses along the lateral wall of the sphenoid sinus, just superior to the opticocarotid recess (▶ Fig. 11.1). The astute surgeon should be aware that the optic

canal can be located within a posterior ethmoid or Onodi cell, which can be identified on preoperative CT scan. In such cases, widely opening the Onodi cell is an important step to provide adequate surgical exposure. An image-guidance system may be used at the surgeon's discretion to assist with the identification and verification of the location the optic canal.

The lamina papyracea should be cleaned of all adjacent ethmoid air cells and their attachments. A spoon curette is then used to fracture the skeletonized lamina papyracea approximately 1 cm anterior to the face of the sphenoid sinus. The lamina is removed in a posterior direction to expose the underlying periorbita. The surgeon should be careful to avoid penetration of the periorbita, as herniation of orbital fat may obscure visualization of the surgical field. As dissection continues in a posterior direction, the underlying periorbita forms a thick white fascia corresponding to the annulus of Zinn, from which the extraocular muscles originate and through which the optic nerve passes.

As the optic canal is approached, the thin lamina is replaced with the thick bone of the optic ring at the entrance to the optic canal. This bone is thinned using a long-handled drill with a diamond burr and removed using a spoon curette or rongeur. The same drill is used methodically to thin bone in a more posterior direction along the medial surface of the optic canal (▶ Fig. 11.2). While drilling, care must be taken to prevent contact of the drill bit with the prominence of the carotid artery located just inferior and posterior to the optic canal. After the bone is appropriately thinned, it is carefully lifted in a medial direction, away from the underlying optic nerve, with a microcurette or spoon. The ophthalmic artery typically runs in the inferomedial quadrant of the optic canal and should be avoided during bone removal. Bony fragments are removed with small Blakesley forceps (▶ Fig. 11.3). In most patients, removal of bone for a distance of 10 mm posterior to the face of the sphenoid sinus is sufficient to provide adequate nerve decompression

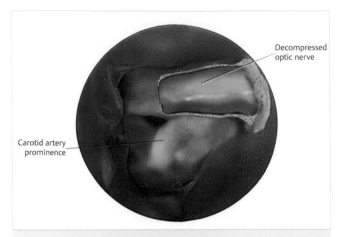

Fig. 11.4 View of the decompressed optic nerve at the completion of surgery. (Reproduced with permission of Metson R. Optic nerve decompression. In: Kennedy D, Myers E, eds. Masters Techniques in Otolaryngology: Head and Neck Surgery. Rhinology. 1st ed. New York, NY: Wolters Kluwer; 2016.)

(▶ Fig. 11.4). In patients with anatomic compression of the nerve (e.g., from fibrous dysplasia or neoplasm) located more proximally along the optic canal, additional bone must be removed until the region of compression is released.

Incision of the optic nerve sheath is not generally recommended, as bony decompression is usually sufficient to relieve pressure along the nerve and achieve the desired clinical benefits. Furthermore, incision of the sheath increases the risk of damage to the underlying nerve fibers and ophthalmic artery, as well as intraoperative cerebrospinal fluid (CSF) leak. Nevertheless, in certain patients, such as those with a suspected intrasheath hematoma or marked papilledema, opening of the optic nerve sheath may play a beneficial role. In such cases, a sickle knife is used to incise the sheath starting just anterior to the annulus of Zinn. The incision in the sheath is continued in a posterior direction with a sickle knife or microscissors along the length of the exposed nerve.

## 11.6 Complications

Intraoperative and postoperative complications are similar to those for routine endoscopic sinus surgery and include bleeding, infection, and CSF leak. If intraoperative bleeding is encountered, it should be controlled with traditional methods such as bipolar cautery or topical agents. Formal packing is typically avoided given the concern for further compression of the exposed optic nerve. Some studies have shown that the rate of CSF leak is higher in optic nerve decompression compared to orbital decompression or endoscopic sinus surgery. If an intraoperative leak is detected, this should be repaired at the time of initial surgery using a combination of cartilage grafts, mucosal grafts, absorbable agents, or intranasal pedicled flaps if appropriate.

Complications that are particularly germane to optic nerve decompression include diplopia, loss of vision, and even blindness. The rate of new-onset diplopia appears to be much greater if concomitant orbital decompression is performed. In cases where double vision persists for more than 2 months, referral to an ophthalmologist for extraocular muscle repositioning surgery should be considered. In the event of decreased visual acuity postoperatively, intravenous steroid therapy can be continued in order to decrease perineural edema and associated neural injury.

## 11.7 Postoperative Care

- Because the optic nerve is exposed, no packing is placed at the conclusion of surgery.
- Patients are observed overnight with hourly vision checks. If stable, they are discharged home the following day.
- Discharge medications include an oral antistaphylococcal antibiotic and steroid taper.
- Twice-a-day nasal saline irrigations are continued until the first postoperative visit 1 week after surgery.
- The sinonasal cavity should be carefully debrided following surgery to assist with mucosal healing and decrease infection rates.
- Repeat ophthalmologic examination is documented 1 day, 1 week, and 1 month following surgery.

## 11.8 Outcomes

The majority of patients who undergo optic nerve decompression for compressive nontraumatic optic neuropathy will have improvement in visual acuity. In a study of 10 consecutive optic nerve decompressions performed for nontraumatic optic neuropathy, Pletcher[10] reported no intraoperative complications. Mean visual acuity improved from 20/300 to 20/30 following decompression. The one patient with no light perception preoperatively from an invasive meningioma did not recover any vision following decompression.

## References

[1] Kennedy DW, Goodstein ML, Miller NR, Zinreich SJ. Endoscopic transnasal orbital decompression. Arch Otolaryngol Head Neck Surg. 1990; 116(3):275–282

[2] Michel O, Bresgen K, Rüssmann W, Thumfart WF, Stennert E. Endoscopically-controlled endonasal orbital decompression in malignant exophthalmos. Laryngorhinootologie. 1991; 70(12):656–662

[3] Metson R, Pletcher SD. Endoscopic orbital and optic nerve decompression. Otolaryngol Clin North Am. 2006; 39(3):551–561, ix

[4] Cook MW, Levin LA, Joseph MP, Pinczower EF. Traumatic optic neuropathy. A meta-analysis. Arch Otolaryngol Head Neck Surg. 1996; 122(4):389–392

[5] Levin LA, Beck RW, Joseph MP, Seiff S, Kraker R. The treatment of traumatic optic neuropathy: the International Optic Nerve Trauma Study. Ophthalmology. 1999; 106(7):1268–1277

[6] Kountakis SE, Maillard AA, El-Harazi SM, Longhini L, Urso RG. Endoscopic optic nerve decompression for traumatic blindness. Otolaryngol Head Neck Surg. 2000; 123(1, Pt 1):34–37

[7] Rajiniganth MG, Gupta AK, Gupta A, Bapuraj JR. Traumatic optic neuropathy: visual outcome following combined therapy protocol. Arch Otolaryngol Head Neck Surg. 2003; 129(11):1203–1206

[8] Li KK, Teknos TN, Lai A, Lauretano AM, Joseph MP. Traumatic optic neuropathy: result in 45 consecutive surgically treated patients. Otolaryngol Head Neck Surg. 1999; 120(1):5–11

[9] McDonald WI. The symptomatology of tumours of the anterior visual pathways. Can J Neurol Sci. 1982; 9(4):381–390

[10] Pletcher SD, Metson R. Endoscopic optic nerve decompression for nontraumatic optic neuropathy. Arch Otolaryngol Head Neck Surg. 2007; 133 (8):780–783

# 12 Primary Neoplasms of the Orbit

*Sophie D. Liao and Vijay R. Ramakrishnan*

## Abstract

Orbital neoplasms represent a large proportion of orbital diseases. A thorough understanding of clinical presentation, workup, and management options is required given the rather broad spectrum of tumors that occur in this space. Primary orbital neoplasms are less common than those that arise from adjacent structures, and wide range of tumors can occur given the numerous histologic entities in the orbit and periorbital region. Tumor location, in addition to tumor histology, imparts a particular significance in the clinical management and treatment sequelae of the individual disease. In this chapter, we will review the presentation, workup, and management of common primary orbital neoplasms.

*Keywords:* primary orbital neoplasm, lacrimal gland tumor, EMZL, idiopathic orbital inflammation, hemangioma

## 12.1 Introduction

Orbital neoplasms constitute 20 to 25% of all orbital diseases. Primary orbital neoplasms are less common than secondary masses that arise from adjacent periorbital and other structures. They comprise a range of benign and malignant diseases that can be either space occupying or infiltrative. They may arise from cells of bony, vascular, muscular, neural, lymphoid, or connective tissue origin. Primary tumors within the orbit may be categorized according to the tissue of origin, location, and benign or malignant behavior. The most common neoplasms seen are of vasculogenic, cystic, and lymphocytic origin. Orbital neoplastic diseases can cause widely variable symptoms, depending on their growth patterns and characteristics (▶ Table 12.1). Since the orbit is anatomically unique, with many important structures packed into a relatively tight space, tumor location imparts particular significance in its clinical sequelae and thus its management. A complete ophthalmic examination should be documented for all patients with an orbital mass. This should include measurement of visual acuity, confrontation visual fields, pupils, intraocular pressure, extraocular motility, exophthalmometry, color vision, and a slit-lamp anterior segment as well as dilated fundus examination. The presence of orbital pathology should prompt formal visual field testing and consideration of nerve optical coherence tomography

**Table 12.1** Signs and symptoms of orbital neoplasms

| |
|---|
| Proptosis |
| Globe dystopia |
| Pain and/or restriction with eye movement |
| Resistance to globe retropulsion |
| Cranial nerve V1 or V2 numbness |
| Decreased vision of visual field |
| Asymmetric ptosis |
| Asymmetric periocular edema or erythema |
| Binocular diplopia |

(OCT). Documenting a thorough patient history and clinical examination should also focus on elements that may help characterize the mass and narrow the differential diagnosis. Proptosis is measureable using an exophthalmometer such as a Hertel device, and should also be clinically characterized by noting whether the patient exhibits axial or abaxial proptosis. Pain should be noted, as this may indicate perineural invasion of the tumor. Periorbital signs such as erythema, swelling of eyelid or conjunctival tissue, telangiectasis or vascular dilatation, or pain to touch may point to inflammatory lesions. Palpable resistance to retropulsion of the globe or a palpable periorbital mass should be documented. Timing of progression of symptoms and signs, if present, should be recorded. Rapidity of onset points toward inflammatory, infectious, or traumatic etiologies, while slower onset over months is more characteristic of slow-growing tumors.

## 12.2 Lymphocytic and Leukemic Lesions

### 12.2.1 Ocular Adnexal Lymphoma

Lymphomas arising in the orbit, lacrimal gland, eyelids, or conjunctiva are termed ocular adnexal lymphoma (OAL). The vast majority of these are primary extranodal tumors, although a minority develop secondary to disseminated diseases. These tumors are almost always extranodal non-Hodgkin's lymphoma (NHL), comprising about 2% of all NHL. The most common subtype is extramarginal zone B-cell lymphoma (EMZL), sometimes called MALToma because it arises from mucosa-associated lymphoid tissue. EMZL accounts for 80% of OAL, followed by follicular lymphoma and diffuse large B-cell lymphoma (DLBCL). The remainder are rare and include mantle cell, small lymphocytic, and lymphoplasmacytic lymphoma.[1,2] Only a handful of primary T-cell lymphoma and Hodgkin's lymphoma cases have been documented. Although often focal, OAL may be bilateral or multicentric or disseminate via the regional lymph nodes. These tumors tend to mold to adjacent structures, only invading into adjoining bone and involving the sinuses or intracranial contents in advanced cases. Risk factors include immunosuppression and ultraviolet irradiation, as well as chronic antigen stimulation with inflammation and possibly infection with *Chlamydia psittaci*.[3,4] Patients typically present in the sixth or seventh decade with a less than a year history of painless eyelid or orbital swelling and proptosis. No sex predilection has been reported. Examination may reveal a pink, "salmon-patch" lesion of the conjunctiva in conjunctival lymphoma (▶ Fig. 12.1). Orbital computed tomography (CT) or magnetic resonance imaging (MRI) with contrast should be ordered to delineate the extent of the tumor. CT scan will demonstrate a homogeneously enhancing, well-circumscribed mass that molds to surrounding structures. Bone erosion is not typical. On MRI, lymphoma is usually isointense to the extraocular muscles on T1 and T2 phases and enhances with gadolinium.[4] If lymphoma is suspected, a biopsy should be performed, with tissue sent both in formalin and fresh for flow cytometry. Once the diagnosis is

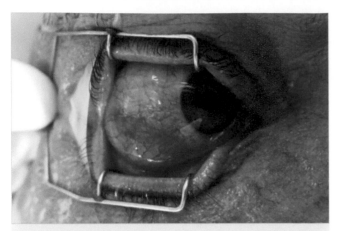

**Fig. 12.1** Classic "salmon-patch" appearance of a conjunctival lymphoma.

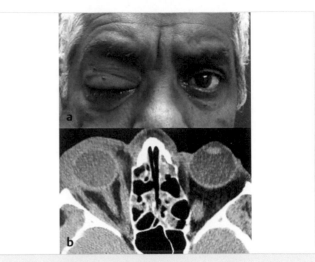

**Fig. 12.2** Nonspecific orbital inflammation of the right lacrimal gland. (a) Periorbital erythema, edema, and ptosis. (b) Axial noncontrast CT (computed tomography) showing enlarged right lacrimal gland and overlying eyelid edema.

confirmed, positron emission tomography CT (PET-CT) of the chest, abdomen, and pelvis should be performed to evaluate for metastases and stage the disease. Blood testing including complete blood count, protein electrophoresis, lactate dehydrogenase, beta-2-microglobulin levels, complete metabolic panel, hepatitis C and HIV testing, and bone marrow evaluation are typically performed by the oncologist. Isolated orbital lesions may be treated with irradiation or systemic chemotherapy, while systemic involvement requires chemotherapy/immunotherapy. Prognosis varies depending on the lymphoma subtype. EMZL has a generally good prognosis, with 90% survival in the long term, unless certain factors, such as aggressive histologic subtype, advanced age, and systemic dissemination, are present. Mantle cell lymphoma is more aggressive, with overall disease-free survival of only 50% at 5 years, although survival has improved with rituximab-based regimens.[5] Follicular lymphoma is typically also aggressively treated, as transformation to DLBCL may occur. Radiotherapy is the treatment of choice, with addition of chemotherapy if DLBCL is present.[6] Follicular lymphoma has an overall mortality rate of about 25%, while DLBCL has about 45% mortality rate. T- and NK-cell lymphomas are very rare as primary orbital lesions. They are much more aggressive and may have up to 100% mortality.

## 12.2.2 Idiopathic Orbital Inflammation

Idiopathic orbital inflammation (IOI), also termed orbital pseudotumor, as well as reactive lymphoid hyperplasia, lies on the benign end of the lymphoproliferative spectrum of orbital lesions. They deserve special mention because these lesions are seen fairly often and may be mistaken for malignant lymphoma or, if the extraocular muscles are primarily involved, may be confused with thyroid eye disease. These lesions often present with rapidly progressive orbital inflammatory signs, including eyelid edema and erythema, conjunctival chemosis and hyperemia, and sometimes severe orbital pain (▶ Fig. 12.2). Progressive inflammation may cause restrictive strabismus with associated diplopia, proptosis, ocular hypertension, and even vision loss. Diagnostic workup includes testing to rule out associated systemic disease including ESR (erythrocyte sedimentation rate), CRP (C-reactive protein), and selective serologic testing depending on review of systems. First-line treatment is high-

dose oral corticosteroids with a slow taper. In cases with optic neuropathy, urgent intervention may be required, including use of IV (intravenous) corticosteroids or surgical decompression. Masses that respond poorly to steroids should be biopsied. If the diagnosis of IOI is confirmed, and there is poor response to corticosteroid therapy, alternative treatments may be considered such as rituximab or other immune modulatory drugs, or external beam radiation therapy.

## 12.2.3 Orbital Leukemia

Leukemia in childhood may occasionally involve the orbit due to extension from involvement of surrounding structures. The two most frequent subtypes are acute lymphoblastic leukemia and acute myelogenous leukemia. Leukemic orbital lesions are also known as granulocytic sarcoma, myeloblastoma, myeloid sarcoma, or chloroma. Children may present with acute onset of proptosis and eyelid swelling that may be mistaken for orbital cellulitis. Neuroimaging of the orbit should be performed, which will show a homogeneous, mildly enhancing mass without bone erosion.[7] Biopsy should be performed and once the diagnosis is confirmed, treatment is nonsurgical, with chemoradiation by an oncologist.

# 12.3 Vasculogenic Neoplasms

## 12.3.1 Infantile Hemangioma

Capillary hemangiomas, also called infantile hemangiomas, are the most common benign vascular pediatric tumors of the orbit. Infantile hemangiomas are congenital hamartomas that progress through an initial proliferative phase during which lesions grow most rapidly, then enter an involutional phase during which the lesions often regress significantly. Infantile hemangiomas present within and grow over the first year of life, and typically regress from 1 to 5 years of age.[8] Superficial hemangiomas typically present as reddish, elevated skin lesions, while deeper hemangiomas appear bluish or violaceous. They are most commonly seen in the superior orbit or upper eyelid. If large enough to cause amblyopia from mechanical ptosis or other etiologies such as induced astigmatism, treatment is indicated. Smaller lesions that are not amblyogenic may be observed without treatment. If found to be very large or involve adjacent facial areas, workup should be performed for the PHACE (posterior fossa malformation, facial hemangioma, arterial lesion, cardiac anomalies, eye abnormalities) syndrome.

Diagnostic evaluation by ultrasound or MRI of the orbits may be performed to confirm a suspected diagnosis and define the extent of the lesion in order to plan treatment. CT imaging should be avoided in young children due to the risks of radiation. Infantile hemangiomas have variable features on neuroimaging, with some lesions appearing more well defined and others poorly defined, and they may appear across multiple spaces within the orbit and lids. They enhance with contrast on MRI scans, and appear heterogeneous on T1- and T2-weighted imaging.[4]

First-line treatment involves beta blockers such as propranolol, which can be administered orally or, if there is a superficial orbital/eyelid component, topically in the form of timolol gel.[9] Timolol topical treatment has been shown in a handful of small case series to induce regression in even deeper orbital infantile hemangiomas.[10] Beta blocker treatment may be complicated by bradycardia, hypoglycemia, hypotension, or bronchospasm and should be closely supervised by a pediatrician. Alternative treatments include use of pulsed-dye laser, Nd:YAG (neodymium:yttrium aluminum garnet) laser, irradiation, interferon alpha-2, and oral or injectable corticosteroids.[11,12] Treatment is continued as long as the lesion is large enough to cause amblyopia. Surgery is only rarely indicated for capillary hemangiomas refractory to medical treatment that are threatening the vision.

## 12.3.2 Cavernous Hemangioma

Cavernous hemangiomas are the most common benign primary orbital tumors in adults. These tumors typically appear between 20 and 60 years of age with a female predominance, and present as painless, slowly progressive proptosis over months to years. They are composed of large vascular spaces separated by fibrous septa surrounded by a pseudocapsule.[4] The majority of these lesions lie intraconally, although larger lesions may extend extraconally. Tumors are typically detected either incidentally, on neuroimaging performed for unrelated reasons, or when the hemangioma is large enough to cause discernable proptosis, visual disturbance, or diplopia. Vision changes may include hyperopic shift, binocular gaze-induced diplopia, visual field deficit gaze-evoked amaurosis secondary to optic nerve compression, or loss of visual acuity. Diagnosis requires orbital imaging. CT and MRI with contrast demonstrate a well-circumscribed lesion that enhances diffusely with a mottled pattern and may rarely contain hyperdense flecks of intralesional calcification.[13] The tumors can be observed unless visual disturbance is significant enough to justify surgery, at which point complete surgical excision is indicated.[14]

## 12.3.3 Lymphangioma

Lymphangiomas are congenital lymphovascular choristomatous malformations that typically present within the first two decades of life with painless, progressive proptosis that may be rapid or insidious (▶ Fig. 12.3). Rapid onset of proptosis may

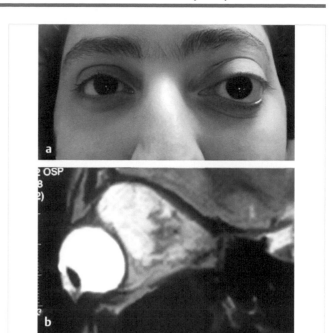

**Fig. 12.3** (a) Orbital lymphangioma presenting with left hypoglobus and proptosis. (b) Sagittal T2-weighted, postcontrast MRI (magnetic resonance imaging) demonstrating a large, heterogeneously enhancing intraorbital mass that crosses the intra- and extraconal space.

occur with an episode of intralesional hemorrhage, which can be posttraumatic or spontaneous. Enlargement of lesions can also occur rapidly during upper respiratory infection. Significant enlargement may cause pain, extraocular motility restriction with diplopia, compressive optic neuropathy, and vision loss. These malformations are infiltrative and may be present in both the intraconal and extraconal spaces with extension superficially into the eyelids or conjunctiva. Workup should include a thorough review of systems as there may be multiple lesions present systemically. Diagnostic orbital imaging should be performed to help verify the diagnosis and extent of lesions. CT imaging will demonstrate a poorly defined, heterogeneously enhancing, multicystic lesion. Fluid–fluid levels and blood of different ages may be identifiable on MRI. The infiltrative nature and risk of significant intraoperative bleeding cause difficulty during attempted surgical resection. Most commonly, lesions are monitored without intervention or treated by a team approach including an interventional radiologist and orbit surgeon. The use of multiple sclerosing agents such as bleomycin, OK-432 (picibanil), onyx, sodium tetradecyl sulfate, ethanol, doxycycline, and others have been described in the literature. Injection of these agents directly into the macro- and microcysts under radiographic guidance is performed and the sclerosant induces collapse of the cyst walls, effectively decreasing the lesion size.[15] A handful of pediatric lymphangiomas have also been successfully treated with oral sildenafil, but larger studies are needed.[16] Surgery should generally be undertaken sparingly given the risk for these tumors to bleed intraoperatively and enlarge aggressively postoperatively. Injection of hardening agents such as cyanoacrylate and Ethiodol into selected lesions prior to resection may lessen hemorrhage during surgery.[17]

## 12.3.4 Varix

Orbital varices are congenital dilated venous channels that may present with progressive proptosis or may be visible and present from birth superficially on the eyelids or ocular surface. These lesions may thrombose, resulting in orbital pain, motility restriction, or, rarely, vision loss. Valsalva maneuver and prone positioning will characteristically cause enlargement and temporarily worsen proptosis. Workup should include diagnostic orbital imaging. CT imaging will show a hyperdense, ovoid, or cylindrical lesion in the orbit that enhances heterogeneously with contrast. MRI demonstrates a lesion that is isointense on T1 imaging and variable intensity on T2 imaging that increases visibly in size with Valsalva during dynamic imaging.[18] Treatment generally involves observation unless there is visual compromise, in which case a combination of surgical drainage and excision is undertaken.[4] In some cases, endovascular embolization or sclerotherapy may be attempted.[19,20]

Other extremely rare vasculogenic orbital lesions include angiosarcoma, Kaposi's sarcoma, angiomyoma, and hemangioendothelioma.

# 12.4 Lacrimal Gland Neoplasms

Lacrimal gland lesions comprise 10% of all orbital masses. Of these, 20% are epithelial and the remaining 80% are nonepithelial. About half of primary epithelial lacrimal gland tumors are benign and half are malignant.[21] Malignant epithelial lacrimal gland tumors tend to present in young to middle-aged adults, with equal frequency in men and women. Presenting symptoms may include pain if there is bony or nerve invasion, as well as increasing proptosis, inferotemporal globe displacement, motility restriction, and ptosis over the course of several months.

Benign epithelial lacrimal gland tumors also present with proptosis and inferotemporal globe displacement, but the time course of progression tends to be greater than that in malignant tumors.

## 12.4.1 Adenocarcinoma

Primary lacrimal gland adenocarcinoma is an extremely rare malignant epithelial tumor that presents with an enlarging, firm, nonmobile mass of the superotemporal orbit. Ptosis, hypoglobus, diplopia, and vision changes may occur as the mass enlarges. Pain may occur with perineural invasion. This aggressive neoplasm may have distant metastases or regional invasion upon presentation. Orbital CT and MRI should be performed and will reveal a homogeneously enhancing lacrimal gland mass with poorly defined margins and bony remodeling of the lacrimal gland fossa.[4] Biopsy is performed to confirm the diagnosis, and staging should be performed with PET-CT evaluation for lymph node or distant metastases. Treatment is surgical with wide margins or orbital exenteration, with the addition of neoadjuvant or adjuvant chemotherapy and adjuvant orbital irradiation. However, recurrence rates are high and prognosis for survival is poor.

## 12.4.2 Adenoid Cystic Carcinoma

Adenoid cystic carcinoma is the most common malignant epithelial tumor of the lacrimal gland, comprising about 60% of primary epithelial lacrimal gland tumors. This rare neoplasm

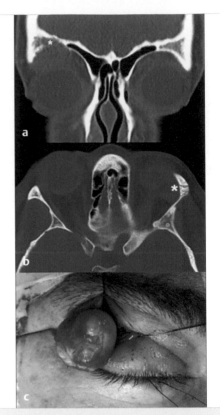

**Fig. 12.4** Noncontrast CT (computed tomography) bone windows can help distinguish a malignant from a benign lacrimal gland mass. **(a)** Adenoid cystic carcinoma of the right lacrimal gland with bony erosion through the orbital roof (*asterisk*). **(b)** Benign mixed tumor of the left lacrimal gland with characteristic scalloping of the lacrimal fossa (*asterisk*). **(c)** Bosselations visible on the surface of the tumor.

presents typically between ages 40 and 60 years and may have a biphasic age peak with a cohort of patients 25 years younger, without any sex predilection. Patients present with several months of progressive proptosis and hypoglobus with pain due to a high rate of perineural invasion. Ptosis, diplopia, and visual disturbance may occur as the mass enlarges. Orbital imaging should be ordered to identify and further characterize the mass. CT should be reviewed to evaluate for bone invasion and destruction, which occurs frequently, and will demonstrate an irregular lacrimal gland mass that may have flecks of calcification (▶ Fig. 12.4). MRI demonstrates an irregularly bordered mass with enhancement with contrast. Anterior orbitotomy with biopsy of the mass should be performed to confirm the diagnosis, followed by rapid referral to an oncologist for staging workup. Treatment modalities are currently quite controversial and are still evolving due to the poor prognosis of this tumor, which confers 20% survival at 10 years. Traditionally, orbital exenteration, followed by irradiation was recommended and is still the most commonly utilized treatment despite not improving survival rates. A newer modification to this protocol that adds neoadjuvant intra-arterial chemotherapy administered via the lacrimal vasculature has been recently espoused. Ten-year data for a series of 19 patients treated with this protocol demonstrated improved survival rates of 50 to 100%.[22]

Other extremely rare malignant lacrimal gland tumors include mucoepidermoid carcinoma, epithelial–myoepithelial carcinoma, malignant mixed tumor, oncocytoma, Warthin's tumor, myoepithelioma, and poorly differentiated carcinomas.

## 12.4.3 Benign Mixed Tumor

Benign mixed tumor, also known as pleomorphic adenoma, is the most common benign epithelial tumor of the lacrimal gland. This neoplasm presents with progressive, painless proptosis and hypoglobus, with onset of symptoms typically noted for over a year. Patients may additionally exhibit ptosis, diplopia, and vision disturbance with a firm, palpable nontender mass. The age at presentation is typically between the second and fifth decades with a slight male predilection.[4] Orbital CT and MRI reveal well-circumscribed enlargement of a portion or all of the lacrimal gland, and CT may demonstrate bony expansion of the lacrimal gland fossa (▸ Fig. 12.4). Enhancement with contrast may be homogeneous or heterogeneous. Treatment is complete surgical excision, ideally with the pseudocapsule intact, as spilled tumor cells may seed the surrounding tissues, resulting in recurrence with or without transformation to malignant mixed tumor at a rate of 10% per decade.[4]

## 12.5 Cystic Lesion: Dermoid Cyst

Dermoid cysts are the most common cystic orbital lesions of childhood. They typically present as a slowly enlarging subcutaneous area of firm, painless swelling, and most commonly appear in the superotemporal orbit (▸ Fig. 12.5). Dermoid cysts arise at bony suture lines, most frequently at the frontozygomatic suture, but can also appear at the frontoethmoid, sphenozygomatic, or frontolacrimal sutures. They may take on a "dumbbell" bilobed configuration with extension into the orbit. Diagnosis is generally clinical, but imaging may be considered if there is a diagnostic dilemma or to rule out orbital involvement. MRI will show a well-circumscribed rim-enhancing lesion, filled with homogeneous material and often surrounding molding of the bone. The cyst contents will be hypointense on MRI T1 and hyperintense on T2 sequences, with isointensity to vitreous or fat.[23] Occasionally, dermoid cysts may rupture due

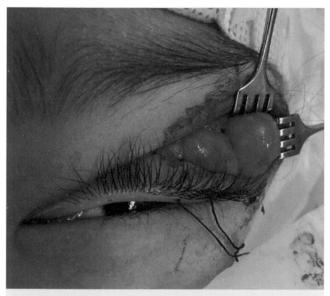

**Fig. 12.5** Dermoid cyst arising at the left frontozygomatic suture.

to mild trauma, resulting in significant inflammation surrounding the mass. Treatment is surgical excision, with intraoperative irrigation with saline, water, or steroid solution if cyst contents are exposed to the surrounding tissues to decrease the postoperative inflammatory response.

Rarer cystic masses that may appear primarily in the orbit include simple epithelial cysts, which may occur congenitally or secondarily to trauma or surgery, colobomatous cysts, and teratoma with cysts.

## 12.6 Mesenchymal Tumors

### 12.6.1 Solitary Fibrous Tumor

Solitary fibrous tumor (SFT) is a nonencapsulated benign spindle cell tumor that typically presents with painless, slow proptosis in middle-aged patients, although they can be diagnosed in any age group. New histopathologic techniques have led to increased recognition of these tumors in the orbit.[24] Clinically, patients may experience eyelid edema, extraocular motility restriction, globe displacement, or compressive optic neuropathy if the lesion is large or posterior. CT or MRI show a well-circumscribed mass, iso- to hypointense on MRI T2-weighted imaging, with heterogeneous enhancement.[25] Calcification may be seen on CT, as well as bony erosion in chronic lesions. Complete surgical excision is recommended, as in rare cases malignant transformation has been reported. Often complete excision is not possible because of tumor location or extent, and repeat debulking or proton beam radiation therapy may be considered in these cases.

### 12.6.2 Fibrous Histiocytoma and Hemangiopericytoma

Fibrous histiocytoma and hemangiopericytoma are other spindle cell tumors that can be confused with SFTs histopathologically. Given morphologic similarities, many "fibrous histiocytomas" in past literature have since been reclassified as SFTs, and some believe these lesions should be combined into a single category.[26] Fibrous histiocytomas were once considered the most common orbital mesenchymal tumor, but this is less clear now. Fibrous histiocytomas, like SFTs, are thought to arise from pluripotential mesenchymal cells of the soft tissue in middle-aged adults. Patients present with progressive proptosis, ptosis, eyelid and conjunctival edema, motility restriction and, in some cases, pain. These neoplasms most commonly appear superonasally but can be located anywhere in the orbit. On neuroimaging, the tumor is homogeneous, encapsulated, and well circumscribed with either smooth or irregular borders, and may enhance homogeneously or heterogeneously.[27] Less commonly, the tumor can be invasive locally or undergo malignant degeneration, so treatment involves excision. Malignant tumors require wide resection. Even benign lesions have a tendency to recur, however, and may require repeat resection.

### 12.6.3 Fibrous Dysplasia

Fibrous dysplasia is a hamartomatous congenital lesion found within the orbital bones, most commonly frontal, causing thickening and mass effect on orbital contents and frontal bossing.

Onset may occur in childhood or young adulthood. Affected patients note facial asymmetry that progresses slowly. Orbital volume can decrease due to bone thickening, causing ptosis, proptosis, and globe dystopia. More severe sequelae include lagophthalmos with corneal exposure, orbital apical compression, vision loss from optic canal obstruction, nasolacrimal duct obstruction, and compromise of cranial nerves V1, V2, and V3 from foraminal narrowing. In the polyostotic form, the McCune–Albright syndrome, multiple bones may be involved. CT imaging of the orbits should be performed. Debulking surgery is necessary in cases of progressive proptosis or foraminal obstruction causing clinical symptoms of vision loss, sensory loss, corneal exposure, or strabismus. Dacryocystorhinostomy may be required in cases of nasolacrimal obstruction. Radiation treatment is avoided due to an increased risk of malignant transformation into sarcomatous tumors.[28]

### 12.6.4 Fibrosarcoma

Fibrosarcomas are mesenchymal tumors that rarely arise primarily in the orbit or more commonly invade secondarily from the sinuses. They may arise at any age, although they appear most commonly in young to middle-aged adults. Radiation treatment to the orbital area predisposes to formation of these neoplasms. Patients present with subacute, often painful, progressive proptosis, and may also have ptosis, motility restriction, orbital pain, globe dystopia, and vision compromise. On neuroimaging, the tumor appears as well-circumscribed lytic areas within bone with areas of erosion, necrosis, and hemorrhage. Surgical excision with wide frozen-section margins is the treatment of choice given propensity to recur. Adjuvant radiation therapy can be considered as well. Locoregional spread is of primary concern as metastatic rates are low.[4]

### 12.6.5 Juvenile Xanthogranuloma

Juvenile xanthogranuloma (JXG) is a benign non-Langerhans cell histiocytosis that presents within the first several years of life with orange cutaneous nodules and single or multiple masses involving any body part including the orbit. The most common ocular sign is iris nodules, but JXG lesions can appear in the orbit, conjunctiva, optic nerve, or elsewhere. Orbital lesions are commonly anterior and may be palpable; systemic workup should be performed as 5% of patients may have involvement elsewhere. Neuroimaging of orbital tumors demonstrates a poorly circumscribed, infiltrative appearing mass with some enhancement. Management of nonclinically significant lesions is by monitoring as they often involute over several years. Tumors causing amblyopia may be treated with corticosteroids or surgery.

Rarely, lipoid mesenchymal tumors such as lipomas, liposarcomas, and myxofibrosarcomas appear primarily in the orbit.

### 12.6.6 Rhabdomyosarcoma

Rapidly progressive proptosis over days to weeks in a child should always trigger concern for presence of a rhabdomyosarcoma (▶ Fig. 12.6). This is a malignant neoplasm that arises from pluripotent mesenchymal cells, typically presenting within the first 10 years of life. It is the most common mesenchymal orbital

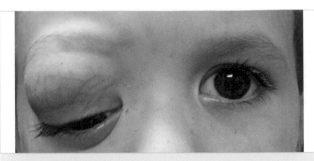

**Fig. 12.6** Right orbital rhabdomyosarcoma most commonly occurs within the first decade of life and must be considered in any child presenting with rapidly progressive proptosis.

tumor in the pediatric population, comprising about 4% of all pediatric orbital masses.[4] Although these masses can grow anywhere in the orbit, they most commonly originate in the superonasal quadrant, causing nonaxial proptosis in the direction opposite to the mass. Clinically, patients may appear to have periorbital edema that is erythematous or ecchymotic, which may be mistaken for cellulitis. There may be associated mechanical ptosis, extraocular muscle restriction, and proptosis. Neuroimaging shows an enhancing well-circumscribed, irregular, typically extraconal mass that may have intraconal extension. There may be adjacent bony destruction as well as intralesional hemorrhage. Bone involvement is best appreciated on a CT scan, while MRI may be required to detect intracranial extension. An urgent biopsy should be performed to confirm the diagnosis, systemic workup performed to rule out metastasis, and treatment begun immediately with chemoradiation therapy. Surgical debulking of the tumor should be undertaken whenever possible, preferably at the time of initial biopsy, as this alters the treatment protocol. The prognosis is generally very good with treatment, but is dependent on the subtype and tumor extent. Pleomorphic or embryonal rhabdomyosarcoma comprise the vast majority of cases and portend a 90% survival rate,[4] but the less common inferior alveolar subtype confers a worse prognosis particularly if there is metastatic spread.

Rare myogenic/mesenchymal lesions include leiomyoma, leiomyosarcoma, rhabdomyoma, and malignant rhabdoid tumor.

## 12.7 Neurogenic Tumors

### 12.7.1 Primary Central Nervous System Tumors

#### Optic Nerve Glioma

Optic nerve gliomas are slowly progressive, benign tumors of childhood. They enlarge painlessly, causing progressive axial proptosis that can eventually lead to vision loss and intracranial extension. Neuroimaging shows a fusiform enlargement of the optic nerve, often with cystic degeneration and a characteristic kink that is virtually pathognomonic for optic nerve glioma. About 20% of optic nerve gliomas are associated with neurofibromatosis type I,[29] and these patients may have bilateral gliomas. MRI of the orbit and brain should be performed in an effort to determine the posterior border of the tumor and for serial monitoring. Management of these tumors depends on

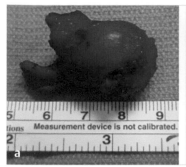
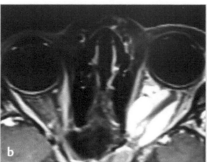

**Fig. 12.7** **(a)** Excised optic nerve glioma including intracanicular tumor. **(b)** Corresponding axial T1-weighted, postcontrast MRI (magnetic resonance imaging) demonstrating a large fusiform mass arising from the left optic nerve extending into the optic canal.

their growth. Tumors that grow slowly and do not reach the optic canal should be monitored with serial neuroimaging, while those that breach the optic canal should be excised (▶ Fig. 12.7).[30]

## Optic Nerve Meningioma

Slowly progressive, painless vision loss in a middle-aged patient presenting with axial proptosis should raise concern for an optic nerve sheath meningioma. These rare, benign neoplasms arise from the optic nerve meningeal arachnoid villi, in the same fashion as the more common intracranial meningiomas. Vision is progressively compromised due to optic nerve compression by tumor growth. The slow pace of growth often leads to formation of optociliary shunt vessels on the optic disc, as well as pallid optic nerve edema. Neuroimaging may show calcification within the tumor, optic nerve enlargement, and "tram-tracking," parallel linear radiodensities along the periphery of the optic nerve that are a pathognomonic sign of optic nerve meningioma. Biopsy of these tumors is not advised, since the optic nerve and tumor share the same blood supply, and biopsy can lead to profound visual loss. Because of this, treatment is usually nonsurgical involving stereotactic radiotherapy.[31,32]

## 12.7.2 Primary Peripheral Nerve Sheath Tumors

### Schwannoma

Schwannomas are encapsulated, benign Schwann cell neoplasms arising from peripheral nerves, and may occur in the orbit, typically in young and middle-aged adults. They appear most commonly along the supraorbital and supratrochlear nerves and may cause pain or sensory deficits. If large, these neoplasms may cause globe displacement, dysmotility, or optic neuropathy. Neuroimaging shows an enhancing, well-circumscribed fusiform mass within the intraconal or extraconal space along the pathway of a peripheral nerve. There may be cystic degeneration or calcification within the mass. Tumors may be monitored with serial imaging or excised if symptomatic.[4,33]

### Neurofibroma

Neurofibromas are nonencapsulated, benign Schwann cell neoplasms that also arise from peripheral nerves within and

around the orbit. They are the most common facial hamartomatous lesions. They can take many forms and may be focal, diffuse, or plexiform, and are associated with neurofibromatosis. Plexiform neurofibromas are indicative of underlying neurofibromatosis, and classically cause an **S**-shaped deformity of the eyelid. Clinical symptoms depend on the area of involvement but may include diplopia, ptosis, pain, and proptosis. Neurofibromas are infiltrative lesions, making complete excision nearly impossible. Hence, observation is the treatment of choice. Debulking surgery is undertaken if extensive eyelid involvement affects the visual field or, in the pediatric patient, causes occlusive or astigmatic amblyopia.

### Malignant Peripheral Nerve Sheath Tumor

Malignant peripheral nerve sheath tumor is a rare tumor that may arise from malignant degeneration of a neurofibroma, particularly in adult patients with neurofibromatosis or in a previously irradiated orbit. They may grow along any peripheral or cranial nerve sheath, although they appear most commonly along the supraorbital nerve. These tumors present with similar symptoms as their benign counterparts, but are highly aggressive with more rapid onset of symptoms. They tend to be focal rather than infiltrative, having an irregular fusiform appearance, and may spread intracranially or metastasize to lymph nodes and lungs. Neuroimaging may show bony erosion of a heterogeneously enhancing mass.[34] Treatment is by wide surgical resection or palliative debulking, but recurrence rates are high and the prognosis poor.[33]

## 12.8 Osseous and Fibro-osseous Neoplasms

### 12.8.1 Osteoma

Osteomas are the most common tumors of paranasal sinus bone and less commonly present primarily in the orbit. They typically occur in young to middle-aged adult males. The vast majority of osteomas affect the sinuses alone, causing complaints of chronic sinusitis, but some arise primarily in the orbit causing proptosis, diplopia, pain with eye movement, vision loss, or gaze-evoked amaurosis. Most commonly, inferolateral globe displacement is seen due to involvement of the frontal or ethmoid sinuses. CT imaging is most helpful to delineate the extent of involvement. Patients presenting with multiple osteomas should be evaluated for Gardner's syndrome, which may include adenomatous colon polyps, desmoid tumors, or lipomas. Symptomatic patients, presenting with vision loss or other sequelae, require excision or debulking surgery, along with orbital reconstruction.[35]

## 12.8.2 Ewing Sarcoma

Ewing sarcoma arises from neuroectodermal cells, and presents classically in Caucasian male elementary-aged children. It is extremely rare in the orbit as a primary tumor or metastasis, but may present with slowly progressive, painful double vision, ptosis, and proptosis. Bony destruction is evident on CT imaging. Biopsy confirms the diagnosis, and treatment involves chemotherapy, radiation, and surgical debulking.[4,36]

## 12.8.3 Aneurysmal Bone Cyst

Aneurysmal bone cysts of the orbit are unusual, benign fibro-osseous lesions that are more typically found in the long bones or vertebrae, with fewer than 30 orbital cases reported in the literature. Two-thirds are primary orbital lesions and the remainder are secondary. Most cases present prior to the age of 20 years as a rapidly expanding orbital mass causing proptosis, motility restriction, and vision loss. MRI and CT show a heterogeneously enhancing mass that exhibits bony erosion of the adjacent orbital walls and may extend into adjacent sinuses or intracranially. These are important to distinguish from lymphangiomas, which also comprise multicystic lesions with fluid–fluid levels on imaging. Histopathology demonstrates a spindle-cell mass with sinusoidal vascular spaces separated by fibrous stroma, without malignant features. Workup should rule out associated disorders such as fibrous dysplasia, osteoblastoma, and neurofibromatosis type 1, which can all prompt growth of secondary orbital lesions.[37,38]

## 12.8.4 Other Benign and Malignant Osseous Tumors

Uncommon benign osseous lesions include osteoblastoma and ossifying fibroma, both of which involve the shared bones of the orbit and adjacent sinuses. Excisional surgery is typically performed when these lesions are identified because they may grow rapidly and cause compression of orbital contents, and if only partially resected may recur.

Osteosarcoma is the most common malignant orbital bony tumor, although it is almost always a secondary tumor presenting with invasion from the sinuses. Rarely, it may represent an orbital metastasis from a distant primary tumor. It may also uncommonly arise primarily within an area of orbital fibrous dysplasia, particularly after radiation treatment.[4] Treatment involves wide excision, chemotherapy, and radiation.

## References

[1] Stefanovic A, Lossos IS. Extranodal marginal zone lymphoma of the ocular adnexa. Blood. 2009; 114(3):501–510

[2] Ferry JA, Fung CY, Zukerberg L, et al. Lymphoma of the ocular adnexa: a study of 353 cases. Am J Surg Pathol. 2007; 31(2):170–184

[3] Collina F, De Chiara A, De Renzo A, De Rosa G, Botti G, Franco R. Chlamydia psittaci in ocular adnexa MALT lymphoma: a possible role in lymphomagenesis and a different geographical distribution. Infect Agent Cancer. 2012; 7:8

[4] Black ENF, Calvano C, Gladstone G, Levine M, eds. Smith and Nesi's Ophthalmic Plastic and Reconstructive Surgery. 3rd ed. New York, NY: Springer; 2012

[5] Rasmussen P, Sjö LD, Prause JU, Ralfkiaer E, Heegaard S. Mantle cell lymphoma in the orbital and adnexal region. Br J Ophthalmol. 2009; 93(8): 1047–1051

[6] Rasmussen PK, Coupland SE, Finger PT, et al. Ocular adnexal follicular lymphoma: a multicenter international study. JAMA Ophthalmol. 2014; 132 (7):851–858

[7] Bidar M, Wilson MW, Laquis SJ, et al. Clinical and imaging characteristics of orbital leukemic tumors. Ophthal Plast Reconstr Surg. 2007; 23(2):87–93

[8] Haik BG, Karcioglu ZA, Gordon RA, Pechous BP. Capillary hemangioma (infantile periocular hemangioma). Surv Ophthalmol. 1994; 38(5):399–426

[9] Chambers CB, Katowitz WR, Katowitz JA, Binenbaum G. A controlled study of topical 0.25% timolol maleate gel for the treatment of cutaneous infantile capillary hemangiomas. Ophthal Plast Reconstr Surg. 2012; 28(2):103–106

[10] Semkova K, Kazandjieva J. Rapid complete regression of an early infantile hemangioma with topical timolol gel. Int J Dermatol. 2014; 53(2):241–242

[11] Tawfik AA, Alsharnoubi J. Topical timolol solution versus laser in treatment of infantile hemangioma: a comparative study. Pediatr Dermatol. 2015; 32 (3):369–376

[12] Ni N, Guo S, Langer P. Current concepts in the management of periocular infantile (capillary) hemangioma. Curr Opin Ophthalmol. 2011; 22(5):419–425

[13] Davis KR, Hesselink JR, Dallow RL, Grove AS, Jr. CT and ultrasound in the diagnosis of cavernous hemangioma and lymphangioma of the orbit. J Comput Tomogr. 1980; 4(2):98–104

[14] Harris GJ, Jakobiec FA. Cavernous hemangioma of the orbit. J Neurosurg. 1979; 51(2):219–228

[15] Shiels WE, II, Kang DR, Murakami JW, Hogan MJ, Wiet GJ. Percutaneous treatment of lymphatic malformations. Otolaryngology–head and neck surgery: official journal of American Academy of Otolaryngology-. Head Neck Surg. 2009; 141(2):219–224

[16] Gandhi NG, Lin LK, O'Hara M. Sildenafil for pediatric orbital lymphangioma. JAMA Ophthalmol. 2013; 131(9):1228–1230

[17] Malhotra AD, Parikh M, Garibaldi DC, Merbs SL, Miller NR, Murphy K. Resection of an orbital lymphangioma with the aid of an intralesional liquid polymer. AJNR Am J Neuroradiol. 2005; 26(10):2630–2634

[18] Magrath GN, Wright HE, Proctor CM. Dynamic MRI of an orbital varix. Ophthal Plast Reconstr Surg. 2015; 31(3):e78

[19] Kumar RR, Singh A, Singh A, Abhishek. Embolization of a deep orbital varix through endovascular route. Indian J Ophthalmol. 2015; 63(3):270–272

[20] Vadlamudi V, Gemmete JJ, Chaudhary N, Pandey AS, Kahana A. Transvenous sclerotherapy of a large symptomatic orbital venous varix using a microcatheter balloon and bleomycin. J Neurointerv Surg. 2016; 8(8):e30

[21] Shields JA, Shields CL, Scartozzi R. Survey of 1264 patients with orbital tumors and simulating lesions: the 2002 Montgomery Lecture, part 1. Ophthalmology. 2004; 111(5):997–1008

[22] Tse DT, Kossler AL, Feuer WJ, Benedetto PW. Long-term outcomes of neoadjuvant intra-arterial cytoreductive chemotherapy for lacrimal gland adenoid cystic carcinoma. Ophthalmology. 2013; 120(7):1313–1323

[23] Jung WS, Ahn KJ, Park MR, et al. The radiological spectrum of orbital pathologies that involve the lacrimal gland and the lacrimal fossa. Korean J Radiol. 2007; 8(4):336–342

[24] Bernardini FP, de Conciliis C, Schneider S, Kersten RC, Kulwin DR. Solitary fibrous tumor of the orbit: is it rare? Report of a case series and review of the literature. Ophthalmology. 2003; 110(7):1442–1448

[25] Yang BT, Wang YZ, Dong JY, Wang XY, Wang ZC. MRI study of solitary fibrous tumor in the orbit. AJR Am J Roentgenol. 2012; 199(4):W506–11

[26] Furusato E, Valenzuela IA, Fanburg-Smith JC, et al. Orbital solitary fibrous tumor: encompassing terminology for hemangiopericytoma, giant cell angiofibroma, and fibrous histiocytoma of the orbit: reappraisal of 41 cases. Hum Pathol. 2011; 42(1):120–128

[27] Dalley RW. Fibrous histiocytoma and fibrous tissue tumors of the orbit. Radiol Clin North Am. 1999; 37(1):185–194

[28] Ricalde P, Magliocca KR, Lee JS. Craniofacial fibrous dysplasia. Oral Maxillofac Surg Clin North Am. 2012; 24(3):427–441

[29] Listernick R, Ferner RE, Liu GT, Gutmann DH. Optic pathway gliomas in neurofibromatosis-1: controversies and recommendations. Ann Neurol. 2007; 61(3):189–198

[30] Shriver EM, Ragheb J, Tse DT. Combined transcranial-orbital approach for resection of optic nerve gliomas: a clinical and anatomical study. Ophthal Plast Reconstr Surg. 2012; 28(3):184–191

[31] Turbin RE, Thompson CR, Kennerdell JS, Cockerham KP, Kupersmith MJ. A long-term visual outcome comparison in patients with optic nerve sheath meningioma managed with observation, surgery, radiotherapy, or surgery and radiotherapy. Ophthalmology. 2002; 109(5):890–899, discussion 899–900

[32] Lesser RL, Knisely JP, Wang SL, Yu JB, Kupersmith MJ. Long-term response to fractionated radiotherapy of presumed optic nerve sheath meningioma. Br J Ophthalmol. 2010; 94(5):559–563

[33] Sweeney AR, Gupta D, Keene CD, et al. Orbital peripheral nerve sheath tumors. Surv Ophthalmol. 2017; 62(1):43–57

[34] Kim HY, Hwang JY, Kim HJ, et al. CT, MRI, and 18F-FDG PET/CT findings of malignant peripheral nerve sheath tumor of the head and neck. Acta Radiol. 2017; 58(10):1222–1230

[35] Wei LA, Ramey NA, Durairaj VD, et al. Orbital osteoma: clinical features and management options. Ophthal Plast Reconstr Surg. 2014; 30(2):168–174

[36] Alfaar AS, Zamzam M, Abdalla B, Magdi R, El-Kinaai N. Childhood Ewing sarcoma of the orbit. J Pediatr Hematol Oncol. 2015; 37(6):433–437

[37] Menon J, Brosnahan DM, Jellinek DA. Aneurysmal bone cyst of the orbit: a case report and review of literature. Eye (Lond). 1999; 13(Pt 6):764–768

[38] Johnson TE, Bergin DJ, McCord CD. Aneurysmal bone cyst of the orbit. Ophthalmology. 1988; 95(1):86–89

# 13  Open Management of Primary Orbital Neoplasms

*Susan Tonya Stefko, Paul A. Gardner, and Carl Snyderman*

**Abstract**

Tumors may affect the orbit from within. The chief complaints of these patients include protrusion of the eye (proptosis), double vision (diplopia), and pain. The surgical approach to the tumor ideally is determined by the relationship of the mass to the important neurovascular structures of the orbit. A surgeon must be able to offer anterior orbitotomies for those masses anterior to the equator of the eyeball. Approaches including osteotomies are appropriate for growths which are posterior to the equator and lie lateral and/or inferior and superior to the optic nerve. It is critical to think through the goal of surgery (biopsy, debulking, or resection), and plan the approach with the greatest likelihood of success and safety.

*Keywords:* orbit, tumor, orbitotomy

## 13.1  Introduction

Primary neoplasms of the orbit include a wide range of pathology, and these differ between children and adults. The position of the neoplasm in the orbit in relation to the optic nerve, extraocular muscles, blood vessels, and other cranial nerves, perhaps more so than the type of neoplasm, will determine whether the mass is suitable for an open surgical approach or an endoscopic endonasal approach. As surgeons, we have traditionally been taught surgical approaches by those in our own specialties, and this sometimes limits the choices we offer the patient. Our patients benefit from multidisciplinary care; depending on the approach, the surgical team may include ophthalmology, otolaryngology, neurosurgery, plastic surgery, and maxillofacial surgery.

## 13.2  Patient Selection and Indications

Adults with orbital masses will be found to harbor a malignant tumor in about one-third of cases[1,2] In children, the incidence of malignancy is a bit lower, about one in four.[3] The most frequently encountered type of tumor is vasculogenic, with cavernous hemangioma and lymphangioma (lymphovenous malformation) representing the majority of these. Cavernomas are recognizable by their smooth exterior, (sometimes late) contrast enhancement, and slow growth. These should be resected when the risk–benefit ratio is favorable, as many can be observed. Lymphovenous malformations are very low flow lesions that often have multiple cysts and a bright appearance on T2-weighted magnetic resonance imaging (MRI) sequences. These are not generally amenable to resection and should be sent for sclerotherapy or embolization. In the event of an acute bleed into a lymphovenous malformation with severe pain or optic neuropathy, these may be decompressed from an anterior approach by aspiration. Even in adults, dermoid cysts are the most commonly encountered cystic mass. These should be excised intact, but computed tomography (CT) is necessary to

evaluate the adjacent bone for defect, either with extension of the cyst or with encephalocele.

Other common primary orbital malignancies include lymphoma, sarcoma, and lacrimal gland malignancies.[4] In several series, lymphoid neoplasms comprise about 10% of orbital space occupying lesions and about half of lacrimal gland masses. Incisional biopsy is indicted in many cases, but care should be taken preoperatively to characterize lacrimal gland lesions, as some should be excised in toto (benign mixed tumor/pleomorphic adenoma). The tissue should be sent both in formalin and fresh for possible cell sorting, and the receiving lab should be notified of the surgeon's clinical suspicion. Metastatic masses in adults represent about 3% of all orbital masses, and breast, prostate, and lung are the most common of these. Bilateral orbital masses suggest systemic disorders or metastasis.

## 13.3  Diagnostic Workup

The most common presenting complaints of a patient with an orbital mass will be proptosis (increased projection of the eye) and double vision. Others may include pain, dryness or irritation of the eye, or tearing. Decreased vision is often a late symptom or sign.

The patient's medical and surgical history, particularly regarding autoimmune disorders and malignancies, must be first discussed. Medications, with attention to anticoagulants, must be assessed. A complete physical examination of the orbit, preferably by an ophthalmologist experienced in orbit surgery, must be performed, including documentation of visual function, proptosis, strabismus, and examination of the posterior segment of the eye. If indicated, an examination of the head and neck with particular attention to the nose, paranasal sinuses, and lymph nodes, should be performed. Nasal or sinus endoscopy may be indicated.

The first radiologic study in a patient's workup is usually CT of the orbits. CT is helpful in delineating the size and location of the lesion and is also important for assessing whether and how the bone is involved in the pathologic process. There may be bony deformity or expansion, frank destruction, or no bony change, which may be of significance in elucidating the diagnosis. When working up a likely orbital mass, intravenous (IV) contrast can be very helpful in its characterization. If the patient is allergic to contrast, pretreatment with antihistamine or corticosteroid may allow for contrast use. MRI of the orbits with and without contrast is very helpful in delineating soft-tissue detail. Even without contrast, the orbital fat acts as natural contrast for the other orbital structures, so it is important to look at both fat-suppressed and non-fat-suppressed images. Additional radiologic considerations may be found in Chapter 3.

In patients with suspected malignancy (infiltrative or destructive mass, bilateral orbital tumors, lymphadenopathy) or history of cancer, a thorough evaluation for a primary tumor and metastases should be performed. Options include CT scans of the neck, chest, and abdomen, or positron emission tomography (PET). Serum markers associated with any known primary tumors may also be helpful.

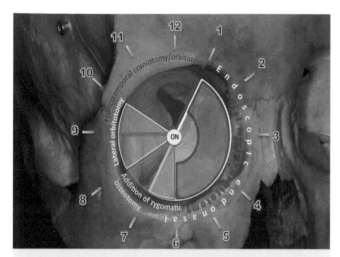

**Fig. 13.1** Clock model of the orbit summarizing how the different approaches fit together and overlap.[5] ON, optic nerve.

## 13.4 Surgical Anatomy

For neoplasms in the anterior half of the orbit (anterior to the equator of the eye, where the extraocular muscles insert), an anterior approach is appropriate. For pathology farther posterior, some osteotomy will likely be required. Though it is attractive to approach posterior pathology without bone removal, orbital fat and other soft tissues obscure the view and must be retracted deep in the orbit, greatly narrowing the corridor. As depicted in ▶ Fig. 13.1, the medial and inferomedial posterior orbit are amenable to endoscopic approaches. The inferolateral, lateral, and superior portions of the orbit require either a lateral orbitotomy or a supraorbital craniotomy for good access.

The lateral orbitotomy as originally described by Kronlein[6] is the workhorse approach for pathology of the lacrimal gland, the lateral and inferior intraconal spaces, and some limited pathology in the superior orbit. This is performed through a crow's foot incision, which is cosmetically pleasing and safe for the temporal branches of the facial nerve, which pass at least 2.4 cm posterior to the bony lateral canthus at the midpupil level. The inferior extent of the osteotomy in this approach will be at the zygomatic arch. The zygomaticofacial neurovascular bundle (sensory only) emerges on the lateral surface of the zygoma superior to the arch. When operating intraconally in this area, it is important to remember that the ciliary ganglion lies between the lateral rectus muscle and the optic nerve, about 1 cm posterior to the globe, and may be quite diaphanous in some patients (▶ Fig. 13.2).

To reach the posterosuperior orbit, a traditional supraorbital craniotomy using a hemicoronal or pterional incision is generally done. It is important to dissect the temporalis muscle planes carefully, and perform an interfascial dissection to spare the motor branch to the frontalis muscle. The supraorbital notch (or foramen) often marks the lateral-most extent of the frontal sinus and generally provides more than adequate access to the orbital roof. The extent of the sinus should be considered when planning the craniotomy, and image guidance is often used for this purpose in addition to lesion localization; avoidance makes the reconstruction simpler and less likely to become infected. The

supraorbital neurovascular bundle should be identified and preserved as much as possible during this approach. In addition to a standard supraorbital craniotomy, an "eyebrow approach" or supraorbital keyhole craniotomy can provide very similar access, though with limited frontal lobe retraction.

When approaching pathology in the medial orbit, such as with a transcaruncular approach, care must be taken to understand the relationship of the lacrimal drainage system to the incision. When opening conjunctiva and dissecting to the posterior lacrimal crest, the lacrimal drainage system stays safely anterior. The inferior oblique muscle arises from the periosteum of the maxilla just lateral to the entrance of the nasolacrimal duct. This should not be transected, but may be elevated by dissecting in a subperiosteal plane at its origin. Likewise, the trochlea, which should be mobilized by elevating it along with underlying periosteum from the bone, will be found just inside the orbital rim at the superomedial corner of the orbit. Neither muscle need be sutured back or fixated in any way when reconstructing. The anterior ethmoidal artery will be found at the level of the frontoethmoidal suture about 2.5 cm posterior to the anterior lacrimal crest in the adult orbit, and may be cauterized with bipolar electrocautery and divided if necessary. The posterior ethmoidal artery will be found about 1 cm posterior to this and may be treated in the same manner. The optic canal may then be less than 0.5 cm away and great care must be exercised.

## 13.5 Surgical Technique

### 13.5.1 Lateral Orbitotomy

The patient is positioned supine and the area from above the brow, back to the hairline, and down to the nasal ala is prepped and draped. The lateral canthus is injected with local anesthetic with epinephrine, if desired. A corneal protective lens lubricated with ointment may be sutured to the eyelids. A tenotomy scissors is used to carefully perform a lateral canthotomy. This is extended posteriorly for about 2 cm. An inferior cantholysis (and limited superior cantholysis) is performed by distracting the lid with forceps, strumming across the deep tissue between conjunctiva and skin (actually the orbital septum), and cutting along the rim until the lid is very loose.

Blunt retractors are used to hold skin edges and a malleable retractor is placed just inside the orbital rim to protect the orbital contents. Needle-tip electrocautery on low power is used to score periosteum in a superoinferior direction on the anterior surface of the orbital rim, as far superiorly as the zygomaticofrontal (ZF) suture, and as far inferiorly as the zygomatic arch. Dissection of the periosteum from the exterior surface of the rim is performed with an elevator such as a Penfield 1 or Cottle. The zygomaticofacial and zygomaticotemporal vessels should be cauterized and divided. Temporalis muscle should be peeled away from the external surface of the wall with cautery, as there is not a good subperiosteal plane. A relaxing incision in the periosteum parallel to the skin incision will make the dissection and the reconstruction easier. Dissection of the periorbita from the interior surface of the lateral wall now proceeds, keeping the periorbita as intact as possible.

A wide malleable is now placed between periorbita and bone, and the skin edge is retracted carefully so that a reciprocating saw can make two anteroposterior cuts in the lateral rim, one

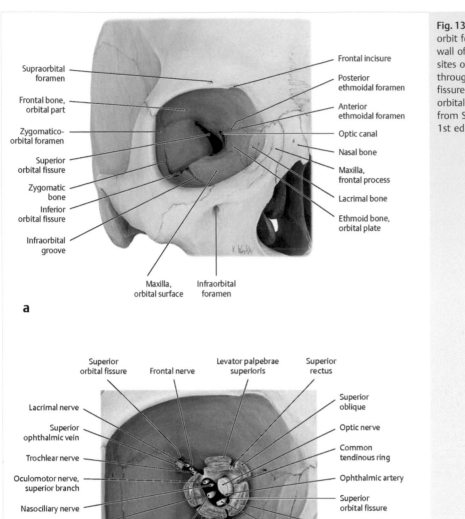

Supraorbital foramen
Frontal bone, orbital part
Zygomatico-orbital foramen
Superior orbital fissure
Zygomatic bone
Inferior orbital fissure
Infraorbital groove

Frontal incisure
Posterior ethmoidal foramen
Anterior ethmoidal foramen
Optic canal
Nasal bone
Maxilla, frontal process
Lacrimal bone
Ethmoid bone, orbital plate

Maxilla, orbital surface
Infraorbital foramen

a

**Fig. 13.2 (a)** Anterior view: opening in the right orbit for neurovascular structures. **(b)** Posterior wall of the orbit: common tendinous ring and sites of passage of neurovascular structures through the optic canal and superior orbital fissure—right orbit, anterior view with most of the orbital contents removed. (Used with permission from Schuenke et. al. Theime Atlas of Anatomy 1st ed. New York, NY: Thieme 2007.)

Superior orbital fissure
Frontal nerve
Levator palpebrae superioris
Superior rectus

Lacrimal nerve
Superior ophthalmic vein
Trochlear nerve
Oculomotor nerve, superior branch
Nasociliary nerve
Lateral rectus
Inferior orbital fissure

Superior oblique
Optic nerve
Common tendinous ring
Ophthalmic artery
Superior orbital fissure
Medial rectus
Oculomotor nerve, inferior branch

Abducent nerve
Inferior ophthalmic vein
Inferior rectus

b

just superior to the zygomatic arch and one just superior to the ZF suture. The inferior cut ends in the inferior orbital fissure. A rongeur placed at the lateral canthus now outfractures the wall and this bone is removed after clearing remaining temporalis muscle from its exterior surface with electrocautery. If the wall is too thick to fracture easily, a vertical groove may be drilled with a small drill bit such as an M8. This bone is kept safely in saline for later replacement. A rongeur or drill may be used to drill the sphenoid bone posteriorly until adequate exposure is obtained.

When opening periorbita, the incision should be made in an anteroposterior direction if possible, to avoid injury to the lateral rectus muscle. Resection of tumor and hemostasis are undertaken (▶ Fig. 13.3 and ▶ Fig. 13.4).

If a drain is to be used, it is often best placed after replacement of the lateral wall, so that undue traction is not placed on the drain. The lateral wall is replaced with two small, low-profile titanium plates, usually a dogbone plate superiorly at the ZF suture, and either a "y" or a box plate at the inferior osteotomy. It is not necessary to reconstruct the periorbita or the posterolateral orbital wall. The lateral wall may also be fixated with suture passed through angulated drilled holes created in the ends of the bone flap and adjacent fixed bones. A 5-0 braided nonabsorbable suture is passed through the tarsus of the upper lid and the lower lids (kept in the plane of the tarsus) laterally. The upper and lower lids may be resuspended from a drill hole in the lateral wall near Whitnall's tubercle, but prior to tightening these knots, a horizontally buried 6-0 Vicryl

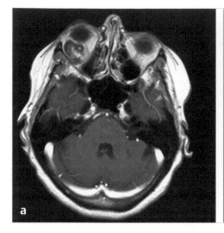
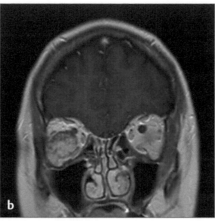

Fig. 13.3 (a) Axial T1-weighted magnetic resonance imaging (MRI) with contrast showing typical patchy contrast enhancement and smooth external contour of orbital cavernous hemangioma. (b) Coronal T1-weighted MRI with contrast of lesion in (a) showing intraconal location and later more intense uptake of contrast.

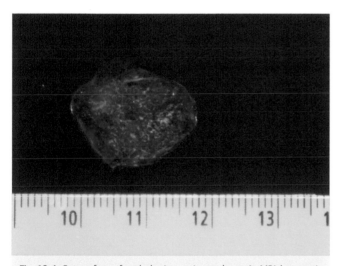

Fig. 13.4 Cut surface of pathologic specimen shown in MRI (magnetic resonance imaging) from ▶ Fig. 13.3.

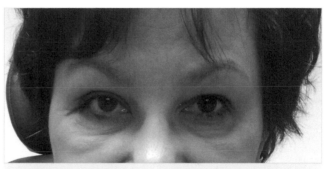

Fig. 13.5 External appearance of a patient 1 month postoperative from right lateral orbitotomy to remove lesion shown in ▶ Fig. 13.3 and ▶ Fig. 13.4.

suture is placed precisely at the lateral commissure of the lids to reappose them (in the coronal plane).

The lateral deep tissue, including periosteum, is now closed with deep 5–0 absorbable suture, and the dermis with 6–0 absorbable suture. The skin may be closed with 7–0 absorbable or nonabsorbable suture in a running fashion. The drain, if used (0.25-inch Penrose or similar), will emerge from the incision line, and this should be sutured with a 6–0 nylon purse string that can be tightened after removal of the drain the following morning (▶ Fig. 13.5).

## 13.5.2 Transconjunctival Approach for Inferior Pathology

The patient is positioned supine and the area from above the brow, back to the hairline, and down to the nasal ala is prepped and draped. The inferior conjunctival fornix is injected with local anesthetic with epinephrine, if desired. A corneal protective lens lubricated with ointment is placed, and a Desmarres retractor is used to hold back the lower eyelid. The assistant should toe in with this retractor to keep the lid anterior to the

inferior orbital rim. A malleable retractor holds back the orbital contents, and needle-tip electrocautery on low power is used to open the conjunctiva in the inferior fornix. If the mass is subperiosteal, this is deepened until the periosteum along the rim can be scored with the cautery and elevated posteriorly. If the mass is within the fat or intraconal, careful blunt dissection around the inferior rectus and inferior oblique muscles will be required. Neurosurgical cottonoids (0.5 × 3 inch) are often helpful for control of orbital fat and orientation during intraorbital dissection. If the operation is expected to last more than about an hour, or if difficulty is encountered in having enough exposure because of the margin of the lower lid, a relaxing canthotomy and cantholysis should be performed. This may be reconstructed easily at the conclusion of the case, and spares the delicate lid margin and canaliculus from undue traction.

After resection or biopsy and hemostasis, the fat may be gently reposited in the orbit. The conjunctival incision is not closed. If a drain is desired, a 0.25-inch Penrose or similar may be inserted into the surgical site and brought out to the external surface of the lid and sutured there with a loose drain stitch. If a canthotomy was performed, the lower lid is now resuspended by precise placement of a 6–0 braided absorbable stitch, buried laterally, at the lateral commissure. Skin is closed with 7–0 interrupted absorbable suture. The lower lid is now put on stretch overnight by placing a 5–0 nonabsorbable monofilament through the skin and muscle just inferior to the lower lashes and taping to the brow with Mastisol and Steri-Strips. This is removed with the drain the following day and helps align the cut edges of the conjunctiva without any introduction of foreign body such as suture. The eye is covered lightly with an absorbent dressing.

## 13.5.3 Transcaruncular Approach for Medial Pathology

This approach is suitable for pathology that is medial to the medial rectus muscle or subperiosteal. The patient is positioned supine and the surgical field (eye and lids) is prepped and draped. The medial conjunctival fornix is injected with local anesthetic with epinephrine, if desired. A protective contact lens lubricated with ointment may be placed, but often it will be difficult to maintain in position. While an assistant retracts the upper and lower lids, needle-tip electrocautery is used to open the sulcus between the plica semilunaris and the caruncle. This is carefully deepened by directing the needle tangential to the eye and medially, and extended superiorly and inferiorly in the conjunctival fornix. Blunt curved tenotomy scissors are now directed posteromedially at an angle of about 45 degrees, again tangential to the globe, toward the posterior lacrimal crest. This will be felt as a vertically oriented ridge on the medial wall of the orbit. The scissors are spread until the posterior lacrimal crest is reached, then periosteum is opened with the cautery and subperiosteal dissection is carried out posteriorly, superiorly, and inferiorly, as needed.

The anterior ethmoidal artery will be found at the level of the frontoethmoidal suture about 2.5 cm posterior to the anterior lacrimal crest in the adult orbit, and may be cauterized with bipolar electrocautery and divided if necessary. The posterior ethmoidal artery will be found about 1 cm posterior to this and may be treated in the same manner. The optic canal may then be less than 0.5 cm away and great care must be exercised. This is also the level in most patients of the cribriform plate, and rough dissection or retraction superiorly may violate the skull base.

After resection and hemostasis, the orbital tissues are gently reposited and ointment is placed in the eye. There is no closure required, nor any dressing.

## 13.5.4 Transconjunctival Approach for Intraconal Pathology

Most often, the transconjunctival approach will be used for pathology between one of the rectus muscles and the globe, which lies relatively anterior. This approach is also used for optic nerve sheath fenestrations.

An eyelid speculum is placed, and the cornea is lubricated with ointment. The surgeon and assistant must remain vigilant to replenish the ointment periodically to prevent damage to the cornea. The conjunctiva is opened with a limbal peritomy spanning 90 degrees, and radial relaxing incisions may be made at its edges. The medial, inferior, or lateral rectus muscle is

isolated on a Jameson muscle hook, limiting the dissection around it except at its insertion in order to use the surrounding connective tissue to retract orbital fat. A double-armed 6–0 braided absorbable suture on spatulated needles is used to fix the muscle tendon in any one of a number of strabismus stitches. The muscle is then carefully detached from the surface of the eye with Westcott scissors, and the sutures clamped with a bulldog clamp. A malleable retractor may now be inserted along the axis of the muscle, and another along the external surface of the globe, and the area between the globe and the muscle gently explored. Retraction of the eye laterally is facilitated by carefully passing a running stitch on a spatulated needle through the tendon stump of the muscle, without violation of sclera. If significant herniation of intraconal fat occurs, this may be controlled either with gentle irrigating bipolar cautery when away from the optic nerve, or by moist neurosurgical cottonoids.

When the biopsy or resection has been completed and the area found to have hemostasis, the rectus muscle is reattached to the surface of the eye with partial-thickness scleral bites. Care is taken neither to advance nor to recess the muscle so as not to induce strabismus. The conjunctiva is closed with two inverted sutures of absorbable suture at either end of the peritomy.

## 13.6 Supraorbital Craniotomy

Transcranial approaches to the orbit are rarely needed, but can be irreplaceable for very posterior lesions in the superior orbit (superior to the optic nerve). A large supraorbital craniotomy can be performed via a hemicoronal incision, a more medially limited supralateral craniotomy through a pterional craniotomy, and a minimally invasive supralateral craniotomy through a keyhole, "eyebrow" approach. Prior to surgery, the eye should be sutured closed after placement of ointment.

For maximal exposure and access, a hemicoronal incision is made down through galea from the contralateral superotemporal line to the skin crease immediately anterior to the ipsilateral tragus. Rainey clips are applied to the scalp and then careful subperiosteal elevation of the scalp (differential flap from temporalis) is performed, including interfascial dissection over the anterior temporalis muscle to protect the frontalis branch of the facial nerve. Varying degrees of temporalis muscle elevation are performed, from simple exposure of the pterion "keyhole" to entire muscle elevation and inferior retraction, depending on the amount of lateral orbital exposure needed. A standard frontotemporal craniotomy is then performed, with or without orbitotomy, which is generally only needed for lesions extending to the globe.[7]

The eyebrow approach, or supraorbital craniotomy, provides a minimally invasive "keyhole" approach to a similar, though slightly limited, region, and is generally all that is necessary for most superior orbital lesions. An incision is made just inferior to the superior border of the eyebrow, taking care to bevel the incision about 15 degrees from perpendicular in order to parallel in the hair follicles. Subcutaneous coagulation is avoided to preserve the follicles as well.

Needle-tip monopolar cautery is then used to dissect down to the pericranium. Superior dissection is performed deep to the frontalis muscle and medial and inferior to the frontalis branch of the facial nerve. A small, inferiorly based, "U-shaped" pericranial flap is elevated and used to retract the brow inferiorly. Hook retractors are placed on the upper part of the incision as superiorly as possible. The temporalis muscle is dissected away from the pterion "keyhole" and a single burr hole made. Careful epidural dissection is performed and a craniotome used to make a single osteotomy flush with the orbital roof. This is connected to an osteotomy that arches in line with the maximal superior skin retraction. The small bone flap is then dissected from the dura. A critical step to maximize access is the drilling of the posterior cortex of the orbital rim flush with the orbital roof. The orbital rim can also be removed as needed as a second piece or as one with the craniotomy. Care should be taken, if possible, to avoid entering the frontal sinus, as repair options are limited.

With either approach, the frontal dura is then elevated from the orbital roof, as far posteriorly as the optic canal and/or superior orbital fissure. The bone of the orbital roof is then removed with drill and/or rongeur to expose the entire superior orbit. The lateral orbit can be included with a standard craniotomy.

## 13.7 Orbital Exenteration with Temporalis Flap Transposition

This technique is used for malignancies (or selected benign pathology) in which the eye is blind and/or painful, or in which the eye constitutes one margin of a possible complete resection. Surgical margins are marked. A suture tarsorrhaphy is usually helpful. If the exenteration is to be a lid-sparing technique, an incision line several millimeters proximal to the eyelid margins and parallel to them is marked. A knife is used to cut through skin and orbicularis, and blunt dissection in the pretarsal/preseptal plane is then carried out to the level of the orbital rim. Periosteum is incised, and the surgery proceeds as described in the following text.

If the skin is to be included in the resection, the excision margins are drawn at the orbital rim and at least 1 to 2 cm from the cutaneous lesion. The marked areas may be infiltrated with local anesthetic with epinephrine to help with hemostasis. A no. 15 scalpel is used to cut through skin to the periosteum. Bleeding should be expected at the supraorbital vessels. The periosteum is elevated with a Cottle or Freer elevator, beginning at the superotemporal portion of the orbit where the bone is thickest. Dissection in this plane continues circumferentially and posteriorly, with cautery of the zygomaticofacial and zygomaticotemporal vessels encountered in the lateral wall. Resistance will occur in the area of the trochlea (superomedially) and at the canthal ligaments and may require sharp dissection in these areas. The posterior limb of the medial canthal tendon should be elevated from bone, and the lacrimal sac should be divided at its junction with the nasolacrimal canal. The inferior oblique muscle originates just lateral to the sac and should be elevated with the periosteum. Dissection proceeds posteriorly toward the orbital apex.

Special care should be directed to the following areas. Elevation of the periosteum over the lamina papyracea must be carried out very gently to avoid entry into the ethmoid sinuses. The ethmoidal vessels must be divided and bleeding controlled

with bipolar electrocautery. Areas of the orbital roof, particularly posteromedially, are often quite thin or contain frank dehiscences.

The contents of the superior and inferior orbital fissures and the apical stump must now be divided, which may be accomplished with a curved knife, curved enucleation scissors, or a snare. The latter is tightened to a soft stop and tightened sequentially over a period of several minutes to assist with hemostasis. The snare may then be tightened completely to transect the apical stump, or curved scissors may be used to cut just anterior to it. The orbit should immediately be packed with gauze and pressure applied for 5 to 10 minutes. The apex should then be explored cautiously with suction and bipolar electrocautery to localize and control any bleeding.

If the orbit is to heal by granulation, it should now be lined with a nonadherent dressing such as Telfa followed by Xeroform gauze, packed with fluffed gauze, and bandaged tightly. A small pledget of cellulose (Surgicel) or other hemostatic agent may be placed over the apical stump.

If the lid skin has been spared, it is draped over the rim and spread posteriorly as far as possible. The remainder of the orbit may be left to granulate or may be covered with a split-thickness skin graft. If a split-thickness graft is used, it is harvested from a non-hair-bearing area of the inner surface of the thigh or the abdomen and the donor site covered with an adherent dressing. Dimensions of the graft are approximately 5 × 10 cm before meshing. The graft is carefully draped into the orbital cavity, with care taken to ensure that the epithelial side remains exterior. The graft is sutured in place at the rim with interrupted 7–0 chromic gut or silk suture. The wound is then dressed as discussed earlier.

When flap reconstruction is not used, the pressure dressing remains undisturbed for 3 to 5 days. During this time, the patient should have antibiotic coverage. After this time, the pressure dressing is gently removed, and the area is soaked with saline. After 5 to 10 minutes, the lining layer (nonadherent dressing such as Telfa or Xeroform) may be gently loosened from the underlying tissue. Minimal debridement should occur at this stage because areas of skin that appear devitalized may heal surprisingly well. The area is coated lightly with antibiotic ointment, and the patient and family are instructed to repeat the application of ointment twice daily. Ointment should also be applied to the light dressing placed over the orbit to prevent adherence. Vigorous cleaning of the area should be avoided.

Transposition of the temporalis muscle (or its anterior half) through a defect created in the lateral orbital wall (either by removing the rim or by drilling through the wall) can be used to create a shallower cavity and provide a better surface for skin grafting. If the anterior half is used, the posterior half may be moved forward to prevent temporal hollowing. A right hemicoronal incision is marked out and the incision extends to the underlying skull superior to the superotemporal line and superficial to the deep temporal fascia over the temporalis muscle laterally. Upon elevating the skull flap over the temporalis muscle, the superficial fat pad superior to the zygomatic arch is identified, incised, and elevated with the flap. The root of the zygoma is identified and electrocautery is used to incise the periosteum along its superior aspect in a posterior to anterior direction to the lateral orbital rim. Periosteum overlying the zygoma is then elevated, combined with elevation over the lateral orbital rim until full exposure is obtained. Temporalis muscle is now elevated from the temporal fossa and completely mobilized. This is divided approximately in half in a vertical fashion so as to preserve the proximal blood supply to both aspects of the muscle. A window in the lateral orbital wall is drilled out if the rim has not been resected, so that the muscle flap may be passed into the orbit. If the muscle is too bulky, the orbital rim is removed. The muscle is placed into the orbit and tacked into place using 3–0 braided absorbable sutures. Any lid tissue is draped over this, and a light bandage placed. Exposed muscle may be covered with a small skin graft. The scalp incision is closed in layers using 2–0 absorbable galeal sutures after placement of a drain (no. 7 flat Jackson–Pratt drain). Skin may be closed with staples.

## 13.8 Complications

The most feared complication of orbital surgery is unexpected postoperative blindness, usually thought to be caused by excessive manipulation or traction on the optic nerve, with damage to the perfusion of the optic nerve. The incidence of vision loss from orbital surgery is likely less than 0.5%.[8] Risk of postoperative hematoma and resulting compartment syndrome causing loss of vision can be minimized by meticulous hemostasis, leaving a drain after surgery if necessary, and strict bed rest and Valsalva precautions. A recent review of orbital surgeries showed about a 1% postoperative hematoma rate, all occurring within the first 6 hours post-op and none causing vision loss.[9]

Other complications of surgery include restrictive or paralytic strabismus causing diplopia, infection, and eyelid malposition (ptosis, or turning inward or outward of the lid margin relative to the globe). Reassure patients that after orbital surgery, the eye may "swell shut" in the first few days post-op, and that this is not necessarily a cause for alarm. This is concerning only in the setting of severe pain or pressure sensation, loss of vision, or proptosis.

## 13.9 Postoperative Care

Patients are admitted for observation overnight after orbital surgery. They are administered the remainder of a 24-hour course of IV antibiotics if alloplastic material was used for reconstruction. Most patients are given steroid (e.g., Decadron 4 mg IV every 6 hours) during the admission to help control any vasogenic edema. They are kept at bed rest with the head of the bed elevated, and allowed bathroom privileges.

Drains are removed the following morning and the patient discharged home with appropriate pain medications, with strict instructions not to bend below the waist or strain for 3 days. They are to return to the ER (emergency room) immediately for any sudden decrease in vision, severe pain, or pressure sensation. Antibiotic–steroid ophthalmic ointment is used over the wounds twice a day until follow-up. Nonabsorbable sutures are removed at 5 to 7 days in the outpatient clinic.

## References

[1] Bonavolontà G, Strianese D, Grassi P, et al. An analysis of 2,480 space-occupying lesions of the orbit from 1976 to 2011. Ophthal Plast Reconstr Surg. 2013; 29(2):79–86

[2] Hassan WM, Bakry MS, Hassan HM, Alfaar AS. Incidence of orbital, conjunctival and lacrimal gland malignant tumors in USA from Surveillance, Epidemiology and End Results, 1973–2009. Int J Ophthalmol. 2016; 9(12): 1808–1813

[3] Kodsi SR, Shetlar DJ, Campbell RJ, Garrity JA, Bartley GB. A review of 340 orbital tumors in children during a 60-year period. Am J Ophthalmol. 1994; 117(2):177–182

[4] Kügel J, Sixta A, Böhme M, Krönlein A, Bode M. Breaking degeneracy of tautomerization-metastability from days to seconds. ACS Nano. 2016; 10 (12):11058–11065

[5] Paluzzi A, Gardner PA, Fernandez-Miranda JC, et al. "Round-the-clock" surgical access to the orbit. J Neurol Surg B Skull Base. 2015; 76(1):12–24

[6] Kronlein R. Zur Pathologic und Behandlung der Dermoidcysten der Orbita, Beitrage zur Klin. Chir.. 1888; IV:149

[7] Seiichiro M, Yoshinori H, Kentaro H, Naokatu S. Superolateral orbitotomy for intraorbital tumors: comparison with the conventional approach. J Neurol Surg B Skull Base. 2016; 77(6):473–478

[8] Bonavolontà G. Postoperative blindness following orbital surgery. Orbit. 2005; 24(3):195–200

[9] Guyot L, Thiery G, Salles F, Dumont N, Chossegros C. Post-operative orbital haematomas over a 12-year period. A description of three cases among 280 orbital procedures. J Craniomaxillofac Surg. 2013; 41(8):794–796

# 14 Endoscopic Management of Primary Orbital Neoplasms

Benjamin S. Bleier

## Abstract

Historically, orbital tumors have been approached via external approaches. Endoscopic sinus and skull base techniques have been progressively adapted to the management of orbital tumors, providing improved visualization while eliminating the need for globe retraction. The historical progression of these approaches, relevant surgical anatomy of the medial orbit, and surgical methodologies are discussed in this chapter. While endoscopic orbital surgery remains a nascent field, it has already demonstrated improved access to the medial orbital apex with decreased morbidity relative to external approaches. As the cumulative global surgical experience increases beyond high-volume centers, the indications for this approach are likely to continue to expand.

*Keywords:* endoscopic orbital surgery, intraconal space, cavernous hemangioma, medial rectus muscle, oculomotor nerve, ophthalmic artery

## 14.1 Introduction

Classic external approaches to the orbit include the frontotemporal craniotomy with orbitozygomatic osteotomy, transcutaneous or transconjunctival orbitotomy, and lateral orbitotomy.[1] Despite this multiplicity of options, lesions located in the medial or inferior aspect of the orbital apex have posed a significant challenge as the dissection cavity is deep, poorly illuminated, obscured by orbital fat, and often requires considerable globe retraction. Consequently, transantral approaches were introduced in an attempt to improve visualization and access to this region. Unfortunately, this approach was associated with significant morbidity including oroantral fistula, hypesthesia, and enophthalmos.[2]

Endoscopic sinus surgery was first introduced in the 1980s and its potential to improve approaches to the peri-sinonasal structures including the orbit was quickly recognized. The endoscope provided a magnified, highly illuminated view as compared to a headlight or binocular microscope. Kennedy et al[3] was among the first to apply these new endoscopic techniques to peripheral orbital structures in their early description of the endoscopic orbital decompression. These techniques continued to proliferate as more complex pathologies of the sino-orbital interface were tackled such as sinonasal tumors with orbital extension and compressive optic neuropathy.[4] In recent years, endoscopic techniques have begun to breach the sino-orbital boundary by extending into the medial extra and intraconal spaces to access primary orbital neoplasms. Thus, current state-of-the-art methods of endoscopic orbital surgery have subtended an evolutionary arc from open to endoscopic-assisted techniques and finally to purely endoscopic techniques.

## 14.2 Indications

A wide range of space occupying lesions can present in the orbit. These occur at a rate of 3 to 5 tumors per year per 1 million people, and there are no clear differences in rate based on race or gender.[5] The most common lesions are vasculogenic, constituting approximately 17% of orbital masses. Among those, cavernous hemangiomas are the most common. Other common benign lesions include optic nerve glioma (4%) and pseudotumor (8%).[5] The most common malignant lesion is non-Hodgkin's lymphoma (8%), followed by orbital metastases.

## 14.3 Diagnostic Workup

All patients presenting with an orbital tumor should be evaluated by a multidisciplinary team including an otolaryngologist and ophthalmologist. Neurosurgical consultation is not mandatory but should be considered if an adjunctive craniotomy approach may be required. All patients require a full ophthalmological examination including formal visual field testing. Patients should additionally undergo a high-resolution computed tomography (CT) scan to assess the bony structures as well as a magnetic resonance imaging (MRI) with contrast to assess the character of the lesion. Moreover, the contrast-enhanced MRI will help the surgeon assess whether the ophthalmic artery crosses above or below the optic nerve. Three-dimensional reconstruction can often help delineate the exact relationship between the lesion and the optic nerve; however, this is not mandatory (▶ Fig. 14.1). Angiography is not generally required; however, this may help differentiate primary orbital lesions from ophthalmic artery dolichoectasia in select cases.

The decision as to whether an endoscopic approach is suitable for a specific tumor depends on the location, morphology, and anticipated histology. An endoscopic approach is suitable for orbital lesions inferior or medial to a plane between the nares and the long axis of the optic nerve. Lesions that extend lateral to the nerve but remain inferior to this plane are still candidates for an endoscopic approach as the tumor may be delivered without requiring nerve retraction.

## 14.4 Surgical Anatomy

The medial orbit is separated from the sinus contents by the lamina papyracea. The lamina is derived embryologically from the ethmoid bone and extends from the sphenoid bone posteriorly to the lacrimal bone anteriorly. Immediately lateral to the lamina is the periorbita, which surrounds the orbital structures and is penetrated superiorly by the ethmoid neurovascular pedicles. The orbital contents within the periorbita can be separated into extraconal and intraconal compartments. The medial extraconal space consists of the orbital fat and its lateral limit from an endonasal perspective is the medial rectus muscle. This region is relatively devoid of important neurovascular structures other than the ethmoidal neurovasculature, which cross from lateral to medial over the superior border of the medial rectus muscle and the medial ophthalmic vein.[6]

The medial intraconal space is bounded by the medial and inferior rectus muscles and contains a complex and rich neurovascular arcade, which makes this region particularly

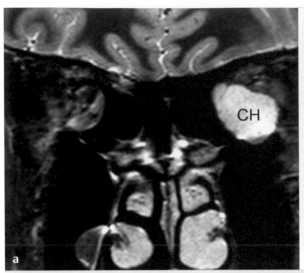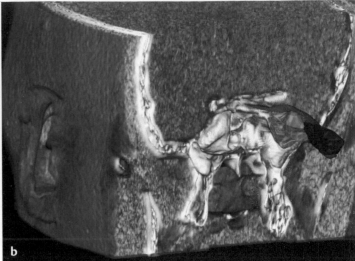

**Fig. 14.1** (a) T2-weighted coronal MRI (magnetic resonance imaging) demonstrating the classic appearance of a large extraconal cavernous hemangioma (CH) in the left orbital apex. (b) Three-dimensional reconstruction of the same patient demonstrating the relationship between the cavernous hemangioma (green), the medial rectus muscle (red), and the optic nerve (blue).

challenging to address (▶ Fig. 14.2). The lateral boundary is the optic nerve, ophthalmic artery, nasociliary nerve, and the long ciliary artery and nerve. The superior boundary is the anterior and posterior ethmoid artery and nerve. The oculomotor nerve enters this space and branches almost immediately into superior and inferior rami. A branch of the inferior ramus inserts along the posterior third of the lateral aspect of the medial rectus muscle. Similarly, an inferomedial muscular trunk arborizes from the ophthalmic artery and sends multiple arterioles to supply the medial rectus muscle approximately 1 cm anterior to the sphenoid face. These vascular pedicles divide the medial intraconal compartment into three conceptual compartments of increasing technical difficulty.[6] Zones A and B lie anterior to the inferomedial muscular trunk and are differentiated by an imaginary line dividing the upper and lower halves of the medial rectus muscle belly. Lesions within the more superior zone B are therefore more challenging to address due to their proximity to the ethmoid vasculature and the necessity to work above the medial rectus. Zone C represents the potential space posterior to the takeoff of the inferomedial muscular trunk. This region is the most technically challenging to access due to the small space and proximity to the optic nerve[6](▶ Fig. 14.3). While the ophthalmic artery usually crosses superior to the optic nerve, it may cross inferiorly in 16 to 33% of cases.[7] This variant brings the artery in even closer proximity to a zone C lesion and thus the course of the ophthalmic artery should generally be identified on preoperative imaging.

## 14.5 Surgical Technique

An endoscopic approach begins with wide exposure of the lamina by opening the adjacent maxillary, ethmoid, and sphenoid sinuses. For mid-orbit and posterior lesions the frontal outflow air cells may be preserved to protect the frontal recess from secondary obstruction. Adequate bony exposure including total removal of the lamina and drilling of the superior pterygoid

process and optic canal is critical to enable adequate bimanual dissection. While wide exposure of the periorbita is desired, a hockey stick incision through the periorbita is carefully placed just anterior to the lesion in order to prevent unnecessary prolapse of extraconal fat into the endoscopic visual cavity. With lesions that extend inferolaterally, the orbital process of the palatine bone may be further drilled to allow for more lateral exposure and enhance the ability to dissect inferior to the lesion (▶ Fig. 14.4).

The decision to proceed with a uni- versus bi-narial approach depends on multiple factors including location and size of the tumor as well as the preference of the surgical team.[8,9,10,11] While most extraconal tumors may be resected through a single nostril, intraconal lesions often require more difficult dissection, which is facilitated by using three or four hands through a bi-narial, trans-septal approach.[12] This method enables dynamic retraction of the medial rectus, intraconal fat retraction, and careful suctioning of pooled blood.[12] Additionally, the trans-septal trajectory improves dissection of the lateral aspect of the lesion due to the increased working angle from the contralateral side.

### 14.5.1 Methods of Medial Rectus Muscle Retraction

The medial rectus muscle represents the gateway to the medial intraconal space and thus access demands effective and atraumatic retraction.[13,14] Multiple external and endoscopic techniques for medial rectus muscle retraction have been described. External methods include disinsertion of the muscle via a transconjunctival incision or external placement of a vessel loop.[1,14] However, several endoscopic retraction techniques have been reported, which provide excellent access to the intraconal space while avoiding external incisions. These options include transchoanal retraction using a vessel loop placed around the muscle endoscopically,[15] trans-septal retraction using a suture or vessel

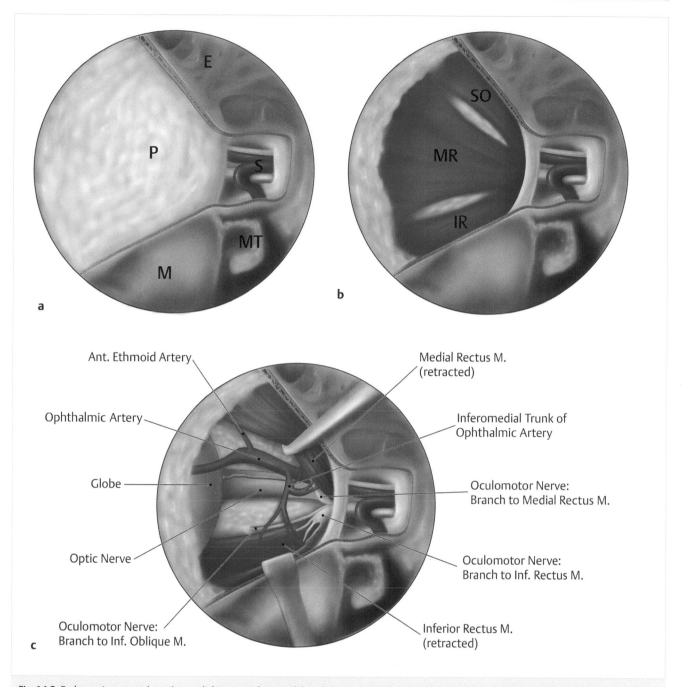

**Fig. 14.2** Endoscopic approach to the medial intraconal space. **(a)** Endoscopic view of right orbit following complete opening of the sinuses (E, ethmoid roof; S, sphenoid sinus; M, maxillary sinus), resection of the middle turbinate (MT), and removal of the lamina papyracea to expose the periorbita (P). **(b)** Same view after removal of the periorbita to expose the medially positioned extraocular muscles (SO, superior oblique; MR, medial rectus; IR, inferior rectus). **(c)** Endoscopic view of the right medial intraconal neurovascular structures after removal of the intraconal fat and extraocular muscle retraction.

loop passed through a septal window,[13] and finally trans-septal retraction using an instrument such as the double-ball probe (▶ Fig. 14.5).

When comparing the methods of retraction, both trans-septal techniques offer the greatest area exposure of the intraconal space.[16] The double-ball probe method offers some benefits over a vessel loop in that it provides dynamic retraction and reduces the risk of traction injury to the oculomotor nerve or ophthalmic arterial branches to the medial rectus muscle. Potential downsides of this method include the fact that a larger

septal window is needed and it occupies one of the surgical hands for the duration of the procedure.

## 14.5.2 Surgical Dissection Techniques for Intraconal Lesions

After the lesion is identified, blunt dissection through the surrounding orbital fat is performed to isolate the tumor. One surgeon will hold the endoscope, while the other will

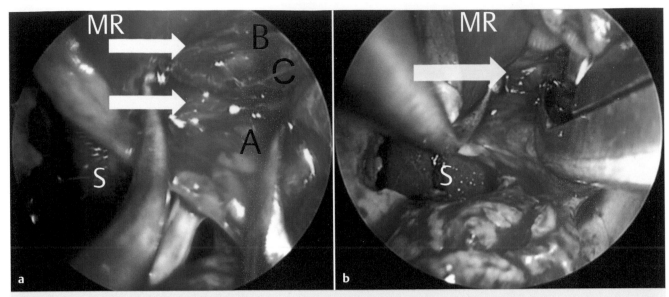

Fig. 14.3 (a) Intraoperative endoscopic view of the left intraconal space demonstrating several branches of the inferomedial muscular trunk of the ophthalmic artery (*white arrows*) inserting on the medial rectus muscle (MR; S, sphenoid sinus). These branches divide the medial intraconal space into three conceptual zones A, B, and C as illustrated. (b) Same intraoperative view as in (a). Here the oculomotor nerve (*white arrow*) may be seen coursing along the lateral aspect of the medial rectus muscle.

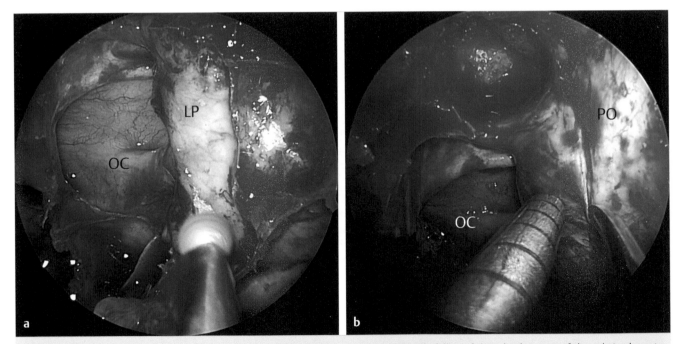

Fig. 14.4 (a) Wide bony exposure of the left lamina papyracea (LP) and optic canal (OC) with drilling of the orbital process of the palatine bone to provide improved access to the inferior aspect of the lesion. (b) Following removal of the lamina, a controlled vertical incision is made in the periorbita (PO) just anterior to the mass in order to minimize extraconal fat prolapse.

use a suction and dissection instrument to gently free the lesion from surrounding structures while keeping the field clear of pooled blood. A fourth hand may be used to assist with tumor retraction when necessary (▶ Fig. 14.6). The lesion should be dissected approximately 270 degrees around the periphery; however, direct dissection between the optic nerve and tumor capsule should be avoided as manipulation of the nerve could lead to direct injury or ophthalmic artery vasospasm. The final maneuver is to gently retract the lesion anteriorly in a plane parallel to the optic nerve in order to lyse the final lateral attachments. Some authors advocate the use of a cryoprobe to grasp the lesion although a small cupped forceps may also be used.[17] If the tumor does not easily break free at this point, this suggests the presence of persistent adhesions, which should continue to be dissected.

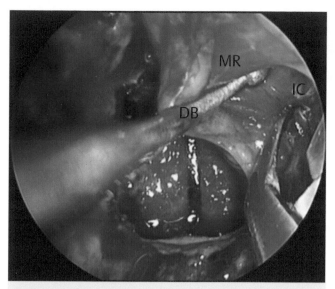

Fig. 14.5 Example of trans-septal endoscopic retraction of the left medial rectus (MR) muscle using a double-ball (DB) probe to gain access to the intraconal (IC) space.

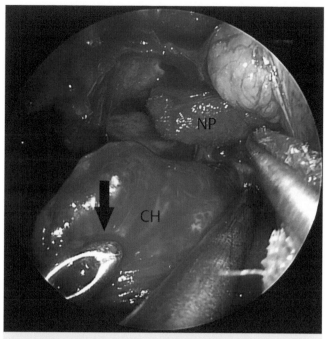

Fig. 14.6 Example of a four-handed technique during endoscopic resection of a left extraconal cavernous hemangioma (CH). The primary surgeon is seen retracting the extraconal fat using a neuropatti (NP) and using a Frazier suction, while a second surgeon holds the endoscope and retracts the tumor via the contralateral nostril using a grasping forceps (*black arrow*).

## 14.5.3 Hemostasis and Management of Orbital Fat Planes

Perhaps the most challenging aspects of performing endoscopic intraorbital surgery are dealing with orbital fat prolapse and management of intraconal bleeding. Although extraconal fat may be reduced with a bipolar electrocautery, this remains controversial. In contradistinction, intraconal fat should neither be cauterized nor resected. However, the retraction of intraconal fat is critical to enable visualization of the intraconal structures. Thus, in order to prevent excessive and potentially traumatic manipulation, use of a saline-soaked patty can be helpful for both fat retraction and blood absorption, providing a cleaner dissection plane (▶ Fig. 14.6). Hemostasis is also challenging in these cases. Both electric current and thermal spread can easily injure the orbital structures and thus monopolar cautery should be avoided. Bipolar cautery may be used safely within the extraconal space if absolutely necessary; however, the lowest setting possible should be employed. Besides the saline-soaked cottonoid, warm water irrigation is also a useful tool to help control bleeding as it promotes activation of platelet aggregation and enhanced coagulation. [18,19]

## 14.6 Postoperative Care

While there are no general criteria for orbital reconstruction following endoscopic orbital surgery, the goals of preserving orbital volume and prevention of extraocular muscle tethering should be considered.[20] The author favors reconstruction for most intraconal lesions given the potential for enophthalmos and secondary diplopia following extensive dissection and exposure of intraconal fat. Methods for reconstruction vary throughout the literature; however, immediate rigid reconstruction should be avoided due to the risk of orbital compartment syndrome. This may occur if the orbital contents cannot expand in the face of postoperative bleeding, fluid transudation,

and swelling of the extraocular muscles. A pedicled nasoseptal flap is preferred by the author as it may be raised at the same time as the creation of the septal window and offers complete coverage of both medial and inferior orbital defects. The flap further permits swelling and blood egress in the immediate postoperative period[13] while conforming to the orbit in a semirigid fashion due to contraction over time (▶ Fig. 14.7).

Once the area is reconstructed, nasal packing directly against the orbit should be avoided due to a similar fear of raising intraocular pressure and inducing ischemic damage.[17,20,21] However, Gelfoam and tissue glues may be used on the nasal surface of the graft in order to support the mucosal flap and minimize the risk of flap migration in the postoperative period.[12]

## 14.7 Outcomes

As with open approaches, the most common reported morbidities are diplopia, enophthalmos, and visual impairment. With respect to diplopia, Dubal et al[22] reported an improvement between the pre- and postoperative periods of 25 to 15%, respectively. Among the intraconal subgroup analyzed by Bleier et al,[23] use of the dynamic medial rectus retraction technique appeared to be protective against the development of new diplopia. Similarly, in this cohort there was no incidence of new visual impairment. A systematic review of 39 articles describing the endoscopic technique found that complete resection was possible in 73 to 100% of intraconal lesions and virtually all extraconal lesions.[1,22,23,24] The findings of Bleier et al[23] confirmed these results noting that intraconal lesions are at a higher risk of incomplete resection as well as greater rates of

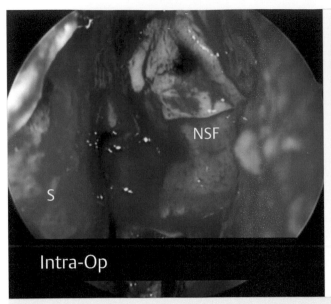 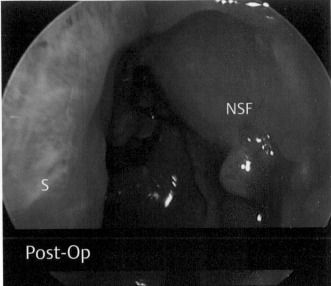

**Fig. 14.7** Intraoperative and 3-month postoperative images of a reconstruction of the left orbit using a nasoseptal flap (NSF; S, septum). Flap contraction and conformation to the orbit may be seen in the postoperative image.

enophthalmos and diplopia relative to extraconal lesions. This likely results from the larger orbitotomy required, coupled with the greater extent of surgical manipulation of the medial rectus and its neurovascular contributions.

A theoretical drawback to endoscopic over open approaches is the potential for incurring sinonasal morbidity. There has been no published literature on the sequelae of instrumenting an otherwise healthy nasal cavity in order to provide access to the orbit. However, a recent study by the author that analyzed 44 patients who underwent endoscopic endonasal dacryocystorhinostomy with no previous nasal symptoms concluded that the surgical manipulation of an otherwise nasal cavity does not result in any long-term decrement in nasal-specific quality of life.

# 14.8 Conclusion

To date, the global surgical experience with endoscopic orbital surgery remains limited due to the lack of widespread collaboration among oculoplastic and skull base surgeons.[23] However, this represents a rapidly advancing field as it provides a less morbid approach to the medial orbit than existing open techniques. A multidisciplinary team approach is essential in order to enhance patient care and optimize surgical outcomes. A better understanding of the indications and techniques for endoscopic intraconal surgery will continue to be refined as surgeons gain more experience with these lesions.

# References

[1] Paluzzi A, Gardner PA, Fernandez-Miranda JC, et al. "Round-the-clock" surgical access to the orbit. J Neurol Surg B Skull Base. 2015; 76(1):12–24

[2] OGURA JH, WALSH TE. The transantral orbital decompression operation for progressive exophthalmos. Laryngoscope. 1962; 72:1078–1097

[3] Kennedy DW, Goodstein ML, Miller NR, Zinreich SJ. Endoscopic transnasal orbital decompression. 1990; 32(1):275–282

[4] Lenzi R, Muscatello L. Considerations about endoscopic endonasal optic nerve and orbital apex decompression. Acta Neurochir (Wien). 2015; 157(4):629–630

[5] Shields JA, Shields CL, Scartozzi R. Survey of 1264 patients with orbital tumors and simulating lesions: the 2002 Montgomery Lecture, part 1. Ophthalmology. 2004; 111(5):997–1008

[6] Bleier BS, Healy DY, Jr, Chhabra N, Freitag S. Compartmental endoscopic surgical anatomy of the medial intraconal orbital space. Int Forum Allergy Rhinol. 2014; 4(7):587–591

[7] Perrini P, Cardia A, Fraser K, Lanzino G. A microsurgical study of the anatomy and course of the ophthalmic artery and its possibly dangerous anastomoses. J Neurosurg. 2007; 106(1):142–150

[8] Signorelli F, Anile C, Rigante M, Paludetti G, Pompucci A, Mangiola A. Endoscopic treatment of orbital tumors. World J Clin Cases. 2015; 3(3):270–274

[9] Kingdom TT, Delgaudio JM. Endoscopic approach to lesions of the sphenoid sinus, orbital apex, and clivus. Am J Otolaryngol. 2003; 24(5):317–322

[10] Murray KP, Mirani NM, Langer PD, Liu JK, Eloy JA. Endoscopic transnasal septotomy for contralateral orbital apex venous angioma resection and decompression. Orbit. 2013; 32(1):36–38

[11] Karaki M, Kobayashi R, Kobayashi E, et al. Computed tomographic evaluation of anatomic relationship between the paranasal structures and orbital contents for endoscopic endonasal transethmoidal approach to the orbit. Neurosurgery. 2008; 63(1) Suppl 1:ONS15–ONS19, discussion ONS19–ONS20

[12] Healy DY, Jr, Lee NG, Freitag SK, Bleier BS. Endoscopic bimanual approach to an intraconal cavernous hemangioma of the orbital apex with vascularized flap reconstruction. Ophthal Plast Reconstr Surg. 2014; 30(4):e104–e106

[13] Tomazic PV, Stammberger H, Habermann W, et al. Intraoperative medialization of medial rectus muscle as a new endoscopic technique for approaching intraconal lesions. Am J Rhinol Allergy. 2011; 25(5):363–367

[14] Wu W, Selva D, Jiang F, et al. Endoscopic transethmoidal approach with or without medial rectus detachment for orbital apical cavernous hemangiomas. Am J Ophthalmol. 2013; 156(3):593–599

[15] Felippu A, Mora R, Guastini L, Peretti G. Transnasal approach to the orbital apex and cavernous sinus. Ann Otol Rhinol Laryngol. 2013; 122(4):254–262

[16] Lin GC, Freitag SK, Kocharyan A, Yoon MK, Lefebvre DR, Bleier BS. Comparative techniques of medial rectus muscle retraction for endoscopic exposure of the medial intraconal space. Am J Rhinol Allergy. 2016; 30(3):226–229

[17] Chhabra N, Wu AW, Fay A, Metson R. Endoscopic resection of orbital hemangiomas. Int Forum Allergy Rhinol. 2014; 4(3):251–255

[18] Bhatki AM, Carrau RL, Snyderman CH, Prevedello DM, Gardner PA, Kassam AB. Endonasal surgery of the ventral skull base: endoscopic transcranial surgery. Oral Maxillofac Surg Clin North Am. 2010; 22(1):157–168

[19] Kassam A, Snyderman CH, Carrau RL, Gardner P, Mintz A. Endoneurosurgical hemostasis techniques: lessons learned from 400 cases. Neurosurg Focus. 2005; 19(1):E7

[20] McKinney KA, Snyderman CH, Carrau RL, et al. Seeing the light: endoscopic endonasal intraconal orbital tumor surgery. Otolaryngol Head Neck Surg. 2010; 143(5):699–701

[21] Castelnuovo P, Dallan I, Locatelli D, et al. Endoscopic transnasal intraorbital surgery: our experience with 16 cases. Eur Arch Otorhinolaryngol. 2012; 269 (8):1929–1935

[22] Dubal PM, Svider PF, Denis D, Folbe AJ, Eloy JA. Short-term outcomes of purely endoscopic endonasal resection of orbital tumors: a systematic review. Int Forum Allergy Rhinol. 2014; 4(12):1008–1015

[23] Bleier BS, Castelnuovo P, Battaglia P, et al. Endoscopic endonasal orbital cavernous hemangioma resection: global experience in techniques and outcomes. Int Forum Allergy Rhinol. 2016; 6(2):156–161

[24] Wang Y, Xiao L, Li Y, Yan H, Yu X, Su F. Endoscopic transethmoidal resection of medial orbital lesions. Zhonghua Yan Ke Za Zhi. 2015; 51(8):569–575

# 15 Endoscopic Management of Skull Base Neoplasms with Orbital Involvement

*Raewyn G. Campbell and Richard J. Harvey*

## Abstract

Skull base neoplasms are rare, yet among skull base malignancies, orbital involvement is not uncommon and often represents advanced disease. Orbital involvement in skull base malignancies portends a poor prognosis. The ultimate aim of treatment is optimal local control that results from gross tumor removal with negative margins and appropriate adjuvant therapy. Endoscopic approaches are often appropriate for tumors medial and inferior to the optic nerve and provide superior cosmetic outcomes when compared to open approaches. This chapter will discuss common pathologies, patient presentations, investigations, surgical anatomy, indications, contraindications, and a step-by-step endoscopic surgical approach for removal of these tumors as well as postoperative management.

*Keywords:* orbital tumors, malignancy, skull base, endoscopy, neoplasm, orbital preservation

## 15.1 Introduction

Skull base neoplasms are rare, yet among skull base malignancies, orbital involvement is not uncommon. Skull base malignancies often present with symptoms that are vague and easily associated with benign pathology such as sinusitis. Therefore, patients with these tumors often present late and/or with a delayed diagnosis and with advanced disease.[1] This is likely due to the fact that neoplasms can expand unhindered in the large sinonasal airspaces before causing symptoms. Therefore, patients often present with involvement of surrounding critical

structures such as the orbit. Likewise, benign neoplasms will often grow with significant orbital involvement and globe displacement but rarely with clinical features of diplopia or vision loss. Adaptation accounts for this lack of clinical symptoms as the neoplasms grow slowly and without invasion (▶ Fig. 15.1).

Orbital invasion is defined as a tumor that has breached/involved the periorbita. These tumors are largely determined by the site of origin and by the histology of the tumor. The orbit may be involved by direct extension from tumors in surrounding areas such as the nasal cavity, paranasal sinuses, mandible, cranial cavity or skull base, or by metastases. Adenocarcinomas and squamous cell carcinomas (SCC) are the most common tumor types involved.[2] Perineural spread is another mode for tumor extension. In particular, SCC and adenoid cystic carcinomas have a propensity for perineural spread.[3,4] SCC has a high propensity for local recurrence[5] and SCC and undifferentiated carcinomas favor the worst prognosis.[6]

Orbital involvement by tumor portends a less favorable prognosis and orbital soft-tissue tumor involvement is an independent risk factor for survival.[7,8,9,10] Indications for orbital exenteration are controversial and no universal criteria exist for the degree of orbital involvement that necessitates exenteration or safe preservation. Ianetti et al devised a grading system for orbital invasion[11]—grade 1: erosion/destruction of the medial orbital wall; grade 2: extraconal invasion of periorbital fat; and grade 3: invasion of the medial rectus muscle, ocular bulb, optic nerve, and/or overlying skin.[5] Currently, grade 3 orbital invasion is the most accepted criteria for exenteration.[12,13] However, other authors also use involvement of intraconal fat or the orbital apex as indications for exenteration.[5,12] Positive orbital margins

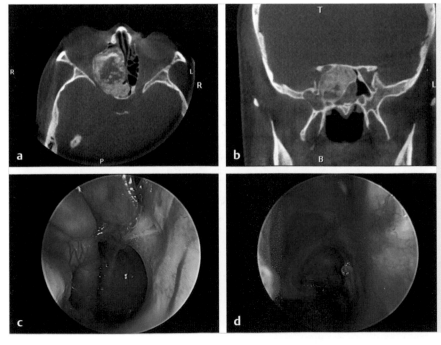

Fig. 15.1 Ossifying fibroma. (a) The degree of orbital displacement is significant enough to create proptosis and a cosmetic deformity. (b) The orbital apex is compressed but springs the optical canal. (c) Previous partial resection performed elsewhere resulted in improvement to nasal airway only and persistent sinus dysfunction. (d) The surgeon needs to be prepared to use reliable fixed landmarks rather than "sinus" anatomy to complete the resection.

are another risk factor for local recurrence and may warrant consideration of exenteration.[5] Essentially, the two considerations are the functional and oncologic outcomes of the preserved orbit.

For tumors medial and inferior to the optic nerve, endoscopic approaches are often appropriate as these provide direct access to the medial orbital wall. These approaches include endoscopic transnasal approaches and endoscopic-assisted approaches such as transcaruncular, transconjunctival,[14,15] transblepharoplasty,[16] transorbital,[17] and trans-supraorbital approaches. When tumor creeps superior and lateral to the orbit, anterior and anterolateral open approaches are more appropriate. This chapter will focus on endoscopic transnasal approaches.

# 15.2 Common Pathology

## 15.2.1 Benign

- Fibro-osseous:
  - fibrous dysplasia.
  - osteoma.
  - ossifying fibroma.
- Invasive fungal disease.
- Inverting papilloma.
- Vascular lesions:
  - hemangioma.
  - hemangiopericytoma.
- Meningioma.
- Foreign body.

## 15.2.2 Malignant

- SCC.
- Neuroectodermal and neuroendocrine tumors:
  - olfactory neuroblastoma.
  - mucosal melanoma.
  - sinonasal undifferentiated carcinoma.

- Rhabdomyosarcoma.
- Lymphoma.
- Salivary gland–type carcinoma:
  - adenoid cystic carcinoma.
  - adenocarcinoma.
  - mucoepidermoid carcinoma.

# 15.3 Patient Selection and Indications

## 15.3.1 Patient Presentation

Skull base neoplasms with orbital involvement commonly present with insidious symptoms such as nasal obstruction, rhinorrhea, epistaxis, headache, facial pain, hyposmia/anosmia, and epiphora. As tumors progress, patients may experience/demonstrate exophthalmos, globe dystopia, chemosis, facial swelling, cheek mass, facial paresthesia, visual field defects, diplopia, reduced visual acuity, or loss of vision. Loss of corneal sensation indicates nasociliary nerve involvement and may present as dry eye and corneal opacification resulting in loss of vision. Involvement of the cavernous sinus may produce diplopia, restricted ocular movement, or pupillary changes such as mydriasis or miosis, due to involvement of the third, fourth, or sixth cranial nerves or the sympathetic nerves within the cavernous sinus. The optic nerve is less often involved[18] and, therefore, pupillary afferent defects are uncommon at presentation without orbital apex compression or involvement. Diplopia or the fixed eye is more common (▶ Fig. 15.2).

## 15.3.2 Indications

Endoscopic orbital surgery is suitable for any pathology medial and/or inferior to the optic nerve (the neural axis).

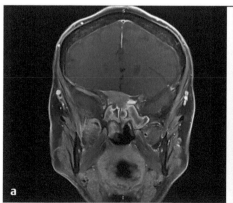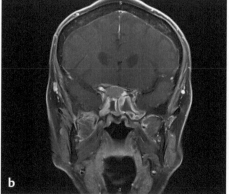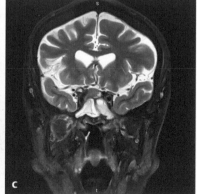

**Fig. 15.2** Squamous cell carcinoma: the posterior extent of orbital involvement is critical. **(a)** These magnetic resonance images demonstrate the right sphenoid and roof involvement. **(b)** The tumor abuts the internal carotid artery, but the lateral opticocarotid recess appears free of disease. **(c)** The optic nerve and the origin of the ophthalmic artery immediately below it appear clear. Tumor was removed and postoperative radiotherapy was given to this area. There was no margin here but to drill bone from the lateral sphenoid wall. Dura was resected over the planum to a free margin. The patient died 4 years postresection from a perineural spread along the third cranial nerve with pontine mass. The local area was otherwise free of gross disease.

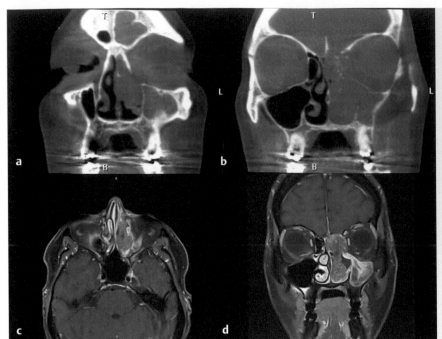

**Fig. 15.3** Squamous cell carcinoma: computed tomography scans are critical for assessing the bone erosion associated with malignancy. The bone surrounding the lacrimal duct and sac is eroded (a) as well as the bone of the medial orbital wall, ethmoid roof and crista galli (b). Magnetic resonance imaging confirms anterior extension (c) and pushing margin (d) that histologically involved the dura but not the periorbita. Both were resected with no gross disease beyond.

### 15.3.3 Contraindications

Endoscopic orbital surgery is contraindicated in the following circumstances:

- Significant tumor lateral or superior to the optic nerve.
- Malignant tumor involving the globe, extraocular musculature, eyelids.
- Tumor involving the optic nerve.

### 15.3.4 Diagnostic Workup

- Multidisciplinary tumor board presentation.
- Ophthalmology assessment. There are four constructs to consider:
  - Afferent visual function: visual acuity, color vision, papillary reaction/afferent defect, automated visual field testing.
  - Ocular motility: ductions, prismatic measurement of strabismus.
  - Lacrimal outflow functional: clinical epiphora, lacrimal irrigation.
  - Cosmesis: exophthalmometry, ptosis/eyelid position measurements
- Consideration of pre-op radiotherapy and/or chemotherapy to reduce tumor size to avoid/minimize injury to vital structures.[19]

### 15.3.5 Imaging

- CT:
  - Predicts lamina papyracea involvement with 91% sensitivity and 55% specificity.[20]
  - Predicts involvement of lacrimal system with 100% sensitivity and 45% specificity[20] (▶ Fig. 15.3).

- MRI:
  - Determines periorbital involvement with 93% sensitivity and 81% specificity.[20]
  - Periorbital thickening less than 2 to 3 mm is usually not a sign of true invasion (▶ Fig. 15.2 and ▶ Fig. 15.3).[21]
  - Consideration for image guidance/stereotactic/neuronavigational imaging and preoperative corticosteroids ± antibiotics (▶ Fig. 15.4).

## 15.4 Surgical Anatomy

The ophthalmic artery initially travels inferomedial to the optic nerve in the canal and then rotates to the inferolateral border as it travels toward the orbit and exits the dura[22,23] (▶ Fig. 15.2). The optic canal is thinnest in the middle segment on the medial wall.[22]

The trochlea is attached to the trochlear fovea or spine on the orbital surface of the frontal bone a few millimeters posterior to the superomedial margin of the orbit.[23]

It is important as it is a common cause of postoperative diplopia with external frontal procedures,[24] and removal of bone in this area will produce loss of function of the superior oblique and a vertical diplopia. The anterior ethmoid artery (AEA) branches from the ophthalmic artery in the orbit and runs in a anteromedial direction as it passes between the superior oblique and medial rectus muscles, and crosses the fovea ethmoidalis from the orbit to the lateral lamella of the cribriform plate. It travels posterior to the bulla ethmoidalis or in the frontal recess when a suprabullar recess is present. The AEA runs in a mesentery below the skull base in up to 43% of patients.[25] The posterior ethmoid artery (PEA), also a branch of the ophthalmic artery, runs approximately 11 mm posterior to the AEA and 7 mm anterior to the optic nerve.[26] The PEA runs more horizontally than the AEA and has a more variable path.[26] It runs

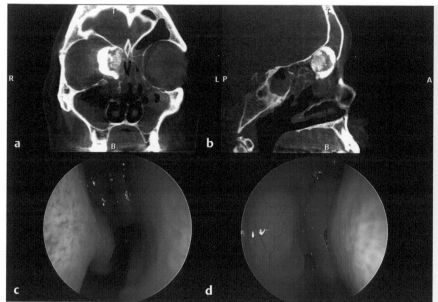

**Fig. 15.4** Osteoma: a classic frontoethmoidal osteoma rarely produces cosmetic abnormalities and is more likely to present with sinus dysfunction **(a)**. Managing the approach to frontal sinus and superior access is important **(b)**. The inflammation around tumors seen in the right nose **(c)** and middle meatus **(d)** can be managed with preoperative corticosteroid to improve the surgical field and hemostasis upon removal.

superior to the superior oblique muscle to cross the ethmoid sinuses a few millimeters anterior to the anterior wall of the sphenoid sinus in the sphenoethmoidal angle.[26]

# 15.5 Surgical Technique

## 15.5.1 Equipment

- Standard endoscopic sinus surgery instruments.
- Zero-degree (angled endoscopes are to be avoided if possible).
- Angled Beaver blade, straight and right-angled keratome blades or dacryocystorhinostomy (DCR) blade.
- A 4- to 5-mm 15-degree diamond burr (DCR burrs are rarely useful in neoplasia cases).
- Bipolar forceps.
- Cottle's elevator.

## 15.5.2 Surgical Steps

1. Total intravenous anesthesia for optimal mucosal hemostasis.[27]
2. Application of 1:1,000 to 2,000 epinephrine and ropivacaine-soaked neuropathies/cotton pledgets.
3. Injection with 1% ropivacaine with 1:100,000 adrenaline to lateral nasal wall and axilla of the middle turbinate.
4. Uncinectomy and wide maxillary antrostomy to ensure the roof of the maxillary sinus/floor of the orbit and infraorbital canal are easily identified.
   a) The maxillary sinus roof may be used as a landmark to remain safely below the skull base and to permit safe entry into the sphenoid sinus.[28]
5. At least a modified medial maxillectomy is utilized for increased access to the floor of the orbit, infratemporal fossa, and control of the internal maxillary artery.

6. Total sphenoethmoidectomy. Identifying the roof as a landmark of the skull base and lateral wall for the optic canal/orbital apex.
   a) This may require dissection of an Onodi cell if one is present.
7. Identify the lateral opticocarotid recess, internal carotid artery, and optic nerve canal in the superolateral wall of the sphenoid sinus (or in the Onodi cell if present).
8. Frontal recess clearance if tumor approaches the AEA and Draf III if the tumor extends anterior to the AEA.
9. Expose and ligate the AEA and PEA with bipolar cautery if exposure more laterally over the orbital roof is required (see above for a description of the anatomy).
10. Clearance of the mucosa off the lamina papyracea.
11. Drill the orbital strut/tubercle (junction of medial orbital wall and lateral sphenoid wall) using an irrigated diamond burr.
12. The optic nerve decompression is performed before incising the lamina papyracea to avoid orbital fat obscuring the view and also avoiding any inadvertent injury to the orbital contents.
    a) This is performed for tumors extending to the medial optic canal.
    b) When incising the optic nerve sheath, the location of the ophthalmic artery must be considered (see above). Incising the sheath in the superomedial quadrant will minimize risk of arterial injury.[22]
13. If tumor involves the nasolacrimal duct, it may be resected with the tumor and the remnant duct marsupialized. If the nasolacrimal sac is involved, then a formal dacryocystorhinostomy is performed and the involved sac is removed. The medial portion of the sac is reconstructed with a free mucosal graft with a central perforation for the common canaliculus. A stent is then placed and a Gelfoam (Pfizer Inc., New York, NY) dressing is used to secure the graft. If the common canaliculus is involved, then this is resected and a glass Jones tube will be required.

14. Removal of lamina papyracea.
    a) This can removed as far superiorly as roof of orbit and as far inferomedially as immediately medial to infraorbital nerve.
    b) One and a half orbital walls can comfortably be removed without reconstruction if the periorbita is intact.
    c) This can be done using a Freer dissector and flaking off the lamina.
15. Incise periorbita if involved by tumor.
    a) This is an important barrier in benign disease and should be preserved to prevent recurrence within the orbit.
    b) For periorbital involvement and/or malignant disease, the periorbita should be removed.
    c) Start the incision posteriorly and inferior at the orbital apex with an angled beaver blade, DCR knife, or keratome blade.
    d) Make two incisions in a **V**-shape with the apex at the orbital apex.
    e) Grasp the periorbita at the apex of the incision and remove anteriorly.
16. Tease out the orbital fat using a ball-tipped seeker probe and ablate it with bipolar diathermy if required. Volume loss will lead to endophthalmitis.
17. Identify the medial rectus muscle. This may require image guidance and/or the assistance of an oculoplastic surgeon to tug on the muscle externally so that its location can be identified/confirmed endoscopically.
18. Excise the lesion.
19. Hemostasis is achieved using a bipolar diathermy on a low setting to avoid collateral damage to vital structures such as the optic nerve.
20. A thin (0.51-mm), soft polymeric silicone (Silastic) sheet is placed over the medial orbital wall.
    a) This sheet may be placed in the middle meatus in an inverted **U**-shape, which will also aid in preventing lateralization of the middle turbinate.
21. Free mucosal grafts may be used to cover any exposed bone.
22. Place absorbable hemostatic packing material in the nasal cavity/middle meatus and consider suturing the middle turbinate to the septum with absorbable suture material to prevent its lateralization.
    a) Avoid placement of bulky, nonabsorbable packing material due to the risk for intraorbital placement or migration.

# 15.6 Postoperative Care

High-volume, low-pressure saline irrigations are used starting day 1 postoperatively if the periorbita remains intact. This prevents adhesions and crusting and enhances healing. If the periorbita has been incised or removed, high-volume irrigations are commenced at days 5 to 7 postoperatively. The Silastic sheet is removed from the periorbita/middle meatus after 3 to 6 weeks. Oral antibiotics are given for 10 days and dexamethasone and antibiotic eye drops are used if there has been any surgery to the lacrimal system. Patients are discharged 1 day postoperatively if no other dural resection has occurred; otherwise, they are discharged between days 5 and 7.

Patients are assessed endoscopically 3 weeks postoperatively and then at 3 months.

A postoperative ophthalmologic assessment is performed 12 weeks postoperatively (earlier in the setting of complications).

# 15.7 Complications
## 15.7.1 Intraoperative

- Extraocular muscle/tendon injury.
- Trochlea injury.
- Cranial nerve injury.
- Retrobulbar hemorrhage.
- Optic nerve injury.
- Incomplete tumor resection.
- Cerebrospinal fluid leak.

## 15.7.2 Postoperative

- Loss of visual acuity.
- Orbital cellulitis.
- Periorbital ecchymosis.
- Enophthalmos.

# 15.8 Outcomes

Functional outcomes of preserved eyes have been graded as follows: grade 1—functional without impairment; grade 2—functional with impairment; and grade 3—nonfunctional.[12] In particular, outcomes such as globe malposition including enophthalmos and hypoglobus, restricted extraocular motility resulting in diplopia, and epiphora must be considered. The impact/outcomes of adjuvant therapy on the eye, particularly radiation therapy, must also be considered when planning treatment as orbital preservation does not necessarily guarantee an intact, functional eye at the conclusion of treatment. Therefore, this must be considered when counseling the patient preoperatively.

Patients with sinonasal tumors with orbital involvement that originated in the nasal cavity and maxillary sinus have better long-term survival and those whose tumor originated in the ethmoid sinuses have the worst survival.[29] Many studies have noted that orbital exenteration provided no survival advantage versus preservation.[10,12] In a series of 66 cases of sinonasal malignancy encroaching upon the orbit, Imola and Schramm noted a local recurrence of 30% in the preservation group and 33% in the exenteration group.[12] However, one retrospective study of 220 patients with a minimum follow-up of 4 years found in favor of exenteration.[6] They found that the actual locoregional control rates were 79% for those who underwent exenteration and 14% for those without exenteration ($p = 0.03$).[6] However, this study also found that orbital extension of tumor was not associated with worse prognosis. These two findings would seem contradictory and warrant further discussion. Optimal local control results from gross tumor removal with negative margins and appropriate adjuvant therapy.[5,20] A recent meta-analysis including 443 patients with paranasal sinus neoplasms with orbital involvement who underwent craniofacial resection with or without orbital exenteration concluded that while the evidence is not robust or definitive, orbital preservation provides a more favorable 5-year survival rate compared to exenteration. However, this effect may be limited to patients with SCC or adenocarcinoma only.

# 15.9 Conclusion

The endoscopic approach to sinonasal tumors with orbital involvement provides exceptional visualization of the anatomy, the tumor, and the tissue planes, and permits directed frozen section biopsies. This can result in the avoidance of more invasive open approaches and provides a superior cosmetic outcome, shorter hospital stay, and faster recovery. The endoscopic approach may also be used as an adjunct to an open approach affording a smaller incision and providing simultaneous access to complex lesions.

# References

[1] Breheret R, Laccourreye L, Jeufroy C, Bizon A. Adenocarcinoma of the ethmoid sinus: retrospective study of 42 cases. Eur Ann Otorhinolaryngol Head Neck Dis. 2011; 128(5):211–217

[2] Reyes C, Mason E, Solares CA, Bush C, Carrau R. To preserve or not to preserve the orbit in paranasal sinus neoplasms: a meta-analysis. J Neurol Surg B Skull Base. 2015; 76(2):122–128

[3] Catalano PJ, Sen C, Biller HF. Cranial neuropathy secondary to perineural spread of cutaneous malignancies. Am J Otol. 1995; 16(6):772–777

[4] Goepfert H, Dichtel WJ, Medina JE, Lindberg RD, Luna MD. Perineural invasion in squamous cell skin carcinoma of the head and neck. Am J Surg. 1984; 148(4):542–547

[5] Rajapurkar M, Thankappan K, Sampathirao LM, Kuriakose MA, Iyer S. Oncologic and functional outcome of the preserved eye in malignant sinonasal tumors. Head Neck. 2013; 35(10):1379–1384

[6] Dulguerov P, Jacobsen MS, Allal AS, Lehmann W, Calcaterra T. Nasal and paranasal sinus carcinoma: are we making progress? A series of 220 patients and a systematic review. Cancer. 2001; 92(12):3012–3029

[7] Suarez C, Llorente JL, Fernandez De Leon R, Maseda E, Lopez A. Prognostic factors in sinonasal tumors involving the anterior skull base. Head Neck. 2004; 26(2):136–144

[8] Ganly I, Patel SG, Singh B, et al. Craniofacial resection for malignant paranasal sinus tumors: report of an International Collaborative Study. Head Neck. 2005; 27(7):575–584

[9] Patel SG, Singh B, Polluri A, et al. Craniofacial surgery for malignant skull base tumors: report of an international collaborative study. Cancer. 2003; 98(6):1179–1187

[10] Lund VJ, Howard DJ, Wei WI, Cheesman AD. Craniofacial resection for tumors of the nasal cavity and paranasal sinuses: a 17-year experience. Head Neck. 1998; 20(2):97–105

[11] Iannetti G, Valentini V, Rinna C, et al. Ethmoido-orbital tumors: our experience. J Craniofac Surg. 2005; 16(6):1085–1091

[12] Imola MJ, Schramm VL, Jr. Orbital preservation in surgical management of sinonasal malignancy. Laryngoscope. 2002; 112(8, Pt 1):1357–1365

[13] Weizman N, Horowitz G, Gil Z, Fliss DM. Surgical management of tumors involving the orbit. JAMA Otolaryngol Head Neck Surg. 2013; 139(8):841–846

[14] Pillai P, Lubow M, Ortega A, Ammirati M. Endoscopic transconjunctival surgical approach to the optic nerve and medial intraconal space: a cadaver study. Neurosurgery. 2008; 63(4) Suppl 2:h:204–208, discussion 208–209

[15] Sillers MJ, Cuilty-Siller C, Kuhn FA, Porubsky ES, Morpeth JF. Transconjunctival endoscopic orbital decompression. Otolaryngol Head Neck Surg. 1997; 117(6):S137–S141

[16] Knipe TA, Gandhi PD, Fleming JC, Chandra RK. Transblepharoplasty approach to sequestered disease of the lateral frontal sinus with ophthalmologic manifestations. Am J Rhinol. 2007; 21(1):100–104

[17] Locatelli D, Pozzi F, Turri-Zanoni M, et al. Transorbital endoscopic approaches to the skull base: current concepts and future perspectives. J Neurosurg Sci. 2016; 60(4):514–525

[18] Ableman TB, Newman SA. Perineural spread of head and neck cancer: ophthalmic considerations. J Neurol Surg B Skull Base. 2016; 77(2):131–139

[19] Zheng JW, Qiu WL, Zhang ZY. Combined and sequential treatment of oral and maxillofacial malignancies: an evolving concept and clinical protocol. Chin Med J (Engl). 2008; 121(19):1945–1952

[20] Christianson B, Perez C, Harrow B, Batra PS. Management of the orbit during endoscopic sinonasal tumor surgery. Int Forum Allergy Rhinol. 2015; 5(10):967–973

[21] McIntyre JB, Perez C, Penta M, Tong L, Truelson J, Batra PS. Patterns of dural involvement in sinonasal tumors: prospective correlation of magnetic resonance imaging and histopathologic findings. Int Forum Allergy Rhinol. 2012; 2(4):336–341

[22] Chou PI, Sadun AA, Lee H. Vasculature and morphometry of the optic canal and intracanalicular optic nerve. J Neuroophthalmol. 1995; 15(3):186–190

[23] McMinn RM, ed. Last's Anatomy, Regional and Applied. 9th ed. Edinburgh, UK: Churchill Livingstone; 2003

[24] Lund VJ. Superior oblique palsy following ethmoidal surgery. J R Soc Med. 1991; 84(11):695

[25] Başak S, Karaman CZ, Akdilli A, Mutlu C, Odabaşi O, Erpek G. Evaluation of some important anatomical variations and dangerous areas of the paranasal sinuses by CT for safer endonasal surgery. Rhinology. 1998; 36(4):162–167

[26] Monjas-Cánovas I, García-Garrigós E, Arenas-Jiménez JJ, Abarca-Olivas J, Sánchez-Del Campo F, Gras-Albert JR. Radiological anatomy of the ethmoidal arteries: CT cadaver study. Acta Otorrinolaringol Esp. 2011; 62(5):367–374

[27] Wormald PJ, van Renen G, Perks J, Jones JA, Langton-Hewer CD. The effect of the total intravenous anesthesia compared with inhalational anesthesia on the surgical field during endoscopic sinus surgery. Am J Rhinol. 2005; 19(5):514–520

[28] Harvey RJ, Shelton W, Timperley D, et al. Using fixed anatomical landmarks in endoscopic skull base surgery. Am J Rhinol Allergy. 2010; 24(4):301–305

[29] Chu Y, Liu HG, Yu ZK. Patterns and incidence of sinonasal malignancy with orbital invasion. Chin Med J (Engl). 2012; 125(9):1638–1642

# 16 Transorbital Approaches to the Sinuses, Skull Base, and Intracranial Space

*Darlene E. Lubbe and Kris S. Moe*

## Abstract

Transorbital endoscopic surgery involves a target-determined group of pathways to provide access to pathology located within the orbit, the adjacent sinuses and skull base, and intracranial structures. These pathways—one for each quadrant of the orbit—provide access to previously difficult-to-reach areas where traditional approaches create significant morbidity by collateral damage. This chapter highlights the current concepts, anatomy, and surgical pathology that can be addressed using minimally disruptive transorbital endoscopic approaches.

*Keywords:* endoscopic, transorbital, orbital, anterior cranial fossa, middle cranial fossa, anterior skull base, minimally invasive, multiportal

## 16.1 Introduction

Transorbital endoscopic surgery of the orbit and intracranial structures is a relatively new field of surgery, with reports of significant experience beginning in the latter half of the last decade.[1,2] The reason for this late development was not lack of technology, but rather the compartmentalization of surgical specialties. In 1979 during the pre-endoscopic era, the American Society of Ophthalmology and Otolaryngology (founded in 1896) split into separate academies. Since then, ophthalmologists and otolaryngologists have focused on separate anatomic regions, with endoscopic procedures gaining in popularity mainly in the latter group. Likewise, neurological surgeons' interests have been focused intracranially. Thus, many of the procedures currently performed in endoscopic orbital and transorbital surgery traverse anatomic boundaries that historically divided specialties. It is the recent improvements in surgical training and cooperation that have facilitated the development of endoscopic orbital and transorbital procedures centered in an area that was previously avoided when possible.

With the recent addition of transorbital approaches to the transnasal, transmaxillary, infratemporal fossa, and supraorbital armamentarium, it is now common that multiple pathways can be used to approach a given target pathology. The choice of surgical pathway has thus become increasingly complex. While this ultimately depends on the surgeon's preference, the pathway selection should be influenced predominately by the location of the pathology and proximity of critical neurovascular structures. Perhaps most importantly, the pathway should be *minimally disruptive*, causing the least possible collateral damage. A minimally disruptive pathway creates the least possible morbidity, loss of function, and scarring; shortest period of hospitalization; most rapid recovery; and least possible disruption of the patient's lifestyle. To achieve this, the pathway should be as short and direct as possible while posing the lowest possible risk to vital structures.[3] In addition, the pathway must provide adequate volume for the deployment of multiple instruments, and provide the appropriate angulation of approach to the target to allow comfortable instrumentation and visualization.

While the extended transnasal approach provides excellent access to much of the skull base, 80% of the anterior cranial fossa (ACF) and much of the middle cranial fossa (MCF) are occupied by the orbits.[1] The orbit may thus conflict with transnasal approaches to some skull base targets. Transorbital approaches enjoy a privileged location for directly accessing those regions. Furthermore, the transorbital approaches often allow direct target manipulation without the use of angulation in instrumentation or endoscopy.

In addition to having a number of options for approaching a target, we can also use two or more pathways at once to treat a lesion (multiportal technique).[4] Operating through a single pathway or paired adjacent pathways (e.g., through both nostrils) can lead to visual obstruction of the target by instruments, or a challenge in instrumenting the target because the endoscope may be in the way. Furthermore, blood and secretions can run down the instruments onto the endoscope, further obscuring visualization. By operating through two or more separated portals, these problems can be avoided with the additional benefits of adding more working room between instruments and hands and the additional perspective of another viewing angle (▶ Fig. 16.1).

Endoscopic procedures involving the orbit involve two primary pathways: transorbital (using approaches through a transcutaneous or transconjunctival orbitotomy) and transnasal. Transorbital surgery can be further categorized to describe targets within the orbit (i.e., endoscopic orbital surgery), targets adjacent to the orbit (i.e., transorbital endoscopic surgery), and neurological targets adjacent to the orbit (i.e., transorbital neuroendoscopic surgery). Transorbital approaches are further categorized by the orbital quadrant that they address (▶ Fig. 16.2 and ▶ Fig. 16.3): superior (typically through a blepharoplasty incision); medial (transconjunctival, precaruncular, transcaruncular); inferior (transconjunctival inferior fornix), and lateral (retrocanthal or lateral blepharoplasty). This chapter will focus on transorbital rather than transnasal approaches to the orbit.

While these approaches are applicable and commonly used to address trauma of the orbit, optic nerve, brain, and adjacent structures, a discussion of transorbital endoscopic trauma surgery is beyond the scope of this chapter.

## 16.2 Patient Selection / Indications

Transorbital endoscopic approaches are indicated for targets within the orbit, or adjacent to the orbit in the paranasal sinuses, maxilla, infratemporal fossa, and adjacent anterior cranial fossa (ACF) and middle cranial fossa (MCF). The pathology must be amenable to an endoscopic or endoscopic-assisted

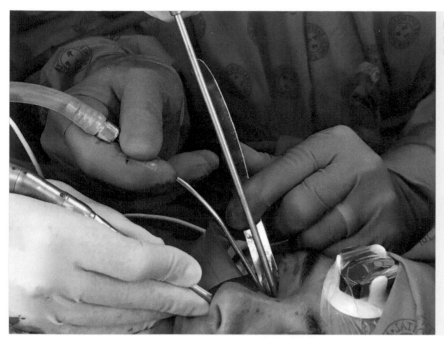

**Fig. 16.1** Multiportal approach using precaruncular and transnasal pathways for optic nerve decompression.

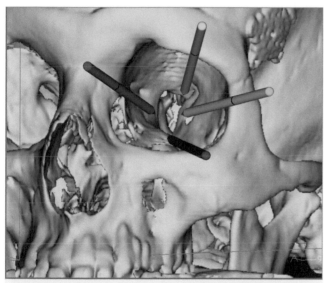

**Fig. 16.2** Trajectory of four quadrant approaches through the orbit.

approach. For tumors invading major vessels such as the internal carotid artery, an open craniotomy should be considered for proximal and distal vascular control in cases of malignant pathology. Transorbital approaches can be used alone or in multiportal combination with other endoscopic portals or as an assistive approach with traditional craniotomies.

Transorbital approaches are contraindicated in patients with recent trauma causing a ruptured globe or hyphema. These approaches should be used with caution for patients who have had intraocular surgery within the last 6 months, or a recent infectious or inflammatory condition of the orbit that has not fully resolved.[5]

## 16.2.1 Superior Approach

The superior and lateral approaches are the workhorse approaches to the ACF and MCF. A combination of the two approaches gives wide access to the superior and lateral orbits to address lesions involving the anterior fossa, middle fossa,

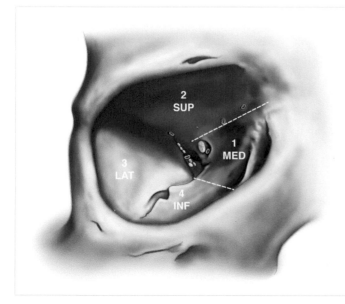

**Fig. 16.3** Bony anatomy of the four quadrants of the orbit.

1 Medial wall
2 Orbital roof
3 Lateral wall
4 Floor

orbit, and structures abutting the superior orbital fissure (SOF) such as the cavernous sinus and Meckel's cave. The superior approach on its own provides good access and visualization to manage orbital, frontal sinus, and ACF lesions. Opening the orbital roof in the floor of the frontal sinus gives access to lateral lesions that are difficult to access with an endoscopic Lothrop procedure, especially bony lesions such as osteomas and fibrous dysplasia. The superior approach is therefore useful during multiportal surgery or in conjunction with a transnasal approach for large lesions extending into the frontal sinus or ACF. The medial aspect of the contralateral frontal sinus and intersinus frontal cells can also be reached through this approach, allowing removal of the intersinus septum if desired. The orbital roof is very thin posterior to the frontal sinus and dura is easily exposed to manage ACF lesions or intracranial collections due to complicated sinusitis. The superior pathway gives wide access up to the orbital apex and SOF. Endoscopic visualization of the posterior/superior orbit is expedient and less disruptive than to a traditional open craniotomy where removal of the orbital roof is required to access posterosuperior orbital lesions. This access route allows neurosurgeons, ophthalmologists, and otolaryngologists to approach orbital lesions, creating an opportunity to close the management gap that exists with regard to orbital pathology. The authors have successfully removed orbital cavernous hemangiomas, neurofibromas, hydatid cysts, and meningoceles using the endoscope through the superior approach.

## 16.2.2 Lateral Approach

The lateral approach provides a wide surgical pathway to the lateral orbit, infratemporal fossa, MCF, greater and lesser wing of the sphenoid, and trigeminal ganglion/lateral cavernous sinus[6,7] and lateral sphenoid sinus.[8] The most common pathology requiring the lateral transorbital route is sphenoid wing meningiomas. The lateral hyperostotic orbital wall can be managed through this approach, obviating the need to remove the orbital rim as with the traditional pterional approach (▶ Fig. 16.4). By removing the lateral orbital wall, temporalis muscle is exposed (▶ Fig. 16.5) and access can be obtained to the infratemporal fossa. Lesions such as angiofibromas or meningiomas extending to the superior infratemporal fossa can be addressed using the lateral pathway as an adjunct during multiportal surgery. After removing the greater wing of the sphenoid bone, a wide surgical pathway is created to the MCF and SOF to manage lesions in these areas. The lateral approach is useful when a two-wall orbital decompression is required in patients with thyroid orbitopathy and can be combined with an

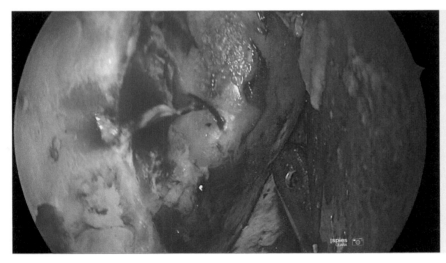

**Fig. 16.4** Lateral pathway showing bony hyperostosis in a sphenoid wing meningioma.

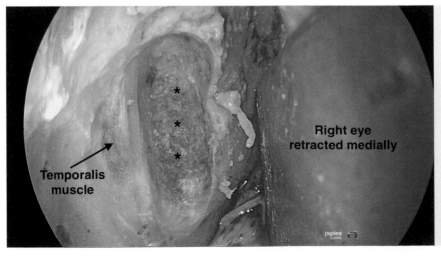

**Fig. 16.5** Lateral approach showing pathway between temporalis muscle (*arrow*) and periorbita of the right eye.

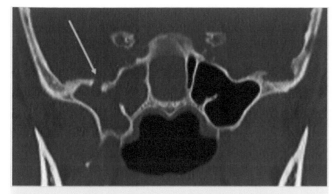

**Fig. 16.6** The Sternberg canal defect in lateral sphenoid sinus.

fluid (CSF) leaks,[9] treatment of orbital and frontoethmoidal mucoceles, orbital and optic nerve decompression, foreign body removal, and resection of tumors of the orbit, ACF, ethmoid and sphenoid sinuses. For tumors involving the ethmoid sinuses and interorbital ACF, we favor this approach due to its ability to provide surveillance of the orbital contents and dura for extent of tissue invasion before resection of the actual mass. Using multiportal technique for tumor resection, the procedure can begin with localization of critical neurovascular structures and then progress toward the sinonasal cavities. We believe this to be safer than working from the nose through tumor into the orbit and cranium. The contralateral precaruncular approach gives excellent access and a direct trajectory to the lateral aspect of a well-pneumatized sphenoid sinus for the repair of Sternberg canal defects and CSF leaks (▶ Fig. 16.6 and ▶ Fig. 16.7).

endoscopic medial decompression that can be performed either transnasally or through a precaruncular approach. Use of the endoscope allows for preservation of the orbital rim, and bone can be removed up to the inferior orbital fissure and SOF during a lateral decompression. Laterally located orbital lesions and the lateral rectus muscle can be accessed via this route. Manipulating the endoscope within an orbital cystic lesion or meningocele is useful since visualization of the posterior attachment of the lesion to vital structures can be appreciated within a cavity that is usually bloodless and free of herniating fat.

## 16.2.3 Medial Approach

The medial approach is used for a variety of pathology ranging from endoscopic ligation of the anterior, posterior, and accessory ethmoid arteries to the repair of complex cerebrospinal

## 16.2.4 Inferior Approach

The inferior transorbital approach accesses the lower orbit through a transconjunctival deep fornix approach. This incision can be extended laterally into a lateral retrocanthal or canthotomy/cantholysis approach depending on access required. Similarly, the incision can be extended medially into a precaruncular approach. An isolated inferior approach is often used to treat pathology of the inferior orbital contents or the infraorbital nerve. In addition, this approach is used in multiportal technique with transnasal and transmaxillary approaches to treat extensive pathology of the maxilla such as juvenile nasopharyngeal angiofibroma (JNA). This technique allows instrumentation and visualization through separate portals, which improves the working space between instruments and moves instruments so they do not obstruct visualization of the pathology.

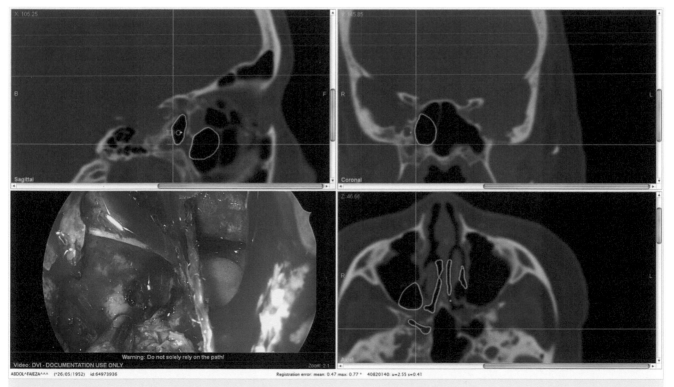

**Fig. 16.7** Contralateral approach to lateral aspect of sphenoid sinus for the Sternberg canal defect repair.

## 16.3 Diagnostic Workup

A multidisciplinary team is required when the transorbital route to orbital, sinonasal, or intracranial lesions is contemplated. Patients should be discussed at tumor board meetings with representatives from ophthalmology, neurosurgery, otolaryngology, and neuroradiology present. The best surgical route and trajectory should be planned using navigation software to compare transnasal, transorbital, transmaxillary, and open approaches alone or in combination. Multiportal or staged surgery may be required for large complex lesions involving multiple areas. An oncologist should provide input in the initial decision making for lesions that may require adjunctive radiotherapy or chemotherapy.

### 16.3.1 Physical Examination

Ophthalmological examination should be thorough since most patients requiring transorbital surgery have some visual loss, cranial nerve fallout, or proptosis. It is therefore imperative to accurately document ophthalmological findings such as visual acuity, visual fields, relative afferent pupillary defect, eye movements, degree of optic atrophy, and proptosis preoperatively. From an otolaryngologist's perspective, it is necessary to evaluate the anatomical configuration and size of the sinuses abutting the orbit, depending on which pathway will be utilized. Sensation in the area of the supraorbital and infraorbital nerves should be tested. All cranial nerves, especially III, IV, $V_1$, and VI, should be evaluated preoperatively because of the risk of tumor invasion through the SOF and because of the risk of traction injury that could occur during surgery. A full neurological examination is always needed for patients with any intracranial tumor component.

### 16.3.2 Laboratory and Radiological Evaluation

Blood tests would depend on patient factors such as age and comorbid diseases. For patients with proptosis, thyroid function tests should be done to exclude thyroid eye disease. Computed tomography (CT) of the orbits, sinuses, and brain, and magnetic resonance imaging (MRI) with and without contrast are required in all cases to delineate tumor extent and assess the degree of bony infiltration. CT and MRI scans should be obtained under navigation protocol. The use of navigation and preoperative surgical route and trajectory planning is important to choose the best approach with maximal exposure but minimal morbidity. Angiography and embolization may be required in some cases to assess and address any feeding vessels.

## 16.4 Surgical Anatomy

It is useful to consider the anatomy of the orbit in four quadrants, which is how we group surgical approaches in target-centered surgical planning. Each quadrant has primary approaches whose pathways transgress it, and unique anatomy to consider when planning a trajectory that involves the region (▶ Fig. 16.8).

The **superior quadrant** is centered between the lacrimal gland and the trochlea of the superior oblique muscle. The superior approach follows the orbital septum to the orbital rim, dissecting deep to the orbicularis oculi muscle. Deep to the septum is the preaponeurotic fat, which provides a buffer zone to protect the levator aponeurosis and muscle during the dissection. At the superior orbital rim, the supraorbital and supratrochlear neurovascular pedicles are identified and preserved, and the plane between the periosteum and the orbital bone is entered (▶ Fig. 16.9). The dissection in the superior orbit is bounded medially by the ethmoid neurovascular bundles at the junction of the ACF with the lamina papyracea. These foramina can be followed posteriorly in a plane posteriorly to the optic nerve, which is the medial boundary of the apical component of this quadrant. The lateral boundary of the apical component is the SOF, through which cranial nerves pass within a periosteal envelope as noted in ▶ Fig. 16.10. Thus, the apex of the dissection is centered between the optic nerve medially and the superior fissure laterally. The extensions of periosteum around these structures function as a landmark and protective layer during dissection.

The **medial quadrant** is bound by the trochlea of the superior oblique superiorly, and the inferior oblique inferiorly (these structures are not typically exposed during the approach). The

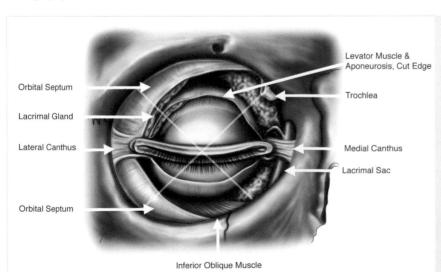

Fig. 16.8 Quadrant-centered approaches to the orbit. In the deep orbit, the lateral approach is separated from the superior and inferior approaches by the superior and inferior orbital fissures, respectively.

Orbital Septum
Lacrimal Gland
Lateral Canthus
Orbital Septum
Levator Muscle & Aponeurosis, Cut Edge
Trochlea
Medial Canthus
Lacrimal Sac
Inferior Oblique Muscle

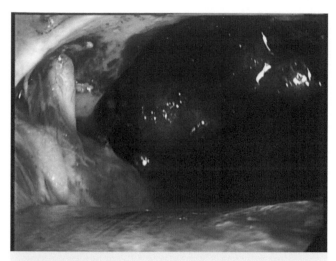

**Fig. 16.9** Supraorbital and supratrochlear neurovascular pedicles within superior quadrant.

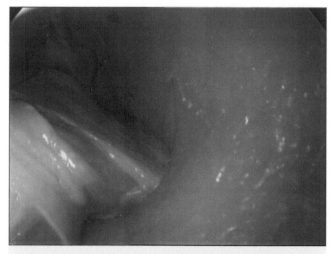

**Fig. 16.10** Superior orbital fissure as viewed through superior quadrant approach.

entrance to this quadrant is created between the caruncle and the medial canthus. The superior and inferior lacrimal canaliculi run through the tarsus between the anterior and posterior limbs of the medial canthal tendon to the lacrimal sac. These structures course superficial to the plane of dissection. The dissection follows the deep side of the posterior limb of the medial canthal tendon back to its insertion on the posterior lacrimal crest, where the subperiosteal dissection plane is opened and entered. The lamina papyracea then forms the medial boundary of the dissection, the periosteum is the lateral structure, the junction of the lamina and the ACF (containing the ethmoid arteries as above) is the superior margin, and inferiorly the dissection proceeds to the junction of the lamina and the orbital floor. The critical structure of this quadrant is the optic nerve, which courses superomedially to enter the optic canal at the superior posterior aspect of the medial wall of the orbit. Navigation is recommended when dissecting toward the optic nerve, and the tighter curvature of the lamina will be noted as the dissection proceeds toward the posterior ethmoid artery and finally the optic canal. Removal of the posterior lamina will allow dissection to continue on the medial aspect of the optic canal within the sphenoid sinus.

The structures of the **inferior quadrant** are located between the attachment of the inferior oblique muscle medially and the junction of the floor and lateral wall laterally. The anatomy is analogous to the superior quadrant, with the lower lid retractors functioning similarly to the levator muscle. The approach is more direct, however, transecting the lid retractors when incising onto the inferior orbital rim. The plane between the periosteum and orbital floor is entered at the orbital rim. As dissection continues posteriorly, care is taken to identify the infraorbital nerve, which typically passes within a canal located within or inferior to the orbital floor, entering the orbit toward the apex as it traverses the posterior aspect of the inferior fissure to enter foramen rotundum. Laterally, the posterior dissection is contained by the inferior fissure. Unlike the superior fissure, however, the inferior fissure contains predominately fibrovascular tissue that can be transected without functional loss if extended access to or from the lateral orbital compartment is desired. The medial border of the dissection is the lamina

papyracea. At the apex of the quadrant, the posterior aspect of the inferior fissure is encountered, and the periosteal attachment to this structure can be followed medially where it lies inferior to the optic nerve at the superior medial aspect of the posterior orbit.

The **lateral quadrant** of the orbit lies between the lacrimal gland superiorly and the junction of the lateral wall with the orbital floor medially. It is accessed through a transconjunctival lateral retrocanthal approach with or without a canthotomy/cantholysis, or a lateral extension of an upper blepharoplasty incision. The lateral canthal tendon inserts on the medial aspect of the lateral orbital wall 1 mm posterior to the rim, just below the frontozygomatic suture. If this structure is disturbed, it must be reconstructed at the end of the procedure to prevent lid dystopia. Once the subperiosteal plane is entered deep to the orbital rim, dissection continues posteriorly bounded by the orbital roof above and the inferior fissure below. As noted, the latter structure can be transected as needed for exposure. Dissecting deeper within the orbit, the pathway narrows as the superior and inferior fissures converge posteriorly. These structures, when preserved, prevent damage to the optic nerve medially. The bone of the lateral orbit divides the orbital contents from the infratemporal fossa and temporalis muscle anteriorly, thickening into the greater wing of the sphenoid posteriorly behind which lies the MCF and temporal lobe dura.

# 16.5 Surgical Technique

## 16.5.1 Anesthesia and Preparation

The anesthesia and preparation is the same in all four approaches. The position of the head may differ according to the approach used and eye to be operated on. We do not recommend pinning the head, but instead use a horseshoe headrest so that the position of the head can be manipulated intraoperatively. The authors prefer total intravenous anesthesia (TIVA) to obtain normotensive anesthesia with a low heart rate. Patients are intubated using a south-facing ray tube secured to the left corner of the mouth to keep the area in front of the nose and eye clear for instrument and endoscope manipulation for a right-handed surgeon standing on the right of the patient. The head of the patient will need to be positioned according to the target area and the approach to be used. Pin fixation may be required in some instances, but being able to manipulate head position during surgery can be beneficial, especially during multiportal surgery. To access the frontal sinus and the anterior aspect of the ACF just posterior to the frontal sinus, the head often needs to be in extension (or 15 degrees of retroflexion) to achieve the optimum endoscope position and trajectory. During the initial part of the surgery, the surgeon creating the surgical pathway holds the endoscope and manages the powered instrumentation. The surgical team may differ from unit to unit and consist of a combination of otolaryngologist, neurosurgeon, or ophthalmologist working in synchrony. Two assistants are usually required to support the main surgeon unless specialized retractors and multifunctional instruments are used. A single hand holding one instrument that can perform three functions, for example, a drill that has irrigation and suction capabilities, can replace three hands with one less assistant needed. For the neurosurgical or intracranial part of the procedure, surgery is similar to transsphenoidal pituitary surgery, with the otolaryngologist manipulating the endoscope and managing the surgical field in order for the neurosurgeon to work bimanually.

## 16.5.2 General Approach

The surgical approach is chosen by the target location, as indicated in the discussion earlier. The appropriate approach is typically that corresponding to the quadrant that is primarily involved by the pathology; at times two transorbital approaches will be used synchronously (e.g., medial and inferior approaches) or transorbital and transnasal approaches may be combined in a multiportal technique[4,10,11] to improve manipulation and visualization. We have found that preoperative computer planning and analysis can be of significant benefit in planning these procedures.[12] As seen in ▶ Fig. 16.11, multiple approaches to each target should be considered. In this

example of an undifferentiated carcinoma invading the orbit, maxilla, and nasal cavity, inferior and medial transorbital approaches are used at the beginning of the case to ascertain adherence of the tumor to intraorbital structures, and to dissect through normal tissues to the interorbital skull base. Before excision of tumor, the dura is inspected and determination of intracranial tumor extent, if any, is made. Once the involvement of adjacent structures has been definitively determined, resection of the tumor begins. Dissection proceeds outward from critical structures—from the orbital contents toward the sinuses and nasal cavity and from the dura inferiorly into the nasal cavity. The transnasal approach is used later for subsequent excision of the intranasal component. By beginning with transorbital dissection, safety of the orbital contents and brain can be assured without dissecting through tumor, moving outward from delicate structures into less critical regions. Accessing these structures from a transnasal approach requires dissection through tumor, which may be risky, particularly when the border between tumor and critical structures is obscured. Preoperative computer-aided surgical planning will help the surgeon determine the optimal number and placement of surgical portals, as well as the proper approach vectors and pathways to ensure successful completion of the surgical goal.

## 16.5.3 Superior Approach

### Incision and Dissection

The incision for the superior approach is identical to that of an upper blepharoplasty as discussed in Chapter 10. The position can be varied somewhat depending on the surgical target; for more anterosuperior targets such as frontal sinus pathology, it is advantageous to have a more superiorly located incision to decrease the amount of skin on the upper flap adjacent to the orbital rim. The incision should be placed well below the eyebrow to prevent a visible scar, however. The incision through skin and subcutaneous tissue will expose the thin layer of

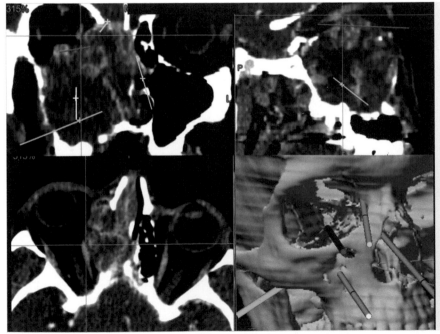

**Fig. 16.11** Preoperative planning and trajectory analysis.

orbicularis oculi muscle, which is incised using a sharp dissecting iris scissors. The orbital septum can then be identified and dissection should remain superficial to this layer to prevent fat herniation and trauma to the levator palpebrae superioris muscle and aponeurosis. Sharp dissection is continued superiorly until the orbital rim is reached. The periosteum is incised on the rim and dissection is continued in a subperiosteal plane using a freer elevator. The entire superior orbit can be exposed from the lacrimal gland laterally to the outflow tract of the frontal sinus medially.

Laterally, the lacrimal gland can be elevated away from the bone since it lies on the orbital side of the periosteum. Medially, injury to the trochlea is prevented by remaining in the subperiosteal plane (the trochlea is lifted with the periosteum, and not typically visualized unless an intraconal approach is being used). The supraorbital and supratrochlear neurovascular bundles must be identified and preserved as the periosteum of the superior orbital rim is elevated. Retraction of the nerves is possible but may require bone around the nerve bundles to be drilled if they lie within a canal, especially when addressing frontal sinus osteomas or fibrous dysplasia. The location of the orbital roof craniectomy depends on the pathology that needs to be addressed. Frontal sinus pathology is easier to address in well-pneumatized frontal sinuses and if the patient's head is placed in extension. For ACF lesions, once the dura has been exposed, surgery can continue with the neurosurgeon and the otolaryngologist/ophthalmologist working together. The ACF up to the lesser wing of the sphenoid can be accessed with dissection being limited by the SOF posteriorly. The anterior, accessory, and posterior ethmoidal arteries can be visualized and cauterized through this approach, but to get better access to structures medially located (intracranially and intranasally), the procedure should be combined with a precaruncular approach.

Any CSF leak needs to be repaired using standard techniques utilizing fat, fascia lata, or other suitable graft material. Reconstruction of the superior orbital wall is usually not indicated but for large craniectomies, reconstruction can be performed using a polydioxanone (PDS) sheet or an orbital plate with screw fixation behind the orbital rim. The patient may initially feel the pulsation of the dura on the orbit, but this sensation usually dissipates within the first few weeks. When dealing with orbital lesions, the superior pathway gives excellent access to tumors located in the posterior orbit. A subperiosteal dissection onto bone is first performed and navigation is useful for lesions that are superficial and closely related to the bony orbit. For deep-lying orbital lesions, navigation is less helpful and ultrasound can be used to determine the exact location of the lesion and periorbital incision site. Once the periorbita has been incised, orbital fat can be contained and the lesion dissected using a suction freer elevator on neurosurgical patties.

## Challenges, Pearls, and Pitfalls

It is critical to dissect superficial to the orbital septum and avoid trauma to the levator aponeurosis. Using surgical loupes greatly facilitates dissection in the correct plane. It is important not to retract the upper eyelid aggressively to avoid traction injury to the levator muscle. If orbital fat is exposed during the early stages of the procedure, dissection may be more difficult. Great care should be taken to prevent orbital fat from being caught in the drill, which could cause damage to the rectus muscles. It is

important to have special drill burrs with less than 2 mm of the shaft of the drill burr exposed beyond the burr tip. Alternatively, ultrasonic bone aspirators have the ability to remove bone, suction, and irrigate at the same time without the presence of a rotating burr. This is particularly useful when operating deep within the orbit. It is important to remember that the bone aspirator handle can become hot, and care must be taken to avoid a thermal injury to the skin around the eye.

## 16.5.4 Lateral Approach

### Incision and Dissection

The choice between three different surgical incisions depends on the procedure being performed and the exposure required. The degree of access may be sequentially increased using the retrocanthal incision, which can be expanded to a lateral canthotomy with cantholysis, and finally an extended upper lid crease incision as described in Chapter 10.

The retrocanthal[13] and lateral canthotomy incisions are ideal if a biopsy or resection needs to be performed in the lateral orbit, infratemporal fossa, or for access to the greater wing of sphenoid bone or MCF. Both incisions give wide access to the lateral orbit with a proximal pathway width of 1 cm at the orbital rim if the orbit is retracted medially using ribbon retractors.[6] The incision can be extended through the conjunctiva as needed to gain greater exposure, though care must be taken not to damage the lateral horn of the levator aponeurosis superiorly. Dissection in the superior orbit may be limited, however, especially to gain adequate access to lesions like sphenoid wing meningiomas where hyperostotic bone often involves the lateral and superior orbital walls. To gain more superior access with a wider pathway, an eyelid crease incision is extended laterally but with preservation of the lateral canthus (▸ Fig. 16.12). Preserving the lateral canthus increases patient comfort postoperatively with more rapid wound healing. This incision is the first author's preference and is used for all lateral resections where there is some involvement of the superior orbital wall. The extended upper lid skin crease incision is started approximately 8 to 10 mm above the upper lid margin. The incision is extended to the natural crease lines above the lateral canthus, and over the lateral orbital rim. Dissection is carried through the underlying orbicularis muscle into the preaponeurotic space. Blunt dissection is performed in a suborbicularis pocket up to the superior orbital rim. Breeching the orbital

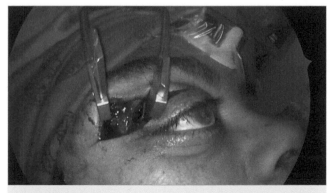

**Fig. 16.12** Eyelid crease incision extending laterally with preservation of the lateral canthus.

septum will cause herniation of orbital fat, making further dissection difficult. The periosteum of the superior orbital rim is incised 10 mm above the arcus marginalis. Dissection is then carried out posteriorly in a subperiosteal plane along the roof and lateral wall of the orbit using a Freer suction elevator. The supraorbital neurovascular bundle should be identified and preserved where it runs just medial to the midpoint of the superior orbital rim. Laterally, periosteum is elevated off the lateral orbital rim. Using instruments with multiple functions such as a drill with suction and irrigation or an ultrasonic bone aspirator allows for ample space for manipulation of the endoscope and instrumentation. The orbit is retracted medially using ribbon retractors, allowing for a wide lateral surgical pathway for the use of an 18-cm, 3-mm, or 4-mm, 0-degree endoscope with two to three other instruments. Adequate space is created by drilling away the lateral orbital wall until the temporalis muscle is visualized, keeping at least 5 mm of orbital rim intact for cosmetic purposes. Two assistants are required without specialized retractors and multifunctional instruments. Again, care must be taken if a rotating burr is used not to damage orbital fat. A bone pathway is drilled through the cancellous bone of the greater wing of the sphenoid bone, leaving a thin wall of bone protecting temporalis muscle laterally and periorbita medially. When treating sphenoid wing meningiomas, it is important to drill away all hyperostotic bone and intraosseous meningioma. As temporalis muscle is exposed posteriorly and the greater wing of the sphenoid is drilled away, the dura of the temporal lobe is encountered posteriorly and laterally. Removal of the orbital roof will expose ACF dura superiorly. The SOF limits dissection posteriorly and the inferior orbital fissure inferiorly. Care should be taken near the SOF as excessive manipulation and traction in this area could lead to a SOF syndrome or damage to cranial nerves III, IV, V$_1$, and VI.

Once the dura of the ACF and MCF is exposed, the intracranial tumor can be removed using a four-handed technique with the assistant holding the endoscope and managing the surgical field in order for the neurosurgeon to perform bimanual surgery. Complete tumor resection is often not possible because of tumor spread through the SOF or encasement of tumor around the middle cerebral artery or cavernous sinus involvement.

A large CSF leak is usually created when intradural pathology is addressed. The defect is repaired using fat and/or fascia lata or synthetic dura although the former is the author's preference. A lumbar drain is not routinely inserted. The lateral wall of the orbit is not reconstructed. In most instances, patients who require a lateral approach present with proptosis, and removal of the lateral wall improves cosmesis. A layer of thin polydioxanone (PDS) sheet may be added if the lateral rectus is exposed or there is concern for scarring or adhesion to the bone.

### Challenges, Pearls, and Pitfalls

Avoiding early exposure of orbital fat is an important factor for successful surgery. Careful dissection in the correct surgical plane is essential. Dissecting onto the lateral aspect of the orbital rim and then dissecting in a subperiosteal plane over the medial aspect of the orbital rim greatly facilitates avoiding early exposure of fat. If orbital fat is exposed, a Silastic sheet or neurosurgical patties are used to contain the fat under ribbon retractors. It is imperative that the eye is intermittently

inspected for a change in pupil size or shape. A dilated or asymmetric pupil indicates increased intraocular pressure, and all retractors and instruments should be removed until the pupil recovers. The surgeon and anesthetist should be aware of the oculocardiac reflex, manifesting as changes in blood pressure or bradycardia due to traction on the extraocular muscles or pressure on the globe. This reflex is mediated by the ophthalmic branch of the trigeminal nerve through the ciliary ganglion and thence the vagal parasympathetics, decreasing output of the sinoatrial node of the heart. If this occurs, intravenous administration of an antimuscarinic acetylcholine antagonist (atropine or glycopyrrolate) may be indicated. Navigation is useful especially to determine the position of the SOF when hyperostotic bone is present or normal anatomy is disturbed by tumor invasion.

### 16.5.5 Medial Approach

The precaruncular approach to the medial quadrant[14] is a versatile, low-morbidity approach to structures within and adjacent to the lamina papyracea. This includes the superior sinonasal structures, ethmoid arteries, skull base and overlying neurologic structures, and the optic nerve. The approach is coplanar with the dissection planes and anatomic structures, which may decrease reliance on angled visualization and instrumentation. It can be extended superiorly as needed, taking care to avoid the levator aponeurosis, and can be extended inferiorly to join a transconjunctival approach to the inferior orbital quadrant.

A precaruncular approach is used as described in Chapter 10. Dissection then continues posteriorly in a subperiosteal plane in the appropriate vector to the target. There is typically a visible groove or delineation at the junction of the lamina papyracea with the skull base, within which the anterior and posterior ethmoid arteries (and accessory middle arteries when present) are located. These neurovascular bundles are carefully cauterized with bipolar forceps and divided. The location of the optic nerve should be ascertained before cautery of the posterior ethmoid artery, as the distance can be quite small and is unpredictable.[15] At this point, dissection can proceed into the medial ACF through a craniectomy, into the frontal/ethmoid/sphenoid regions, or posteriorly for decompression of the orbital apex and optic nerve. We find the medial transorbital approach to be highly effective for optic nerve decompression not only because of the coplanar geometry, but also because it allows visualization of the nerve within the canal, followed by outfracturing or drilling of the bone away from, rather than toward, the nerve.

Reconstruction of the defect at the end of the procedure is directed to the nature of the defect. If a durotomy is created, it should be reconstructed with a graft and fibrin glue, particularly if the construct is supported by the orbital contents. If the dural defect extends over the paranasal sinuses, the use of a pedicled septal mucosa flap should be considered based on volume of flow and pressure of the CSF leak.

Reconstruction of the lamina papyracea should also be considered. Failure to do so may result in enophthalmos, or diplopia if the medial rectus muscle herniates into the defect. While it is difficult to predict whether a lamina defect of given size will cause enophthalmos, we have found that edema typically causes 1 to 3 mm of proptosis at the end of the case. Exophthalmometry can be performed before closing, and if there is less than 2 mm of proptosis bone reconstruction should be strongly considered.

Reconstruction can be performed using resorbable or permanent implants. Defects in the lamina can allow herniation of orbital contents into the ethmoid sinuses, which pose a risk for delayed obstruction, so we use resorbable implants only for small defects. For larger defects, we prefer thin titanium mesh, formed in situ as described earlier. We then line the mesh with thin (0.25-mm PDS) foil as a glide surface. Closure of the precaruncular incision is optional.

## Challenges, Pearls, and Pitfalls

It is critical to avoid damage to the lacrimal canaliculi when creating the precaruncular approach to the lamina papyracea. This can be done by placing lacrimal probes before dissecting to prevent transection, though with experience this is not necessary. It is important to create an adequate conjunctival incision; while the incision is initially centered medial to the caruncle, it can be extended inferiorly without difficulty as needed. It is important to identify the ethmoid arteries; there are often three or more, and each should be cauterized as needed.

## 16.5.6 Inferior Approach

The approach to the inferior quadrant of the orbit that we recommend employs the same transconjunctival incision that is used for lower lid blepharoplasty or orbital floor fracture repair as described in Chapter 10.[1] This approach provides full access to the orbital floor, the overlying orbital contents, the maxilla, and the inferior orbital apex. Within this runs the infraorbital nerve, a common route of metastases from the skin and maxilla to the brain. The lateral floor contains the inferior orbital fissure, which provides a pathway for pathology to transit from the infratemporal and pterygomaxillary fossae. The inferior orbit is thus a common point in the spread of disease from a number of regions and needs to be accessed when performing surgical extirpation. During subperiosteal elevation, care should be taken not to inadvertently damage the infraorbital nerve, which may run in a canal below or within the orbital floor, and courses into the orbital apex posteriorly before entering foramen rotundum. The orbital contents are lifted with a ribbon retractor, and a sheet of thin Silastic may be placed against the orbital contents to protect and prevent herniation of their contents during the procedure. Bone is removed as needed for the procedure.

On completion of the procedure, the orbital floor reconstruction is performed as described earlier, typically with the use of titanium mesh and a glide layer of thin PDS foil. We rarely use resorbable implants alone in this region due to the ongoing need for load bearing. If the pathology does not involve the floor itself, reconstruction is performed by contouring the plate on the floor before bone removal to match the contours precisely. If the pathology prevents this, mirror image overlay (MIO) navigation guidance is used for creation of the implant.[16]

## Challenges, Pearls, and Pitfalls

It is important in creating the incision to avoid the tarsus, and we prefer to dissect posterior to the septum as well. The incision should thus be made at least 3 mm inferior to the tarsus. Adequate retraction of orbital contents is critical to the dissection. This can be provided with malleable ribbon retractors of various sizes alone, or with a thin sheet of transparent Silastic shielding the orbital fat.

# 16.6 Complications and Management

With proper surgical technique and careful surgical dissection, complications from transorbital endoscopic surgery are quite rare.[7] Postoperative lid swelling may be significant, depending on the location and duration of the surgery. Intraoperative intravenous steroid use, possibly with a short course postoperatively, along with the postoperative use of iced compresses for 48 hours will control this. If there is a significant amount of chemosis or proptosis at the end of the case, we place a temporary tarsorrhaphy suture and leave it in place for 3 to 5 days until the swelling subsides.

Detailed knowledge of orbital anatomy is required to avoid any injury to intraconal vessels, nerves, and extraocular muscles during dissection of orbital lesions. Intraoperative CSF leak, if it occurs, can be addressed with graft material as discussed earlier, fixated with fibrin sealant. Watertight closure of the incision is then necessary to prevent leakage of CSF from the wound. As long as there is no route of egress such as through the lamina papyracea into the nose, these leaks do not become problematic, and terminate with re-adherence of the periorbita to the adjacent bone.

With approaches to the superior orbit, excessive traction on the supraorbital or supratrochlear neurovascular pedicles can lead to prolonged forehead numbness. Care should be taken when introducing instruments into the orbit to avoid damage to these structures. Heavy retraction on the levator muscle or aponeurosis can cause postoperative ptosis, though in our experience this resolves spontaneously with time. For some pathology such as osteomas protruding through the orbital roof, the levator muscle or extraocular muscles may actually be involved with the pathology, and require displacement to remove the tumor; in these cases, temporary ptosis and/or diplopia is to be expected regardless of the surgical approach used. This typically resolves in time.

Corneal abrasion is also a risk, though this can be mitigated with meticulous surgical technique. A lubricated corneal protector can also be used, but this necessitates frequent removal to monitor the pupil for dilation or distortion—signs of excessive intraorbital pressure. It is our preference to place a temporary tarsorrhaphy suture at the medial or lateral limbus, which protects the cornea sufficiently while allowing the surgeon to easily separate the lids to visualize the pupil. While we have not had a case of postoperative hemorrhage, this would necessitate an ophthalmology evaluation, tonometry, reopening the incision, possible lateral canthotomy/cantholysis, and evacuation of the hematoma.

Complications of the approach to the inferior quadrant of the orbit are rare. One of the most common complications is postoperative lower lid retraction, which is caused by damage to the lower lid from excessive retraction or from the dissection. We strongly recommend a direct transconjunctival rather than transcutaneous or preseptal approach, as this leaves a thin protective layer of fat on the lid and is less likely to damage the orbital septum.

The attachment of the inferior oblique muscle to the orbital floor is raised with the orbital contents by dissection deep to the periosteum. Dissection within the orbital fat in this region carries a risk of damage to the muscle and subsequent diplopia.

Chemosis (edema of the bulbar conjunctiva) can be problematic after this or any of the orbital approaches.

Complications related to the medial approach itself are rare. As mentioned, monopolar cautery in the region of the lacrimal canaliculi can lead to scarring and postoperative epiphora. Failure to reconstruct the lamina papyracea, if removed, can lead to enophthalmos, ethmoid sinusitis, or mucocele formation, and occasionally may cause diplopia. Until the surgeon is comfortable with the approach, placement of superior and inferior lacrimal probes when establishing the portal will prevent injury to the lacrimal canaliculi.

## 16.7 Outcomes

Transorbital endoscopic surgery is a new and rapidly growing field of surgery. To date, most publications have reported relatively small case series,[11,17,18,19] but larger reports are appearing. Our earlier prospective series that included 107 consecutive patients undergoing transorbital surgery demonstrated the efficacy and safety of transorbital pathways for various orbital, sinus, and intracranial pathologies.[2] In that series, there were no complications related to the surgical approach or use of endoscopy, and no cases of visual loss. We recently reported our outcomes in a series of 45 consecutive transorbital neuroendoscopic skull base cases of various pathology including intracranial and orbital tumors, CSF leak, and intracranial complications of sinogenic infection. All procedures were successful; the complications were limited to one case of temporary ptosis, one case of mild enophthalmos unnoticed by the patient, and one case of epiphora that developed 2 months after surgery and resolved with dacryocystorhinostomy. There were no cases of visual loss, diplopia, stroke, or death in the series.

The safety and efficacy record of orbital and transorbital endoscopic procedures appears to be highly encouraging, and further reports expanding their applications such as robotic[20] and deeper brain surgery[21] are appearing with increasing frequency. Additional studies will be helpful in describing outcomes as the frontiers of these procedures are advanced and new enabling technologies become available.

## 16.8 Conclusion

Using a system of four surgical pathways (one for each quadrant of the orbit), pathology of the orbit as well as the optic nerve, paranasal and cavernous sinuses, anterior and middle cranial fossae, and intracranial space can now be accessed endoscopically with minimally disruptive techniques. Transorbital approaches can be used alone or in a multiportal technique with transnasal, transmaxillary, infratemporal fossa, and supraorbital portals to access adjacent structures. Because the postoperative morbidity associated with traditional approaches is due in large part to extensive collateral destruction of healthy tissue, this disruption can now be avoided by using transorbital pathways, often with improved visualization of the target.

The quadrant-centered endoscopic approaches have allowed management of orbital pathology that was previously difficult to access. Although this surgery has traditionally fallen under the ophthalmologist's domain, the transorbital pathways have gained popularity among otolaryngologists and neurosurgeons, offering new surgical solutions and management options by a multidisciplinary team. A surgical team incorporating three different disciplines can often manage lesions previously deemed inoperable.

## References

[1] Moe KS, Bergeron CM, Ellenbogen RG. Transorbital neuroendoscopic surgery. Neurosurgery. 2010; 67(3) Suppl Operative:ons16–ons28

[2] Balakrishnan K, Moe KS. Applications and outcomes of orbital and transorbital endoscopic surgery. Otolaryngol Head Neck Surg. 2011; 144(5): 815–820

[3] Bly R, Moe KS. Transorbital Endoscopic Skull Base Surgery. In: Lalwani A, Pfister M, eds. Recent Advances in Head and Neck Surgery, 2nd ed. New Delhi: Jaypee Brothers Publishing; 2013

[4] Ciporen JN, Moe KS, Ramanathan D, et al. Multiportal endoscopic approaches to the central skull base: a cadaveric study. World Neurosurg. 2010; 73(6): 705–712

[5] Ellenbogen RG, Moe KS. Transorbital neuroendoscopic approaches to the anterior cranial fossa. In: Snyderman C, Gardner P, eds. Master Techniques in Otolaryngology—Head and Neck Surgery: Skull Base Surgery. Philadelphia, PA: Wolters Kluwer; 2014

[6] Bly RA, Ramakrishna R, Ferreira M, Moe KS. Lateral transorbital neuroendoscopic approach to the lateral cavernous sinus. J Neurol Surg B Skull Base. 2014; 75(1):11–17

[7] Oxford R, Bly R, Kim L, Moe KS. Transorbital neuroendoscopic surgery of the middle cranial fossa by lateral retrocanthal approach. J Neurol Surg B Skull Base. 2012; 22 Suppl 1:68

[8] Moe KS, Ellenbogen RG. Transorbital neuroendoscopic approaches to the middle cranial fossa. In: Snyderman C, Gardner P, eds. Master Techniques in Otolaryngology—Head and Neck Surgery: Skull Base Surgery. Philadelphia, PA: Wolters Kluwer; 2014

[9] Moe KS, Kim LJ, Bergeron CM. Transorbital endoscopic repair of cerebrospinal fluid leaks. Laryngoscope. 2011; 121(1):13–30

[10] Alqahtani A, Padoan G, Segnini G, et al. Transorbital transnasal endoscopic combined approach to the anterior and middle skull base: a laboratory investigation. Acta Otorhinolaryngol Ital. 2015; 35(3):173–179

[11] Dallan I, Castelnuovo P, Locatelli D, et al. Multiportal combined transorbital transnasal endoscopic approach for the management of selected skull base lesions: preliminary experience. World Neurosurg. 2015; 84(1):97–107

[12] Bly RA, Su D, Hannaford B, Ferreira M, Jr, Moe KS. Computer modeled multiportal approaches to the skull base. J Neurol Surg B Skull Base. 2012; 73 (6) B6:415–423

[13] Moe KS, Jothi S, Stern R, Gassner HG. Lateral retrocanthal orbitotomy: a minimally invasive, canthus-sparing approach. Arch Facial Plast Surg. 2007; 9 (6):419–426

[14] Moe KS. The precaruncular approach to the medial orbit. Arch Facial Plast Surg. 2003; 5(6):483–487

[15] Berens A, Davis G, Moe K. Transorbital endoscopic identification of supernumerary ethmoid arteries. Allergy Rhinol (Providence). 2016; 7(3): e144–e146

[16] Bly RA, Chang SH, Cudejkova M, Liu JJ, Moe KS. Computer-guided orbital reconstruction to improve outcomes. JAMA Facial Plast Surg. 2013; 15(2): 113–120

[17] Lubbe D, Mustak H, Taylor A, Fagan J. Minimally invasive endo-orbital approach to sphenoid wing meningiomas improves visual outcomes - our experience with the first seven cases. Clin Otolaryngol. 2017; 42(4):876–880

[18] Ramakrishna R, Kim LJ, Bly RA, Moe K, Ferreira M, Jr. Transorbital neuroendoscopic surgery for the treatment of skull base lesions. J Clin Neurosci. 2016; 24:99–104

[19] Lim JH, Sardesai MG, Ferreira M, Jr, Moe KS. Transorbital neuroendoscopic management of sinogenic complications involving the frontal sinus, orbit, and anterior cranial fossa. J Neurol Surg B Skull Base. 2012; 73(6):394–400

[20] Bly RA, Su D, Lendvay TS, et al. Multiportal robotic access to the anterior cranial fossa: a surgical and engineering feasibility study. Otolaryngol Head Neck Surg. 2013; 149(6):940–946

[21] Chen HI, Bohman LE, Loevner LA, Lucas TH. Transorbital endoscopic amygdalohippocampectomy: a feasibility investigation. J Neurosurg. 2014; 120(6):1428–1436

# 17 Orbital Complications of Sinusitis and Management

*Rodney J. Schlosser, Elliott Mappus, and Zachary M. Soler*

**Abstract**

Infectious and inflammatory rhinosinusitis can involve the orbit and eye given the thin barriers that separate these two anatomic areas. Infectious complications can be acute or chronic and result from direct extension of the bacterial or fungal infection. These complications can be treated medically if caught early or may need surgery in advanced cases. In infectious causes, it is important for the treating physicians to understand the role and treatment of any underlying immune deficiencies. Noninfectious causes can occur from inflammatory conditions, such as mucoceles, allergic fungal rhinosinusitis, or silent sinus syndrome, and usually occur in immunocompetent patients. These conditions are chronic and result due to pressure effect and bone remodeling of the orbital floor, medial wall, or roof. Noninfectious causes that are severe enough to cause bone remodeling respond to medical therapy less often and usually require surgical decompression of the offending sinus pathology in order to avoid permanent orbital complications. Surgical treatment of any orbital complications is more difficult than routine sinus surgery, given the altered anatomy, frequent encounter of acutely inflamed mucosa, and need for care to preserve orbital function. Close collaboration between otorhinolaryngology, ophthalmology, neurosurgery, radiology, and any appropriate medical specialists is required to properly treat patients with orbital complications of rhinosinusitis.

*Keywords:* subperiosteal abscess, orbital abscess, periorbital cellulitis, orbital erosion

## 17.1 Introduction

Given the close proximity of the orbit to the paranasal sinuses, it is not surprising that infectious and inflammatory conditions of the sinuses can involve the orbit. Fortunately, most of these complications respond to medical and/or surgical treatment of the inciting sinusitis without resulting in permanent visual impairment. The time spectrum, infectious agents, and associated inflammatory process involved vary widely. A comprehensive understanding of the differences in patient demographics, underlying host immune status, and anatomic sites involved is critical to the timely management of these patients and avoidance of long-term sequelae.

## 17.2 Types of Orbital Complications and Patient Presentation

Orbital complications can be divided into infectious complications that result from direct extension of bacterial or fungal infections into the orbit (▶ Table 17.1) or noninfectious complications that result from bony remodeling and anatomic changes

due to adjacent sinus pathology causing positive or negative pressure upon the orbit (▶ Table 17.2).

### 17.2.1 Acute Bacterial Rhinosinusitis

Acute bacterial rhinosinusitis (ABRS) can spread to involve the adjacent orbit and is the most common infectious orbital complication of rhinosinusitis. This occurs most often in pediatric patients without any prior history of sinus problems and normal immune function (▶ Fig. 17.1). The onset can be quite rapid and alarming. Chandler has classified the spectrum of acute bacterial complications of rhinosinusitis[1]:

- Preseptal cellulitis: Edema limited to eyelid with normal extraocular motility, painless eye movement, and normal vision. Anatomically, infection is superficial to the fibrous orbital septum and thus excludes the orbital contents.
- Orbital/postseptal cellulitis: Progressive edema, now involving the globe with chemosis, painful or limited extraocular motility, and in rare instances altered visual acuity. Anatomically, infection is deep to the fibrous orbital septum and thus involves the orbital contents.
- Subperiosteal abscess: Defined collection of pus between orbital bone (most often lamina papyracea) and periorbita. Patients may have limited motility and proptosis and an overall clinical picture of postseptal cellulitis; thus, imaging is critical to diagnosis.
- Orbital abscess: Pus within orbit, deep to periorbita, development of ophthalmoplegia.
- Cavernous sinus thrombosis: Intracranial infection with cranial nerve palsies, fever, headaches.

### 17.2.2 Acute Invasive Fungal Rhinosinusitis

Acute invasive fungal rhinosinusitis occurs in patients with suppressed immune systems. This can occur in patients with hematologic malignancies, HIV (human immunodeficiency virus), diabetic ketoacidosis, or those taking immune-modifying medications for transplants or other conditions (▶ Fig. 17.2). Clinical presentation can be quite rapid in patients with extremely suppressed immune systems, such as after a bone marrow transplant, or somewhat indolent and mistaken for a routine viral or sinus infection in patients with more subtle immune deficiencies, such as those on long-term immunosuppressive medications.

### 17.2.3 Chronic Invasive Fungal Sinusitis

Chronic invasive fungal sinusitis occurs most often in patients with normal immune systems or subtle immune suppression. Patients present with a slowly progressive course that is often mistaken for routine chronic rhinosinusitis (CRS) that is refractory to standard antibiotics and steroids. They often have mild inflammatory changes around the orbital apex and can even have endoscopic sinus surgery for presumed CRS that does not resolve normally (▶ Fig. 17.3).

Table 17.1 Infectious orbital complications of rhinosinusitis

| | Acute bacterial rhinosinusitis | Acute invasive fungal rhinosinusitis | Chronic invasive fungal rhinosinusitis |
|---|---|---|---|
| Prevalence of orbital involvement | 5% of patients hospitalized for sinusitis[1]<br>• 50% preseptal cellulitis<br>• 35% postseptal cellulitis<br>• 15% subperiosteal abscess<br>• <1% orbital abscess[9] | 73.5% of AIFS cases[10] | 89.9% of CIFS and granulomatous invasive fungal CRS[10,11] |
| Demographics | More common in children[1]<br>• Preseptal: 3.9-y old<br>• Postseptal: 7.5 y old[12] | Diabetes mellitus<br>Hematologic malignancy<br>Systemic chemotherapy<br>Immunosuppressive drugs<br>AIDS<br>Chronic steroid use[3,11,13] | Can have no known immunosuppression<br>Diabetes mellitus<br>AIDS<br>Chronic steroid use[3,11,13] |
| Immune status | Normal | Compromised[11] | Normal[11] |
| Common organisms | Staphylococcus aureus<br>Streptococcus pneumoniae<br>Haemophilus influenzae<br>Anaerobic species (Peptostreptococcus, Fusobacterium, Bacteroides)[1,9] | Aspergillus spp.<br>Zygomycetes (Rhizopus, Mucor, Rhizomucor)[11] | CIFS: Aspergillus fumigatus[4]<br>Granulomatous variant: Aspergillus flavus[11] |
| Location | Medial or superior orbital wall[9,14] | Medial orbital wall[10] | Medial orbital wall<br>Orbital apex[4] |
| Medical treatment | Preseptal: oral antibiotics<br>Postseptal: IV antibiotics<br>Include anaerobic and MRSA coverage[1,9]<br>Nasal decongestion<br>Elevation of head of bed<br>Serial examinations[9] | IV antifungal<br>Reverse immunocompromised state (i.e., WBC transfusions)<br>Glycemic control in diabetics[4]<br>Discontinuation of steroids[15] | Long term oral antifungals[16]<br>Glycemic control in diabetics[4]<br>Discontinuation of steroids[15] |
| Surgical treatment | Typically performed if one or more are met[1,9]:<br>• Visual impairment<br>• Large abscess (>10 mm on CT)<br>• Failed trial of appropriate medical treatment | Urgent debridement until bleeding, healthy margins[17]<br>May require orbital exenteration[13] | Debride to healthy tissue[4] |
| Prognosis | Excellent for early cases, but if cavernous sinus involved, mortality as high as 30%[1] | Common recurrence[4]<br>Mortality: 50–80%[3] | Inversely related to degree of invasion[4] |

Abbreviations: AIDS, acquired immunodeficiency syndrome; AIFS, acute invasive fungal sinusitis; CIFS, chronic invasive fungal sinusitis; CRS, chronic rhinosinusitis; CT, computed tomography; IV, intravenous; MRSA, methicillin-resistant staph aureus; WBC, white blood cell.

Table 17.2 Noninfectious orbital complications of sinusitis

| | Mucocele | AFRS | Silent sinus | Pneumosinus dilatans |
|---|---|---|---|---|
| Prevalence of orbital involvement | 20% of paranasal sinus mucoceles[5] | Wide variability, 20–93% of AFRS cases[18] | Essentially 100% of silent sinus involve the orbit[7] | Rare[8] |
| Demographics | Elderly (53.1 y old)<br>CRS<br>Previous sinonasal trauma[5,19] | Younger<br>African American males[20]<br>Regions of high humidity[6] | Middle aged (mean 30–50 y)[7] | Idiopathic<br>Meningioma<br>Fibro-osseous disease[8] |
| Immune status | Normal | Atopic[6] | Normal | Normal |
| Common organisms | None | Aspergillus spp. (may present without fungal spores)[6] | None | None |
| Location | Frontal sinus[17]<br>Medial and superior orbital wall[5] | Medial orbital wall[21] | Orbit floor[7] | Most common[8]:<br>• Frontal sinus<br>• Sphenoid sinus<br>• Maxillary sinus<br>• Ethmoid sinus |
| Medical treatment | Typically unresponsive[19] | Oral and topical steroids | Typically unresponsive[7] | Typically unresponsive[8] |
| Surgical treatment | Decompress mass effect[5] | Decompress mass effect[21]<br>Unlikely to need orbital reconstruction as proptosis reverts to normal[2] | Endoscopic maxillary antrostomy[7] | Relief of ocular symptoms by widening of sinus ostium[8] |
| Prognosis | Reduction of symptoms<br>Recurrence rate 25% in patients with orbital complications[5] | Able to control with adjuvant medical therapy, regular follow-ups and monitoring for recurrence[6] | Excellent if sinus remains patent[7] | Reduction of symptoms following surgery[8] |

Abbreviations: AFRS, allergic fungal rhinosinusitis; CRS, chronic rhinosinusitis.

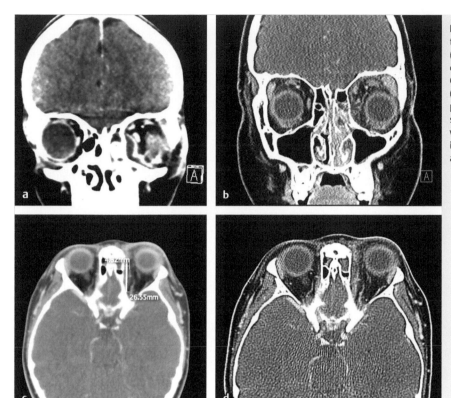

**Fig. 17.1** Coronal soft-tissue computed tomography (CT) of a pediatric patient (a) demonstrates subperiosteal abscess in common location along medial orbital wall. Coronal and axial CT of a different child (b,c,d) demonstrates small defect in lamina papyracea (*arrow*). Patient failed to respond to systemic antibiotics. Endoscopic sinus surgery, with drainage of the abscess resulted in rapid improvement in clinical picture. (These images are provided courtesy of MUSC Rhinology.)

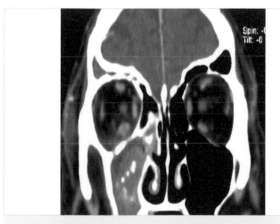

**Fig. 17.2** A transplant patient who presented with 2 to 3 weeks of sinus symptoms and subsequently developed limited extraocular motility. Symptoms were unresponsive to systemic antibiotics. Coronal soft-tissue CT (computed tomography) demonstrates what began as a fungus ball of the maxillary sinus, but eventually became invasive fungal rhinosinusitis with orbital involvement. Endoscopic sinus surgery, with removal of involved tissue down to periorbita and postoperative antifungals, resulted in rapid improvement. (This image is provided courtesy of MUSC Rhinology.)

## 17.2.4 Mucoceles, Polyps, Allergic Fungal Rhinosinusitis, and Pneumosinus Dilatans

Mucoceles, polyps, allergic fungal rhinosinusitis (AFRS), and pneumosinus dilatans can be expansile and cause bone erosion around the orbit without direct invasion. Mucoceles are most often located in the frontal or ethmoid sinuses (▶ Fig. 17.4). AFRS has been reported to have a higher incidence of bone erosion than other polyp subtypes. It occurs primarily in younger patients and is more common in African Americans (▶ Fig. 17.5). Pneumosinus dilatans is a rare condition thought to occur from an obstructed sinus os, but does not result in opacification of the sinus (▶ Fig. 17.6). These expansile conditions often go undetected until patients present with proptosis or changes in their appearance.

## 17.2.5 Silent Sinus Syndrome

Silent sinus syndrome is another rare condition of the sinuses that affects the orbit. Rather than being an expansile process with positive pressure that leads to proptosis, silent sinus consists of negative pressure in the maxillary sinus, leading to enophthalmos (▶ Fig. 17.7) and occasionally double vision.

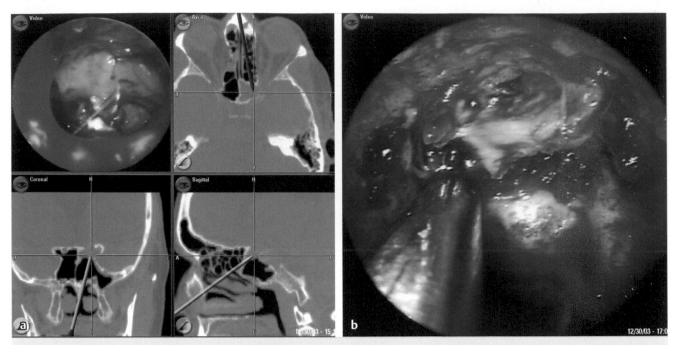

**Fig. 17.3** This elderly patient with no known immune suppression presented with orbital pain, visual loss, and sinus symptoms that were unresponsive to systemic antibiotics and standard endoscopic sinus surgery. Computed tomography (CT; **a**) and endoscopic debridement of orbital apex demonstrate involvement of the optic nerve (**b**). The patient did not recover vision; however, long-term oral antifungals prevented further disease progression. (These images are provided courtesy of MUSC Rhinology.)

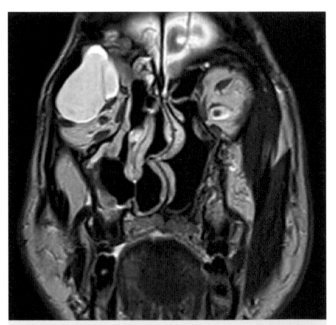

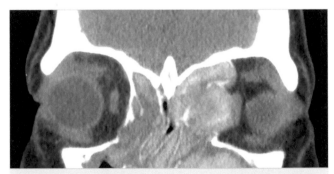

**Fig. 17.5** Coronal soft-tissue CT (computed tomography) demonstrates the classic differential densities noted in AFRS with bony erosion of the medial orbital wall. Endoscopic sinus surgery improved proptosis in this patient. (This image is provided courtesy of MUSC Rhinology.)

**Fig. 17.4** T2-weighted coronal MRI (magnetic resonance imaging) demonstrates the expansile changes of the superior/lateral orbit due to a mucocele. Endoscopic sinus surgery and marsupialization of the mucocele improved the clinical condition. (These images are provided courtesy of MUSC Rhinology.)

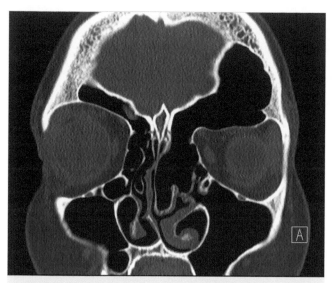

**Fig. 17.6** Coronal bone CT (computed tomography) of a patient with pneumosinus dilatans leading to erosion of orbital roof and proptosis. (This image is provided courtesy of MUSC Rhinology.)

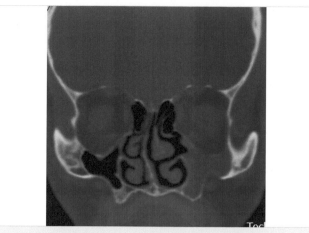

**Fig. 17.7** Coronal bone CT (computed tomography) demonstrates classic silent sinus syndrome with hypoplastic maxillary sinus and collapse of the uncinated process against the medial orbital wall. (This image is provided courtesy of MUSC Rhinology.)

## 17.3 Diagnostic Workup

### 17.3.1 History and Physical Examination

The initial evaluation of any patient presenting to an otolaryngologist with possible orbital complications should include a thorough history, as well as head and neck examination with nasal endoscopy. The history will help determine the patient's underlying immune status, the temporal course of the disease, and prior treatments. The head and neck examination will identify ocular abnormalities, cranial neuropathies, and potential extension of any sinus pathology into the palate, orbit, or skull base. Nasal endoscopy provides a number of benefits. In cases of ABRS, cultures will be useful to guide medical therapy. In cases of acute or chronic invasive fungal rhinosinusitis, endoscopy is used to identify ischemic (white) or necrotic (black) sinonasal tissue that is often insensate. If the diagnosis is in doubt, biopsies with frozen section can be performed to permit rapid surgical intervention if indicated. Tissue should also be sent for fungal cultures. Patients with expansile lesions, such as mucoceles and pneumosinus dilatans often have normal endoscopic examinations, but endoscopy must be performed to rule out other pathologies, including neoplasms, and it will also identify polyps in the case of AFRS causing orbital erosion. Endoscopy in silent sinus cases can identify subtle atelectasis of the uncinate process or retraction of the posterior fontanelle, but may also be normal.

### 17.3.2 Radiographic Imaging

Radiographic imaging is critical in managing patients with orbital complications. Noncontrasted computed tomography (CT) can be useful for processes that remodel but do not otherwise directly involve the orbit, such as mucoceles, AFRS, pneumosinus dilatans, or silent sinus syndrome. A contrast-enhanced CT is preferred for ABRS, which can help differentiate preseptal

from true postseptal orbital cellulitis and can determine if a discrete abscess is present, either subperiosteally or in the orbit proper. If cavernous sinus involvement is suspected clinically, a magnetic resonance imaging (MRI) with and without contrast is also usually obtained, often with specialized protocols such as MR venogram to assess flow through the cavernous sinus.

### 17.3.3 Ophthalmologic Evaluation

Ophthalmologic evaluation is recommended in all patients with possible orbital complications. This provides assessment of visual acuity (including changes in color perception), pupillary reaction, extraocular motility, intraocular pressure, and appearance of the optic nerve. Patients can often present with severe preseptal edema, but as long as visual acuity, pressure, and extraocular movements are intact, a conservative approach may be possible, depending upon the underlying pathology. Regardless of approach, serial ophthalmologic evaluation is critical to ensure disease is not progressing to the point where vision is threatened.

### 17.3.4 Other Multidisciplinary Consultations

Other multidisciplinary consultations depend upon the pathology and extent of disease. Neurosurgical evaluation is useful for possible intracranial or skull base involvement. Correction of underlying immune disorders may require the involvement of hematology-oncology, infectious disease, or endocrine specialists.

## 17.4 Medical Treatment

### 17.4.1 Acute Bacterial Rhinosinusitis

The most common bacteria are listed in ▶ Table 17.1. Empiric broad spectrum oral antibiotics can be used for uncomplicated preseptal cellulitis if patients are followed closely. If postseptal complications of rhinosinusitis are suspected, then patients are typically admitted for intravenous (IV) antibiotics, serial ophthalmologic examination, and contrast-enhanced CT scan. Endoscopically guided cultures can help direct appropriate antibiotics. This is particularly relevant given that between one-third and half of *Staphylococcus aureus* infections related to orbital cellulitis involve methicillin-resistant staph aureus (MRSA). Medical management with intensive observation is typically followed for cases of orbital cellulitis without visual impairment or small subperiosteal abscesses. Several studies have shown that small abscess volumes, perhaps < 1,250 mL, can usually be managed medically, avoiding surgery. This is particularly true if vision is unaffected and stable. However, larger volumes, those that are impacting vision, or those progressing despite medical therapy usually are recommended to have surgery. Orbital abscesses and cavernous sinus thrombosis usually undergo urgent surgery.

### 17.4.2 Acute Invasive Fungal Rhinosinusitis

Reversal of the immunocompromised state is critical to patient outcomes. This may require IV insulin drip for diabetics and hematologic consultation for patients with immune suppression due to leukemia or other malignancies. In cases of life-threatening infection, organ transplant recipients may have to make the difficult decision to discontinue immune-suppressive medications and sacrifice their transplant. Empiric IV antifungals are typically started as well, as cultures often require weeks to be completed.

### 17.4.3 Chronic Invasive Fungal Rhinosinusitis

Correction of any immune suppression is recommended. Typically given the chronic nature of this disease, oral antifungal agents are recommended for an extended period of time, guided by culture data when available.

### 17.4.4 Mucocele

Medical treatment is not typically effective due to complete obstruction of the sinus and the generally noninfectious nature of mucoceles. If there is an acute change due to development of mucopyocele, systemic antibiotics and steroids can be useful for resolution of the secondary bacterial infection and may "cool off" the situation, allowing surgery to be performed on a more elective basis.

### 17.4.5 Allergic Fungal Rhinosinusitis

Oral corticosteroids can often shrink polyps and improve any compressive effects upon the orbit. Topical corticosteroids are generally not effective prior to sinus surgery, due to obstruction by polyps and fungus in the nasal cavity, resulting in limited distribution to the paranasal sinuses.

### 17.4.6 Silent Sinus

Medical therapy is typically not effective due to complete ostial obstruction.

### 17.4.7 Pneumosinus Dilatans

Medical therapy is typically not effective.

## 17.5 Surgical Anatomy and Technique

The surgical approach to any sinus pathology leading to orbital complication is similar to routine endoscopic sinus surgery for CRS. When cases are done urgently in the face of severe inflammation or infection, pretreatment with systemic antibiotics in cases of ABRS and systemic corticosteroids in cases of ABRS or AFRS can optimize the surgical field. Systemic corticosteroids are not used in cases of invasive fungal disease due to the potential for further immune suppression allowing disease progression. Topical epinephrine is useful in decongesting inflamed sinus mucosa and improving visualization. This is particularly useful for cases of ABRS, wherein sinonasal inflammation can be severe and hyperemia with resultant oozing makes otherwise routine sinus surgery challenging.

ABRS most often leads to subperiosteal abscesses along the medial orbital wall with potential extension to the orbital roof. The first goal of surgery is to open the involved sinuses, which clears the purulence, allows directed cultures, and ensures future mucopus does not accumulate under pressure. This generally involves an endoscopic approach, with large maxillary antrostomy and total ethmoidectomy, with sphenoidotomy and occasionally frontal sinusotomy performed when involved. After completion of the maxillary antrostomy and sphenoethmoidectomy, additional steps in the surgical approach are similar to an orbital decompression. The lamina papyracea is removed beginning anteriorly where it is thinnest and furthest away from critical structures such as the medial rectus and optic nerve. Usually this is easiest to perform using an instrument such as a ball-tipped probe or freer elevator to avoid inadvertent entry through the periorbita. The lamina is then removed from anterior to posterior until the abscess is decompressed completely. In cases of superiorly located abscess, an olive-tip suction can be useful to pass between the periorbita and the bony orbital roof to drain the abscess. For isolated superior abscesses that do not have a medial ethmoid component, an external approach via an inferior brow or blepharoplasty incision can provide easy access for drainage. Unless the abscess has progressed to an orbital abscess, the periorbita is left intact. Image guidance is useful in these cases to target the ideal location for decompression. If the periorbita is left intact, the concern for postoperative diplopia is low.

The goals of surgery for acute and chronic invasive fungal rhinosinusitis include (1) obtaining adequate biopsy to confirm the diagnosis (histopathology with specialized fungal stains), (2) providing tissue for fungal-specific cultures, and (3) debridement of ischemic or necrotic tissue back to healthy bleeding tissue. Thus, the extent of surgical resection is determined by the disease present in any individual patient. This may require middle or inferior turbinectomy, medial maxillectomy, septectomy, and resection of other structures not resected in routine CRS cases. Chronic invasive fungal rhinosinusitis appears to have a predilection for the orbital apex and optic nerve decompression may be required with debridement of any fungal debris. Initial surgical approaches for invasive fungal rhinosinusitis typically attempt to preserve the globe/periorbita and dura, which act as natural barriers to fungal spread with prompt institution of IV antifungals and immune system support as needed. Typically, resection of the skull base and intracranial tissues proper is avoided, given that fungal spread directly into the central nervous system is often fatal. The decision to surgically resect the orbit is controversial, as high-level data do not exist proving that aggressive resection confers survival benefit. There appears to be a shift toward more conservative approaches to the orbit, at least upon initial intervention. Close monitoring of any intraorbital or intracranial extension by MRI and/or ocular examination is required and signs of continued extension or when the orbit is clearly irreversibly impacted (i.e., total ophthalmoplegia and complete loss of vision) should prompt more aggressive surgical resection such as orbital exenteration.

Expansile pathologies including mucoceles, AFRS, and pneumosinus dilatans typically require removal/marsupialization of the expansile process, realizing that the anatomy along the orbit can be severely distorted. Image guidance can be useful in these cases. Once the expansile process is addressed, the orbital contents typically return to their native location over time.[2]

Silent sinus is a unique negative pressure phenomenon leading to atelectasis of the uncinate process against the medial orbital wall. It is essential to carefully remove the uncinate process without entering the orbit, which is often dehiscent. This is best performed using ball-tipped probes to reflect the uncinate medially, then resecting it with a back-biter and hand instruments in a retrograde fashion. An anterograde sickle knife technique is best avoided, or at least done using extreme care.

In general, the use of powered instruments around the orbit in cases where there is a sinogenic complication/extension should be done with extreme care. These processes have led to orbital complications due to thinning or destruction of the lamina. When these natural barriers are gone or weakened, the potential for orbital injury increases.

## 17.6 Complications

All infectious orbital complications can lead to visual loss, double vision, and cranial neuropathies, especially with cavernous sinus extension. In cases of invasive fungal rhinosinusitis, these complications are usually permanent. Intracranial extension can often be fatal. Infections can also spread to other adjacent local tissues, such as soft tissue of the cheek and premaxilla, hard and soft palate, Eustachian tube, and nasopharynx.

Noninfectious orbital complications typically do not cause visual impairment or cranial neuropathies due to their slowly progressive time course. They can cause proptosis in cases of mucoceles, AFRS, and pneumosinus dilatans. Silent sinus often leads to enophthalmos and diplopia due to the underlying negative pressure. Successful treatment of the underlying sinus condition in these noninfectious cases usually leads to resolution of the abnormal position of the glove without additional orbital surgery.[2]

## 17.7 Postoperative Care

Standard postoperative care is similar to routine CRS cases and usually consists of saline rinses and periodic endoscopic debridements. Invasive fungal rhinosinusitis patients should be followed clinically to ensure response to medical and surgical treatment. Endoscopy and serial radiographic studies may be useful in monitoring response to medical and/or surgical treatment. In cases where the lamina has been surgically removed or disrupted by the underlying disease process, patients are advised against nose blowing for at least 2 weeks due to the risk of forcing air around the orbit, resulting in sudden and alarming subcutaneous emphysema of the periorbital structures. In all cases, serial ophthalmologic examinations are performed in order to ensure resolution of the potential complication.

## 17.8 Outcomes

ABRS cases that are treated in early stages often respond to antibiotics. Early abscesses respond well to surgical drainage. Once ABRS has progressed to cavernous sinus thrombosis, mortality can be as high as 30%.[1]

Acute invasive fungal rhinosinusitis has fairly poor outcomes due to the underlying immunocompromised state. Recurrence is common and mortality is as high as 80% in some series.[3] However, other modern series show much lower mortality rates. For any specific patient, the morality rate is likely impacted by the extent of involvement at diagnosis and reversibility of the underlying immune status. Those patients whose disease is limited and/or have reversible immune defects should be considered curable, whereas those with intracranial disease and/or irreversible immune defects have a much more guarded prognosis.

Chronic invasive fungal rhinosinusitis is relatively indolent. Cranial neuropathies typically do not recover and survival is related to severity of invasion.[4]

Mucoceles typically have very high success rates, but those with orbital involvement appear to have a higher recurrence rate, as high as 25% in some studies.[5]

AFRS has excellent outcomes with regard to orbital complications, but the underlying polypoid disease frequently recurs unless patients have aggressive surgery and consistent postoperative medical therapy with steroid rinses.[2,6]

Silent sinus has excellent surgical outcomes if the maxillary sinus remains patent.[7]

Pneumosinus dilatans also has excellent orbital outcomes if the sinus remains patent. Unlike AFRS, there is typically not an underlying inflammatory component.[8]

## 17.9 Summary

Orbital complications of rhinosinusitis can vary from acute to chronic, bacterial to fungal and even mucoceles or mass effect from polyps. Medical and surgical management of the inciting sinus condition often resolves any orbital pathology, but a complete understanding of the underlying immunopathology present in each patient is critical. This will guide the timing of surgery versus medical therapy, surgical technique and goals, and relevant anatomy the surgeon can expect to encounter.

## References

[1] Chandler JR, Langenbrunner DJ, Stevens ER. The pathogenesis of orbital complications in acute sinusitis. Laryngoscope. 1970; 80(9):1414–1428

[2]  Stonebraker AC, Schlosser RJ. Orbital volumetric analysis of allergic fungal sinusitis patients with proptosis before and after endoscopic sinus surgery. Am J Rhinol. 2005; 19(3):302–306

[3]  Trief D, Gray ST, Jakobiec FA, et al. Invasive fungal disease of the sinus and orbit: a comparison between mucormycosis and Aspergillus. Br J Ophthalmol. 2016; 100(2):184–188

[4]  Deshazo RD. Syndromes of invasive fungal sinusitis. Med Mycol. 2009; 47 Suppl 1:S309–S314

[5]  Scangas GA, Gudis DA, Kennedy DW. The natural history and clinical characteristics of paranasal sinus mucoceles: a clinical review. Int Forum Allergy Rhinol. 2013; 3(9):712–717

[6]  Marfani MS, Jawaid MA, Shaikh SM, Thaheem K. Allergic fungal rhinosinusitis with skull base and orbital erosion. J Laryngol Otol. 2010; 124(2):161–165

[7]  Annino DJ, Jr, Goguen LA. Silent sinus syndrome. Curr Opin Otolaryngol Head Neck Surg. 2008; 16(1):22–25

[8]  Adams W, Jones R, Chavda S, Pahor A, Taifa K. Pneumosinus dilatans: a discussion of four cases and the possible aetiology. Paper presented at the 16th Congress of the European Rhinologic Society, Ghent, Belgium; September 8–12, 1996

[9]  Bedwell J, Bauman NM. Management of pediatric orbital cellulitis and abscess. Curr Opin Otolaryngol Head Neck Surg. 2011; 19(6):467–473

[10]  Chandrasekharan R, Thomas M, Rupa V. Comparative study of orbital involvement in invasive and non-invasive fungal sinusitis. J Laryngol Otol. 2012; 126(2):152–158

[11]  Chakrabarti A, Denning DW, Ferguson BJ, et al. Fungal rhinosinusitis: a categorization and definitional schema addressing current controversies. Laryngoscope. 2009; 119(9):1809–1818

[12]  Botting AM, McIntosh D, Mahadevan M. Paediatric pre- and post-septal peri-orbital infections are different diseases. A retrospective review of 262 cases. Int J Pediatr Otorhinolaryngol. 2008; 72(3):377–383

[13]  Parikh SL, Venkatraman G, DelGaudio JM. Invasive fungal sinusitis: a 15-year review from a single institution. Am J Rhinol. 2004; 18(2):75–81

[14]  Soon VTE. Pediatric subperiosteal orbital abscess secondary to acute sinusitis: a 5-year review. Am J Otolaryngology. 2011; 32(1):62–68

[15]  Simmons JH, Zeitler PS, Fenton LZ, Abzug MJ, Fiallo-Scharer RV, Klingensmith GJ. Rhinocerebral mucormycosis complicated by internal carotid artery thrombosis in a pediatric patient with type 1 diabetes mellitus: a case report and review of the literature. Pediatr Diabetes. 2005; 6(4):234–238

[16]  Dooley DP, Hollsten DA, Grimes SR, Moss J, Jr. Indolent orbital apex syndrome caused by occult mucormycosis. J Clin Neuroophthalmol. 1992; 12(4):245–249

[17]  Epstein VA, Kern RC. Invasive fungal sinusitis and complications of rhinosinusitis. Otolaryngol Clin North Am. 2008; 41(3):497–524, viii

[18]  Ghegan MD, Wise SK, Gorham E, Schlosser RJ. Socioeconomic factors in allergic fungal rhinosinusitis with bone erosion. Am J Rhinol. 2007; 21(5): 560–563

[19]  Devars du Mayne M, Moya-Plana A, Malinvaud D, Laccourreye O, Bonfils P. Sinus mucocele: natural history and long-term recurrence rate. Eur Ann Otorhinolaryngol Head Neck Dis. 2012; 129(3):125–130

[20]  Ghegan MD, Lee FS, Schlosser RJ. Incidence of skull base and orbital erosion in allergic fungal rhinosinusitis (AFRS) and non-AFRS. Otolaryngol Head Neck Surg. 2006; 134(4):592–595

[21]  Nussenbaum B, Marple BF, Schwade ND. Characteristics of bony erosion in allergic fungal rhinosinusitis. Otolaryngol Head Neck Surg. 2001; 124(2): 150–154

# 18 Management of Iatrogenic Orbital Injury

Joanne Rimmer, Valerie J. Lund, and Geoffrey E. Rose

## Abstract

Orbital complications of endoscopic sinus surgery are rare, and the risks can be minimized with careful preoperative assessment and meticulous surgical technique. The common complications are presented, including breach of the lamina papyracea and orbital periosteum, surgical emphysema, intraorbital hemorrhage, extraocular muscle injury, optic nerve injury, and damage to the nasolacrimal system. The clinical signs suggestive of injury are discussed and management of the complications described, including emergency procedures that may be required to prevent visual loss.

Keywords: orbital injury, endoscopic sinus surgery, orbital hematoma, lamina papyracea, extraocular muscles, diplopia

## 18.1 Introduction

Orbital complications occur in 0.2 to 2.1% of all endoscopic sinus surgical cases,[1,2] and encompass a spectrum of injuries ranging from breach of the lamina papyracea to optic nerve injury and visual loss. Prevention is the key, but if an orbital complication does occur, then prompt identification and appropriate management may prevent severe sequelae.

## 18.2 Prevention

### 18.2.1 Preoperative Considerations

A thorough history should be taken to identify factors that increase the likelihood of orbital injury, such as preoperative abnormality of the lamina papyracea. These factors include previous orbital trauma or surgery, sinonasal tumor, severe nasal polyposis, or expansile lesions such as sinus mucoceles. It is also worth seeking an ophthalmic history of reduced visual acuity, the presence of amblyopia, or prior squint surgery—this provides a baseline if later orbital evaluation is required and will also alert the operator to potential issues. Ophthalmic signs are also relevant should subsequent events occur—such as pupillary dilation due to accidental contact with intranasal sympathomimetics (e.g., cocaine or adrenaline).[3] The normal latent squint during recovery from general anesthesia may be greater after intraoperative muscle relaxants, and thereby engender unwarranted concern for the surgeon.

Examination may reveal orbital signs—such as proptosis, nonaxial displacement of the globe, or restricted eye movements—or confirm the presence of significant sinonasal disease, and any preoperative abnormalities should be carefully documented.

Preoperative imaging with thin-slice computed tomography (CT) of the paranasal sinuses is mandatory before endoscopic sinus surgery, and the surgeon should not proceed with surgery if the images are not available in the operating theater. Scans should be reviewed not only to assess the extent of disease and any previous surgery, but also to evaluate the lamina papyracea and identify anatomical variants that may increase the risk of orbital complications—such as a hypoplastic maxillary sinus, an anterior ethmoid artery on a mesentery (▶ Fig. 18.1a), or a sphenoethmoidal (Onodi) cell (▶ Fig. 18.1b; ▶ Table 18.1).

### 18.2.2 Intraoperative Considerations

Complications are more likely to occur in a poor surgical field, and adequate preparation of the nose with topical adrenaline, Co-Phenylcaine spray, or Moffett's solution (a mixture of adrenaline, cocaine, normal saline, and sodium bicarbonate) provides valuable vasoconstriction of the sinonasal mucosa.[4] Controlled hypotensive anesthesia, with a relative bradycardia, further improves the surgical field[5] and venous oozing is reduced by elevating the head of the operating table or tilting it into the reverse Trendelenburg position. To further improve the surgical field, local anesthetic with adrenaline is sometimes injected into the axilla of the middle turbinate or into the greater

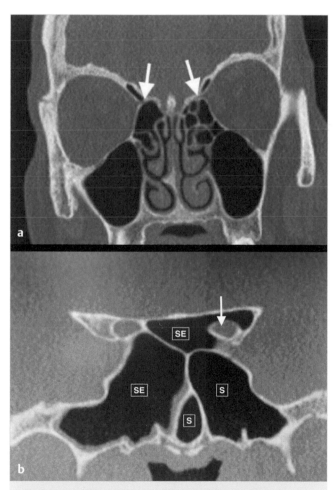

Fig. 18.1 Coronal CT (computed tomography) scans showing (a) bilateral anterior ethmoid arteries on mesenteries (*arrows*) and (b) bilateral sphenoethmoidal cells (SE), with optic nerve running within the left SE cell (*arrow*). "S" denotes sphenoid sinus.

**Table 18.1** Checklist for use when reviewing CT (computed tomography) scans preoperatively

| Anatomical structure | Risks |
|---|---|
| Maxillary sinus | Hypoplastic<br>Infraorbital (Haller) cell |
| Lamina papyracea | Dehiscent |
| Anterior ethmoid artery | On mesentery |
| Sphenoid sinus | Sphenoethmoidal (Onodi) cell<br>Optic nerve dehiscent within lateral wall or within sphenoethmoidal cell |
| Skull base | Cerebrospinal fluid leak |

palatine foramen—but blindness has been reported due to optic nerve ischemia from arterial spasm, or as a result of retrograde flow of injected solutions from the nasal cavity to the retinal artery.[6,7]

The patient's eyes should be left uncovered during endoscopic surgery, with lubricant instilled to prevent corneal erosions; this allows both the surgeon and the scrub nurse to monitor the eye for any intraoperative movement under the eyelid (as would occur if the medial rectus muscle was inadvertently pulled) or for the acute development of proptosis in the case of orbital hemorrhage. The eye should also be balloted under direct vision to assess for dehiscence of the lamina papyracea.

### 18.2.3 Surgical Technique

The nasal endoscope allows excellent visualization of the surgical site, and the tips of surgical instruments should always be visible. Powered instruments, such as microdebriders and drills, are now commonly used in endoscopic sinus surgery and significant injury can occur if they inadvertently enter the orbit through a dehiscent or previously intact lamina papyracea.[8] The microdebrider will suck orbital fat and extraocular muscle into its opening, where the rotating blade cuts at up to 5,000 rpm. Similarly, injudicious use of powered instrumentation in the sphenoid sinus or a sphenoethmoidal cell may lead to optic nerve injury. The blade of such instruments should always be visible, and should be angled away from the orbit to avoid accidentally drawing orbital periosteum or orbital contents into the opening.

The orbital floor is visible through a middle meatal antrostomy, and the lamina papyracea should be identified early, as using these bony orbital walls as anatomical landmarks should help prevent injury. There is some evidence that right orbital injury is more likely with a right-handed surgeon, but equal care should of course be taken on both sides.[9,10]

## 18.3 Management of Orbital Injury

### 18.3.1 Breach of the Lamina Papyracea

This is the most common orbital complication of endoscopic sinus surgery. The lamina papyracea may have a preoperative dehiscence, either from the disease process (▶ Fig. 18.2a) or from previous surgery or trauma (▶ Fig. 18.2b). Such

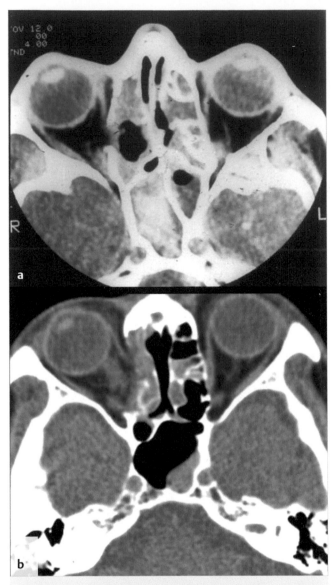

**Fig. 18.2** Preoperative axial CT (computed tomography) scans showing **(a)** breach of the right lamina papyracea due to eosinophilic fungal rhinosinusitis and **(b)** posttraumatic disruption of the right lamina papyracea.

abnormalities do not preclude surgery, but greater vigilance should be taken throughout the procedure—especially with the use of powered instruments—to avoid damage to the underlying orbital periosteum. If the lamina is breached, the extent of the injury should be documented, but surgery can usually be continued without any further injury. The lamina is most commonly injured during anterior ethmoidectomy, or during uncinectomy—particularly if there is a hypoplastic maxillary sinus (▶ Fig. 18.3a) or concha bullosa (▶ Fig. 18.3b) associated with lateralization of the uncinate process.

Periorbital ecchymosis and a large subconjunctival hematoma may be evident after intraoperative orbital hemorrhage (▶ Fig. 18.4a), and serial visual checks should be performed in the early postoperative period. No other specific management is required, but patients should be advised not to blow their

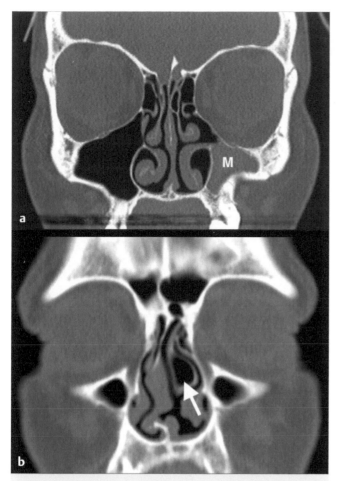

**Fig. 18.3** Anatomical variants that may predispose to orbital injury during endoscopic intranasal surgery. Coronal CT scans showing **(a)** hypoplastic left maxillary sinus (M) with lateralization of the uncinate process. **(b)** Left concha bullosa (*arrow*) associated with narrowing of the middle meatus.

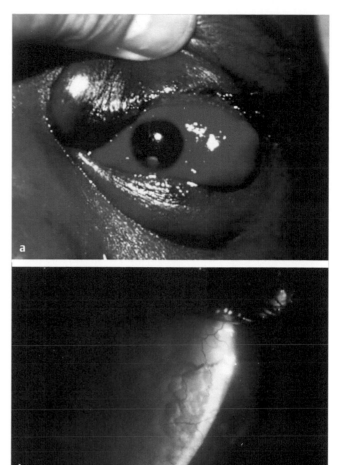

**Fig. 18.4** **(a)** Postoperative orbital hematoma characterized by a tense orbit, reduced eye movements, and a large subconjunctival hemorrhage without visible posterior extent. **(b)** Multiple subconjunctival air bubbles ("emphysema") after nose blowing with a breach of the ethmoid lamina, as viewed on slit-lamp biomicroscopy.

nose for 7 to 10 days after surgery. The risk of developing surgical emphysema of the orbit (▶ Fig. 18.4b) or periorbital region should be explained to them, and they should be advised to seek immediate review if they develop periorbital swelling, pain, or visual symptoms.

## 18.3.2 Surgical Emphysema

Most cases of postoperative surgical emphysema (▶ Fig. 18.4b), usually resulting from a breach in the lamina papyracea, do not require specific management apart from reassurance that it will resolve over several days. If the emphysema is extensive, visual acuity should be checked and ophthalmic review is advisable.

A breach of the lamina papyracea may go undetected, or there may be a natural dehiscence such as that found in the young or elderly. Because of this, oil-based ointments should be avoided within the surgical cavity as they can be forced into the adjacent orbital soft tissues where they may cause a granulomatous reaction, or myospherulosis, which is cosmetically noticeable and difficult to treat.

## 18.3.3 Breach of the Orbital Periosteum

Orbital fat will be visible if the orbital periosteum is breached, and the fat may prolapse into the sinonasal cavity, sometimes associated with periorbital bruising. The eye should be balloted under direct vision to observe for movement of the lateral nasal wall and/or intranasal prolapse of orbital contents. In most cases, a small amount of prolapsed fat will not prevent completion of the procedure, and a neuropatty or piece of Surgicel may be placed over the periosteal breach to prevent further injury. If there is any concern that continued surgery would lead to further orbital injury, then surgery should be stopped on that side.

Surgicel may be laid over any exposed orbital tissues at the end of the operation and nasal packing (absorbable or otherwise) may be considered, depending on the extent of the breach, to minimize surgical emphysema and prevent enophthalmos. Serial visual checks should be performed in the early postoperative period. Patients should be advised to avoid nose blowing for 7 to 10 days after surgery, and they should seek immediate review if they develop periorbital swelling, pain, or visual symptoms. Typically, the injured orbital periosteum heals rapidly and with no long-term sequelae.

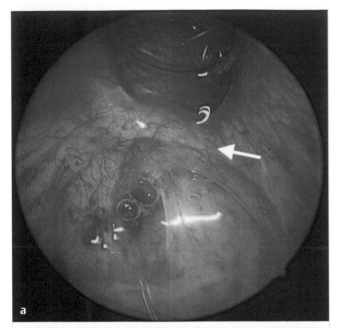

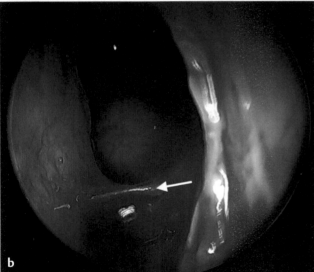

Fig. 18.5 Anterior ethmoid artery (*arrow*; **a**) on the skull base and (**b**) within a mesentery.

## 18.3.4 Intraorbital Hemorrhage

Intraorbital bleeding from a transected anterior ethmoidal artery is regarded as the commonest cause of an iatrogenic intraorbital hemorrhage during endoscopic surgery. The posterior ethmoid artery, running anterior to the face of the sphenoid, is rarely responsible for this complication as it tends to run within the bone of the skull base and mucosa is less often stripped in this region. The anterior ethmoidal artery runs on the skull base in approximately 60% of sinuses and is therefore relatively protected (▶ Fig. 18.5a); when it lies within a mesentery, it is more at risk (▶ Fig. 18.5b).[11] Intraorbital arterial hemorrhage causes pain, with rapid onset of proptosis and increased intraorbital pressure that may cause optic nerve ischemia. The ischemia is probably caused by both compression and stretching of the optic nerve, with consequent blindness if not identified and treated promptly.

Animal studies have reported permanent visual loss after 90 minutes of ophthalmic artery ischemia, but there are clinical reports of this occurring within 1 hour.[8,9]

Venous bleeding can also occur within the orbit, for example, after injury to the lamina papyracea or rupture of orbital veins through excessive manipulation of orbital fat.[7] This tends to present less rapidly—with postoperative swelling, periorbital bruising, and occasionally diplopia—and is usually relatively painless and self-limiting. Although such patients should be closely monitored for visual impairment, this complication is very rare with bleeding of venous origin.[6]

If orbital hemorrhage is diagnosed during surgery, endoscopic medial orbital decompression should be performed immediately, as described in Chapter 7, and, where visible, the offending artery cauterized with bipolar forceps; a prolonged search for a vessel that is not evident should, however, be avoided to minimize further damage to orbital structures. If orbital hemorrhage is recognized after surgery is completed, the patient should be positioned head up, any nasal packing removed, and an ophthalmic opinion requested. Where intraorbital pressure is only mildly elevated—reflected in an intraocular pressure (IOP) of < 30 mm Hg—serial monitoring of orbital signs, visual acuity, and the presence of a relative afferent pupillary defect (RAPD) should be continued.

If orbital pressure continues to rise and the IOP is > 40 mm Hg, with onset of an RAPD, then urgent intervention should be considered. Impairment of ocular blood flow may be visible as changes in the retinal circulation on funduscopy: with normal perfusion, "flashing" of the retinal arteries is seen when digital pressure is applied to the globe to increase the IOP above diastolic pressure. If the IOP is greater than the systolic pressure, this "flashing" phenomenon is lost, and immediate management is required.

Lateral canthotomy and cantholysis should be performed under local anesthetic before returning to the operating theater for definitive management. This maneuver disrupts the orbital septum and temporarily relieves orbital tamponade, and thereby restores perfusion of the optic nerve and globe. The lateral canthal region is infiltrated with local anesthesia and the canthal raphe divided horizontally down to the bony orbital rim (▶ Fig. 18.6a). Using scissors, the upper and lower limbs of the canthal tendon and septum are then divided for about 1 cm along the inside of the orbital rim, allowing prolapse of the orbital contents (▶ Fig. 18.6b).

Intravenous steroids (dexamethasone, 8–10 mg every 8 hours), acetazolamide (500 mg), and/or mannitol (20%, 1–2 g/kg over 30 minutes) may also help reduce the IOP, as can topical timolol drops.[9]

Bleeding from the anterior and/or posterior ethmoid artery usually settles spontaneously, but if it persists or if orbital pressure continues to rise despite emergent treatment, then ligation of the offending vessel(s) should be performed. Endoscopic bipolar diathermy of the ethmoidal arteries is usually possible, but if not, then it may be performed using an external approach (Lynch incision). The Lynch incision is 2 to 3 cm long and placed halfway between the nasal dorsum and the medial canthus, running from the medial end of the eyebrow to just below the level of the medial canthus. The incision is made down to bone, and a Freer elevator is used to elevate the periosteum back to the anterior lacrimal crest; although only a guide, the anterior ethmoid artery, posterior ethmoid artery, and optic foramen

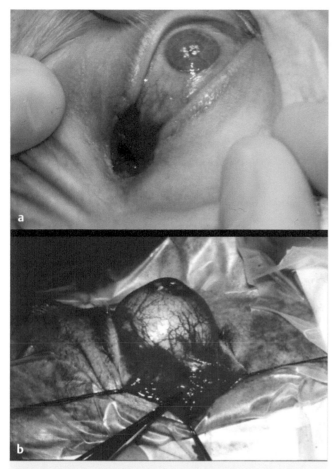

Fig. 18.6 Technique for lateral canthotomy. (a) Initial incision. (b) After lateral canthotomy and cantholysis are completed.

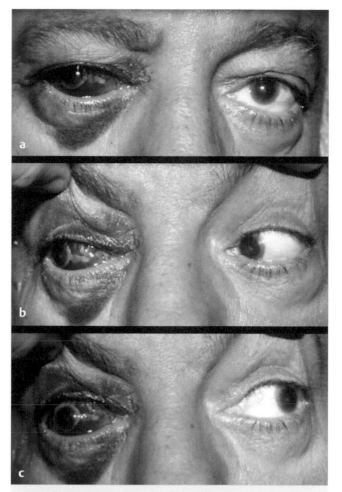

Fig. 18.7 (a) Right proptosis, periocular ecchymosis, and divergent squint after partial avulsion of orbital contents during ipsilateral endoscopic ethmoidectomy. The lack of right horizontal ductions is evident on (b) right and (c) left gaze.

are at an average of 24, 12, and 6 mm (respectively) behind the anterior lacrimal crest.[11] As subperiosteal dissection is continued in this plane, the vessels are identified running medially through the lamina papyracea and can be ligated or cauterized.

## 18.3.5 Damage to the Extraocular Muscles

Orbital penetration may be associated with injury to any structure within it but, lying in close proximity to the lamina papyracea, the medial rectus is the most commonly injured extraocular muscle (▶ Fig. 18.7a).[12] The incidence of medial rectus injury has been reported as 1 in 735 cases in a large series.[13] The inferior rectus is the next most frequently injured, followed by the superior oblique.[14] Four patterns of medial rectus injury have been described: intramuscular contusion or hematoma, complete or near-complete transection of the muscle belly, entrapment of the muscle or orbital fat, and damage to the oculomotor nerve.[13] If muscle injury occurs, or is suspected after surgery—with diplopia, restricted movements or divergent squint (▶ Fig. 18.7b,c)—the orbit should immediately be assessed for other injuries, the orbital pressure noted, and an urgent ophthalmic review sought. Emergency canthotomy and cantholysis should be undertaken

where there is impairment of ocular perfusion due to the commonly associated orbital hemorrhage.

Once the eye is deemed safe, the muscle injury should be addressed as damaged extraocular muscles can have severe long-term effects. The main aim of surgical repair is to re-establish a field of single binocular vision.[12,15] While clinical function of the muscles is a major determinant of treatment, imaging is helpful in planning management. While gadolinium-enhanced magnetic resonance imaging (MRI) is more sensitive than CT in assessing the extent of acute injury, including any edema of the orbital fat and extraocular muscles,[16] thin-slice CT generally has a better structural resolution due to a lack of motion artifact. Orbital exploration is required where there is complete severance of a muscle, or clinical and radiological evidence of entrapment, as early intervention in such cases probably improves prognosis.[12] Where there is clinical evidence of reasonable muscle function—with a moderate squint, some adductive force generation, and imaging shows some intact muscle fibers—then the patient can be observed for improvement over several weeks after the injury.[15,17] Paralysis of the ipsilateral lateral rectus with Botulinum toxin should be considered where there is a large exotropia or where there are only very few muscle fibers remaining intact at the site of damage.[15,17]

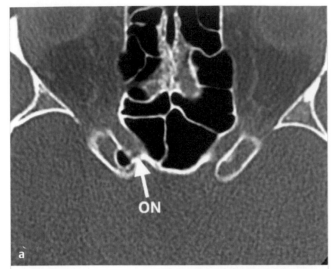

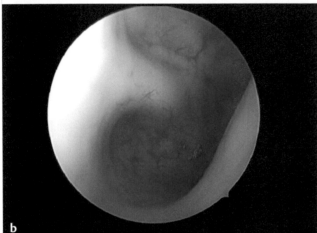

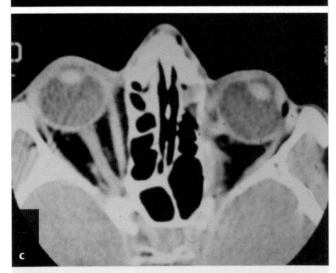

**Fig. 18.8 (a)** Axial computed tomography (CT) demonstrating the optic nerve (ON) canal passing through the right sphenoid sinus. **(b)** Endoscopic view of the right ON passing across the sphenoid sinus. **(c)** Axial CT after avulsion of the left medial rectus and ON during power-assisted endoscopic ethmoidectomy.

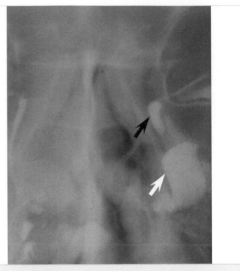

**Fig. 18.9** Dacryocystogram after nasolacrimal duct damage during left intranasal antrostomy. The contrast passes from a shrunken left lacrimal sac (*dark arrow*) into a large cavity within the left maxilla (*light arrow*). Widespread loss of the airspaces within the nose and paranasal sinuses is evident.

Significant loss of muscle can occur with injuries involving the microdebrider, and repair in such cases is difficult, may necessitate a "bridging" suture, and is usually associated with a poor prognosis.[8] Late repair of such squints, with muscle transposition techniques,[14,17] is usually accompanied by persistent and often intractable diplopia.

## 18.3.6 Damage to the Optic Nerve

The optic nerve is most likely to be injured if it traverses a sphenoethmoidal cell (▶ Fig. 18.8a) or is exposed in the lateral wall of the sphenoid sinus (▶ Fig. 18.8b). The intraorbital optic nerve may, however, be injured where there is severe orbital disruption during ethmoidectomy (▶ Fig. 18.8c).[17] If the optic nerve is directly damaged or transected, visual loss is inevitable and there is no proven role for optic nerve decompression in these direct iatrogenic injuries.

## 18.3.7 Damage to the Nasolacrimal System

The lacrimal sac and fossa, lying anteromedially in the orbit, may occasionally be injured during endoscopic sinus surgery.[18] Nasolacrimal duct injury is commoner and usually occurs during endoscopic enlargement of the maxillary ostium, if bone removal is continued anterior to the attachment of the uncinate process; such bone removal should be avoided in routine sinus surgery, but may be unavoidable in more complex cases, such as resection of sinonasal tumors. The nasolacrimal duct may be temporarily retracted to avoid damage during endoscopic medial maxillectomy. Most cases of nasolacrimal duct injury can be left and heal without later epiphora, the defect presumably healing either spontaneously or by draining into the middle meatus or antrum (▶ Fig. 18.9).[18,19] Lacrimal sac massage can be advised after surgery, to encourage resumption of nasolacrimal duct function.

Ophthalmic review is valuable where there is persistent epiphora, and this assessment would typically include dye clearance tests, lacrimal irrigation, and possibly imaging such as dacryocystogram and/or lacrimal scintigraphy (see Chapters 3 and 5). Persistent nasolacrimal duct obstruction is managed with bypass surgery, this being dacryocystorhinostomy that can be performed through an external or endonasal approach (see Chapter 5).

## 18.4 Conclusion

Orbital injury during endoscopic endonasal surgery can generally be avoided with careful preoperative assessment and surgical technique. If injury occurs, prompt recognition and management is important to avoid devastating complications such as blindness or intractable diplopia. Careful postoperative monitoring is required after any complication, assessing both eye movements and vision, and ophthalmic assistance should be sought if there are major concerns.

## References

[1] Hopkins C, Browne JP, Slack R, et al. Complications of surgery for nasal polyposis and chronic rhinosinusitis: the results of a national audit in England and Wales. Laryngoscope. 2006; 116(8):1494–1499

[2] Dalziel K, Stein K, Round A, Garside R, Royle P. Endoscopic sinus surgery for the excision of nasal polyps: a systematic review of safety and effectiveness. Am J Rhinol. 2006; 20(5):506–519

[3] Badia L, Lund VJ. Dilated pupil during endoscopic sinus surgery: what does it mean? Am J Rhinol. 2001; 15(1):31–33

[4] Benjamin E, Wong DK, Choa D. "Moffett's" solution: a review of the evidence and scientific basis for the topical preparation of the nose. Clin Otolaryngol Allied Sci. 2004; 29(6):582–587

[5] Amorocho MC, Fat I. Anesthetic techniques in endoscopic sinus and skull base surgery. Otolaryngol Clin North Am. 2016; 49(3):531–547

[6] Han JK, Higgins TS. Management of orbital complications in endoscopic sinus surgery. Curr Opin Otolaryngol Head Neck Surg. 2010; 18(1):32–36

[7] Stankiewicz JA, Lal D, Connor M, Welch K. Complications in endoscopic sinus surgery for chronic rhinosinusitis: a 25-year experience. Laryngoscope. 2011; 121(12):2684–2701

[8] Graham SM, Nerad JA. Orbital complications in endoscopic sinus surgery using powered instrumentation. Laryngoscope. 2003; 113(5):874–878

[9] Ramakrishnan VR, Palmer JN. Prevention and management of orbital hematoma. Otolaryngol Clin North Am. 2010; 43(4):789–800

[10] Sohn JH, Hong SD, Kim JH, et al. Extraocular muscle injury during endoscopic sinus surgery: a series of 10 cases at a single center. Rhinology. 2014; 52(3):238–245

[11] Lund VJ, Stammberger H, Fokkens WJ, et al. European position paper on the anatomical terminology of the internal nose and paranasal sinuses. Rhinol Suppl. 2014; 24:1–34

[12] Bleier BS, Schlosser RJ. Prevention and management of medial rectus injury. Otolaryngol Clin North Am. 2010; 43(4):801–807

[13] Huang CM, Meyer DR, Patrinely JR, et al. Medial rectus muscle injuries associated with functional endoscopic sinus surgery: characterization and management. Ophthal Plast Reconstr Surg. 2003; 19(1):25–37

[14] Thacker NM, Velez FG, Demer JL, Wang MB, Rosenbaum AL. Extraocular muscle damage associated with endoscopic sinus surgery: an ophthalmology perspective. Am J Rhinol. 2005; 19(4):400–405

[15] Hong JE, Goldberg AN, Cockerham KP. Botulinum toxin A therapy for medial rectus injury during endoscopic sinus surgery. Am J Rhinol. 2008; 22(1):95–97

[16] Bhatti MT, Schmalfuss IM, Mancuso AA. Orbital complications of functional endoscopic sinus surgery: MR and CT findings. Clin Radiol. 2005; 60(8):894–904

[17] Rene C, Rose GE, Lenthall R, Moseley I. Major orbital complications of endoscopic sinus surgery. Br J Ophthalmol. 2001; 85(5):598–603

[18] Cohen NA, Antunes MB, Morgenstern KE. Prevention and management of lacrimal duct injury. Otolaryngol Clin North Am. 2010; 43(4):781–788

[19] Bolger WE, Parsons DS, Mair EA, Kuhn FA. Lacrimal drainage system injury in functional endoscopic sinus surgery. Incidence, analysis, and prevention. Arch Otolaryngol Head Neck Surg. 1992; 118(11):1179–1184

# 19 Anesthetic Technique for Endoscopic Orbital Surgery

*Henry P. Barham and Raymond Sacks*

**Abstract**

There has been a growing trend toward the use of minimally invasive techniques in surgery. With this trend, transnasal endoscopic surgery has become an effective part of the management of chronic rhinosinusitis and tumors of the sinuses, orbit, and anterior skull base. These approaches are also well established for orbital decompression, orbital medial wall fracture repair, and optic canal decompression. Use of the endoscope has also greatly advanced ophthalmologic procedures including endoscopic dacryocystorhinostomy and endoscopic brow lift for both ophthalmologists and otolaryngologists. Nasal endoscopy has been proven useful in the perioperative assessment for lacrimal surgery and probing of the nasolacrimal duct. For the anesthetist, endoscopic surgical procedures provide an interesting challenge with the use of the latest drugs and techniques available to allow an optimal operating field while decreasing the risk of surgery and improve patient safety and satisfaction. Newer drugs such as remifentanil have proven beneficial in improving blood loss and surgical field with minimal side effects. Technological advances have been critical in advancing endoscopic surgical procedures, with the introduction of improved optics and lighting, advanced instrumentation, and image-guided surgical navigation. Hemostatic materials and devices have similarly evolved to assist in the management of the surgical field and the postoperative cavity.

*Keywords:* endoscopic, sinus, rhinology, orbit, dacryocystorhinostomy, anesthesia, orbit

## 19.1 Introduction

In recent years, there has been a growing trend toward the use of minimally invasive techniques in surgery. This is a result of trying to achieve a better cosmetic outcome combined with reducing the morbidity of extensive tissue dissection. Endoscopic surgery exemplifies these attempts and has been enthusiastically adopted by general surgeons, gynecologists, and ear, nose, and throat (ENT) surgeons.

Endoscopic orbital surgery, however, is in its infancy and is performed primarily via sinonasal approaches by ENT surgeons. Transnasal endoscopic approaches are well established for orbital decompression, orbital medial wall fracture repair, and optic canal decompression. The use of a transmaxillary or transnasal endoscopic approach has also been described for repair of orbital floor fractures. The ophthalmologists are familiar with the endoscope primarily in the context of endoscopic dacryocystorhinostomy (DCR) and endoscopic brow lift. Nasal endoscopy has also been proven useful in the perioperative assessment for lacrimal surgery and probing of the nasolacrimal duct. Additional applications in oculoplastic surgery include transcanalicular endoscopy and endoscopic assistance in facelifts and in harvesting fascia lata.

Adverse events are rare, most of which relate to the proximity of the paranasal sinuses to the orbits and brain. Major complications include dura puncture, cerebrospinal fluid leak, meningitis, orbital and optic nerve trauma, and extensive hemorrhage.[1,2] As such, the option for the procedure to be done under general anesthesia offers numerous advantages and the role of the anesthetist in these procedures is undoubtedly significant.

## 19.2 Discussion

The classic endoscopic sinonasal procedure was initially done under topical anesthesia with sedation. In this manner, patients would be conscious and able to signal any kind of pain or discomfort, alerting and allowing the surgeon to minimize trauma and complications.[3,4] In current times, the evolution of surgical technique has allowed surgeons to become much more aggressive with the extent of their resection.

A general anesthetic will allow immobile surgical field, effective airway protection, adequate analgesia, and patient comfort. Currently, local anesthesia is still considered suitable for minor procedures in selected patients, but general anesthesia is preferred for most cases to meet more challenging surgical needs.[5] Maintenance of normothermia is vital for the function of platelets and coagulation factors essential in hemostasis.[6,7]

Depth of anesthesia is important in avoiding any coughing or straining by the patient during a light anesthetic plane, which will result in an increase in intrathoracic pressure and hence impair venous drainage from the head and increase surgical bleeding. The use of muscle relaxants will also effectively prevent such occurrences during the procedure. Intermittent positive pressure ventilation should be adjusted such that the airway pressures are kept to a minimum. Avoidance of the use of positive end expiratory pressure is also helpful via preventing higher intrathoracic pressure.[8,9]

Volatile anesthetic agents cause smooth muscle relaxation and decreases systemic vascular resistance. Tissue perfusion is increased due to vasodilation and may also contribute to surgical bleeding.

Initial studies have suggested that the intraoperative blood loss was reduced with propofol total intravenous anesthesia (TIVA) compared to volatile agents.[10,11,12,13] However, more recent studies do not show significant difference after excluding the effect of concomitant use of remifentanil.[14,15,16] The use of propofol has the advantage of reducing systolic blood pressure via a lesser decrease in systemic vascular resistance.

Hemostasis, both during and after endoscopic procedures, is critical for successful outcomes.[1,17] Intraoperative bleeding, especially in the setting of highly vascular sinonasal tumors and polyposis, remains a common pitfall in performing endoscopic sinus, orbital, and skull base surgery. Although endoscopic bipolar forceps, suction cautery, and newer technologies, such as radiofrequency coblation, are indispensable for producing intraoperative hemostasis, various topical agents are also effective in controlling diffuse bleeding and, in some cases, also provide postoperative benefits.

The primary modality to achieve hemostasis in surgery is the prevention of bleeding. The three steps to improve one's ability to prevent bleeding are patient positioning, proper surgical technique with avoidance of stripped mucosa, and vasoconstriction. The patient's head should be placed in the neutral anatomic position and the operative bed placed in 15- to 20-degree reverse Trendelenburg with total intravenous anesthesia.[2] Proper surgical technique cannot be overemphasized to avoid nuisance bleeding. The stripping of mucosa will cause oozing, which will decrease visualization and is not amenable to topical vasoconstrictors. If persistent bleeding occurs in the absence of mucosal stripping, vasoconstrictors have a significant role in endoscopic sinus, orbital, and skull base surgery.

Epinephrine has been used as a hemostatic agent in various surgical procedures for many years both in topical and injectable preparations. It is inexpensive and has excellent hemostatic properties.[3] The major drawback to its use is the potential for cardiac complications including tachycardia, arrhythmias, hypotension, or hypertension.[4] Hypertension and tachycardia historically are the most commonly observed complications.[5] Recently, use of topical epinephrine in endoscopic sinus and skull base surgery has experienced resurgence as topical preparations provide excellent hemostasis while greatly decreasing the potential for cardiac complications.

The authors' practice routinely uses epinephrine with Naropin (anesthetic benefit) soaked cotton pledgets to aid with hemostasis. Their preferred concentration is 1:2,000, which provides excellent hemostasis with limited side effects. A prospective study evaluating varying concentrations of topical adrenaline including 1:2,000, 1:10,000, and 1:50,000 showed that the 1:2,000 group had a statistically significant decrease in blood loss and shorter operative times.[18]

Hemorrhage decreases visibility of the surgical field during the functional endoscopic sinus surgery (FESS) procedure and is directly related to risk of vascular, orbital, and intracranial complications as well as procedural failure.[18,19] Hence, it is of vital importance to the surgeon as well as anesthetist to minimize surgical bleeding for this operation.[8] Marked hypotension is proven to be induced in a predictable manner, lasting no longer than 4 minutes after local infiltration with epinephrine-containing local anesthetics.[20] Considering the potential for adverse side effects, the effect of topical application of epinephrine 1:100,000 has been studied and it may be able to provide a similar hemostatic effect as intranasal injection during FESS.[6] In a recent study, Cohen-Kerem et al[20] compared the effectiveness of topical 1:1,000 epinephrine versus injected local anesthetic containing 1:100,000 epinephrine during FESS. In this study, it was reported that submucosal injection of local anesthetic with epinephrine facilitated improved surgical condition; however, increased hemodynamic fluctuations were noted after infiltrations.

Bleeding may be difficult to control surgically due to the extensive vascular supply in the sinus region and pathophysiological changes in the patient. Capillary bleeding is the most fundamental problem of note in this procedure, barring any inadvertent trauma to the feeding arterial and venous vessels.[21] Fortunately, bleeding from the capillary circulation may be greatly reduced by decreasing the patient's mean arterial pressure and by local vasoconstriction.

The reverse Trendelenburg 15-degree head up allows for venous decongestion of the upper part of the body by increasing venous pooling of blood in the lower extremities. Every 2.5 cm above the heart correlates to a decrease of 2 mm Hg in arterial blood pressure supply.[22,23] This has been shown to improve the endoscopic field of view.[24]

Injected and topical local anesthetics and vasoconstrictors can help relieve postoperative pain and decrease blood loss and mucosal congestion. Commonly used vasoconstrictors include cocaine, epinephrine, and phenylephrine.[25]

Cocaine has local anesthetic and vasoconstrictor properties. Systemic absorption of these agents may cause hypertension, tachycardia, and other arrhythmias; hence, they should be used with great caution in patients with coronary heart disease, congestive heart failure, malignant arrhythmias, poorly controlled hypertension, and in those taking monoamine oxidase inhibitors.[26]

Hypotension induced by epinephrine under general anesthesia is seldom mentioned, but temporarily able to quickly blunt the sympathetic response to endotracheal tube (ETT) insertion and periods of surgical stimulation. Propofol also decreases cerebral metabolism and hence cerebral blood flow is reduced by autoregulation. This reduces flow via the ethmoidal and the supraorbital arteries, which supply the ethmoid, sphenoid, and frontal sinuses, improving surgical visibility.[27]

Multiple reviews have compared surgical field and blood loss during FESS. Amorocho and Sordillo[28] found propofol general anesthesia improved the surgical field and reduced blood loss, whereas Baker and Baker[29] concluded that propofol general anesthesia improved the surgical field but did not reduce surgical blood loss. A recent Cochrane systemic review found that deliberate hypotension with propofol TIVA did not decrease total blood loss and only improved the quality of surgical field by less than one category on a scale of 0 (no bleeding) to 5 (severe bleeding), with no significant difference in operating times. Although it is of note that only four studies with 278 participants were included in this review, and randomized control trials with good-quality methodology and large sample size are required to investigate the effectiveness of deliberate hypotension with propofol for FESS.[16]

Opioids cause a drop in blood pressure during anesthesia and minimize surges in blood pressure due to surgical pain. Remifentanil has the advantages of being a short acting but potent opioid that can be easily titrated to patient's hemodynamic state.[30] This enables better control of blood pressure to achieve blood pressure targets for hypotensive anesthesia even during sudden surges in surgical stimulation and pain without prolonged effects.

Controlled hypotension refers to a deliberate lowering of the systemic blood pressure to 20% less than the patient's baseline blood pressure. This decreases hydrostatic pressure within capillaries and hence decreased blood loss by capillary ooze. However, there are limitations to controlled hypotension including reduced perfusion to vital organs such as the brain, heart, and kidneys.

Absolute contraindications to controlled hypotension include evidence of cerebrovascular insufficiency, coronary disease, and decompensated heart failure[31]; relative contraindications will include other organ dysfunction (e.g., renal, hepatic, pulmonary), severe anemia, and hypovolemia.

When used judiciously and when no contraindications are present, it has been found to be effective in providing better surgical field without postoperative complications due to intraoperative hypotension.[32] A study by Boezaart et al showed that good operating conditions can be obtained with esmolol-induced hypotension even at mild hypotension with mean arterial pressure more than 65 mm Hg, which was postulated to be in part due to unopposed alpha-adrenergic effect on the mucous membrane vasculature by esmolol.[33]

Choices of agents to maintain controlled hypotension will include glyceryl trinitrate, β-blockers,[34] and α-agonists such as clonidine,[35] magnesium sulphate,[36] and remifentanil.[37] The agent used should ideally be short acting and easily titratable and its effects should not last into the postoperative period.

It is important to be aware of the possibility of local anesthetic toxicity in view of the generous amount that is administered to the patient via packs and injections pre- and intraoperatively by the surgical team and hence effective communication should exist between surgeons and anesthetists.

Remifentanil is effective in controlling the hemodynamic response to surgery by the lowering of heart rate, cardiac output, and blood pressure. In addition to this, it has the added advantage of rapid titratability and faster recovery due to the short half-life non-organ-dependent elimination via nonspecific plasma esterases.[37,38] As the analgesic effect of remifentanil diminishes rapidly after the cessation of infusion, the effects of this will be felt immediately. Hence, there is a need to provide adequate analgesia via longer acting opioids, nonsteroidal anti-inflammatory drugs (NSAID), and acetaminophen to prevent a rebound phenomenon when surgery is concluded. Recent studies considering the effective effect-site concentration of remifentanil for preventing cough during emergence with target-controlled infusion have arrived at 2.94 ng/mL for men after nasal surgery[39] and 2.14 ng/mL for women after thyroid surgery.[40]

An ETT has a cuffed seal that sits below the vocal cords, which helps prevent aspiration and protect the airway and hence is known to be a definitive airway. The oral preformed south-pointing Ring–Adair–Elwyn ETT and armored ETT have the advantage of a lesser tendency to kink versus a standard ETT and is usually positioned either in the midline and secured to the chin or taped at the angle of the mouth, depending on the surgeon's preference and whether software-guided surgical navigation systems such as BrainLab is employed.

In contrast, the laryngeal mask airway (LMA) is a supraglottic device and thus is not traditionally believed to be able to provide airway protection. However, this may not be true as newer evidence has come to show. Blood and secretions can track along the outer surface of the ETT to the level of the vocal cords and subglottis. Direct comparisons of lower airway contamination by fiberoptic examination at the end of nasal surgery have shown that patients on spontaneous ventilation via a flexible LMA have the same or even lower risk of having blood in the airway compared to patients on an ETT.[41,42,43,44,45]

Insertion of the LMA after induction of anesthesia also causes less sympathetic response than tracheal intubation as the larynx is not directly stimulated, hence allowing the further advantage of hemodynamic stability.[46] The LMA also offers added advantage during emergence compared to ETT as it is better tolerated and less stimulating to the airway and hence contributes to reduced bleeding in the immediate postoperative period. As the LMA can be removed in the recovery unit, it may also enable faster turnaround time in a full operating list. However, the switch in responsibility in postoperative airway management of the LMA to the recovery nurse will also mean

that help must be immediately available if airway obstruction is encountered in the recovery area.

The flexible LMA is preferred over the other LMA devices available due to its armored tubing, which allows more flexibility and prevents kinking during taping, thereby avoiding physical obstruction to the surgeons. However, care must be taken to ensure that the LMA sits well and is secured well as the airway is shared in FESS procedure with the surgeon and dislodgment of the LMA is not unknown or uncommon. It is also good practice to determine the seal pressure of the LMA. In addition, LMA removal should only be performed when patients are fully awake and able to open the mouth on command. The LMA should not be deflated prior to removal so that secretions will not flow into the trachea.

The obvious advantage of a smooth emergence will be that of the avoidance of straining and sympathetic release that will increase postsurgical bleeding and decrease the risk of sore throat and patient discomfort.

## 19.3 Author's Practice

The patient's airway is maintained by either an ETT or a laryngeal mask taped to the lower right commissure to allow unimpeded hand mobility for a right-handed surgeon. The patient is prepared topically with 1% ropivacaine and 1:2,000 adrenaline-soaked neurosurgical cottonoids placed within the middle meatus, ethmoid (if previously dissected), and over the inferior and middle turbinates. Endoscopically, the mucosa is injected with 1% ropivacaine and 1:100,000 adrenaline along the inferior border, superior axilla, and anterior head of the middle turbinate. The patient's head is placed in the neutral anatomic position and the operative bed is placed in 15- to 20-degree reverse Trendelenburg with total intravenous anesthesia.[5]

Nasal packing with gauze was routinely used in the postoperative care of the nasal cavity but carries significant drawbacks. Packing can result in pain, rhinorrhea, infection, nasal obstruction, sensation of pressure, alar necrosis, and epistaxis on removal.[8,19,21,22,23] Packing and the removal thereof has been reported as the most uncomfortable portion of the perioperative experience.[22]

Nausea and vomiting are important postoperative complications in all surgical settings. The presence of blood in the stomach, inflammation of the uvula and throat, and the occasional use of opioids for pain control are all contributing factors. Decompression of the stomach with an orogastric tube should be performed prior to extubation. Prophylaxis with ondansetron and dexamethasone should be strongly considered. Should the patient develop severe postoperative nausea and vomiting despite best efforts, rescue intravenous anti-emetics and hydration can be provided and in the worst-case scenario, the patient may need to be admitted for further monitoring.[28,41] The use of TIVA with propofol has also been shown to result in a clinically relevant reduction of postoperative nausea and vomiting compared to traditional volatile anesthesia.[47,48]

The expected postoperative pain from FESS may range from mild to moderate, and is due to surgical trauma as well as nasal packing. Preoperative local anesthetics are used, but are not adequate on their own to alleviate postoperative pain. No differences have been found between infiltrations with long-acting (bupivacaine) and short-acting (lignocaine) local anesthetics.[49,50]Routine analgesic treatment is usually based on nonopioid analgesics with rescue opioids. Oral acetaminophen and an NSAID/cyclooxygenase 2 inhibitor usually provide safe and effective analgesia.

## 19.4 Conclusion

Functional endoscopic sinus, orbital, and skull base surgery has become an effective part of the management of chronic rhinosinusitis and tumors of the sinuses, orbit, and anterior skull base. For the anesthetist, it provides an interesting challenge to use the latest drugs and techniques available to allow an optimal operating field while decreasing the risk of surgery and improve patient safety and satisfaction. Newer drugs such as remifentanil have proven their superiority in multiple trials in improving blood loss and surgical field with minimal side effects. Technological advances have been critical in advancing endoscopic surgical procedures, with the introduction of improved optics and lighting, advanced instrumentation, and image-guided surgical navigation. Hemostatic materials and devices have similarly evolved to assist in the management of the surgical field and the postoperative cavity.

## 19.5 Key Points

- Meticulous mucosal preserving surgical technique.
- Position of patient: 15- to 20-degree anti-Trendelenburg (head up, feet down).
- Local vasoconstriction with both local infiltration and topical vasoconstriction.
- Anesthetic technique: controlled hypotension with bradycardia.
- Mean arterial blood pressure (MABP) ± 60 mm Hg; systolic BP ± 90 mm Hg; and pulse rate ± 60 beats/min.
- Airway maintenance with flexible laryngeal mask.
- Postoperative analgesia.

## References

[1] Cumberworth VL, Sudderick RM, Mackay IS. Major complications of functional endoscopic sinus surgery. Clin Otolaryngol Allied Sci. 1994; 19(3): 248–253

[2] Sharp HR, Crutchfield L, Rowe-Jones JM, Mitchell DB. Major complications and consent prior to endoscopic sinus surgery. Clin Otolaryngol Allied Sci. 2001; 26(1):33–38

[3] Lee WC, Kapur TR, Ramsden WN. Local and regional anesthesia for functional endoscopic sinus surgery. Ann Otol Rhinol Laryngol. 1997; 106(9):767–769

[4] Fedok FG, Ferraro RE, Kingsley CP, Fornadley JA. Operative times, postanesthesia recovery times, and complications during sinonasal surgery using general anesthesia and local anesthesia with sedation. Otolaryngol Head Neck Surg. 2000; 122(4):560–566

[5] Gittelman PD, Jacobs JB, Skorina J. Comparison of functional endoscopic sinus surgery under local and general anesthesia. Ann Otol Rhinol Laryngol. 1993; 102(4, Pt 1):289–293

[6] Schmied H, Kurz A, Sessler DI, Kozek S, Reiter A. Mild hypothermia increases blood loss and transfusion requirements during total hip arthroplasty. Lancet. 1996; 347(8997):289–292

[7] Romlin B, Petruson K, Nilsson K. Moderate superficial hypothermia prolongs bleeding time in humans. Acta Anaesthesiol Scand. 2007; 51(2):198–201

[8] Simpson P. Perioperative blood loss and its reduction: the role of the anaesthetist. Br J Anaesth. 1992; 69(5):498–507

[9] Petrozza PH. Induced hypotension. Int Anesthesiol Clin. 1990; 28(4):223–229

[10] Pavlin JD, Colley PS, Weymuller EA, Jr, Van Norman G, Gunn HC, Koerschgen ME. Propofol versus isoflurane for endoscopic sinus surgery. Am J Otolaryngol. 1999; 20(2):96–101

[11] Eberhart LH, Folz BJ, Wulf H, Geldner G. Intravenous anesthesia provides optimal surgical conditions during microscopic and endoscopic sinus surgery. Laryngoscope. 2003; 113(8):1369–1373

[12] Tirelli G, Bigarini S, Russolo M, Lucangelo U, Gullo A. Total intravenous anaesthesia in endoscopic sinus-nasal surgery. Acta Otorhinolaryngol Ital. 2004; 24(3):137–144

[13] Wormald PJ, van Renen G, Perks J, Jones JA, Langton-Hewer CD. The effect of the total intravenous anesthesia compared with inhalational anesthesia on the surgical field during endoscopic sinus surgery. Am J Rhinol. 2005; 19(5): 514–520

[14] Sivaci R, Yilmaz MD, Balci C, Erincler T, Unlu H. Comparison of propofol and sevoflurane anesthesia by means of blood loss during endoscopic sinus surgery. Saudi Med J. 2004; 25(12):1995–1998

[15] Ankichetty SP, Ponniah M, Cherian V, et al. Comparison of total intravenous anesthesia using propofol and inhalational anesthesia using isoflurane for controlled hypotension in functional endoscopic sinus surgery. J Anaesthesiol Clin Pharmacol. 2011; 27(3):328–332

[16] Boonmak S, Boonmak P, Laopaiboon M. Deliberate hypotension with propofol under anaesthesia for functional endoscopic sinus surgery (FESS). Cochrane Database Syst Rev. 2013; 6(6):CD006623

[17] Senior BA, Kennedy DW, Tanabodee J, Kroger H, Hassab M, Lanza D. Long-term results of functional endoscopic sinus surgery. Laryngoscope. 1998; 108 (2):151–157

[18] Stammberger H, Posawetz W. Functional endoscopic sinus surgery. Concept, indications and results of the Messerklinger technique. Eur Arch Otorhinolaryngol. 1990; 247(2):63–76

[19] Stankiewicz JA. Complications in endoscopic intranasal ethmoidectomy: an update. Laryngoscope. 1989; 99(7, Pt 1):686–690

[20] Cohen-Kerem R, Brown S, Villaseñor LV, Witterick I. Epinephrine/lidocaine injection vs. saline during endoscopic sinus surgery. Laryngoscope. 2008; 118 (7):1275–1281

[21] Jacobi KE, Böhm BE, Rickauer AJ, Jacobi C, Hemmerling TM. Moderate controlled hypotension with sodium nitroprusside does not improve surgical conditions or decrease blood loss in endoscopic sinus surgery. J Clin Anesth. 2000; 12(3):202–207

[22] Enderby GE. Pharmacological blockade. Postgrad Med J. 1974; 50(587):572–575

[23] Larsen R, Kleinschmidt S. Die kontrollierte Hypotension. Anaesthesist. 1995; 44(4):291–308

[24] Hathorn IF, Habib AR, Manji J, Javer AR. Comparing the reverse Trendelenburg and horizontal position for endoscopic sinus surgery: a randomized controlled trial. Otolaryngol Head Neck Surg. 2013; 148(2):308–313

[25] John G, Low JM, Tan PE, van Hasselt CA. Plasma catecholamine levels during functional endoscopic sinus surgery. Clin Otolaryngol Allied Sci. 1995; 20(3): 213–215

[26] Anderhuber W, Walch C, Nemeth E, et al. Plasma adrenaline concentrations during functional endoscopic sinus surgery. Laryngoscope. 1999; 109(2, Pt 1):204–207

[27] Ahn HJ, Chung SK, Dhong HJ, et al. Comparison of surgical conditions during propofol or sevoflurane anaesthesia for endoscopic sinus surgery. Br J Anaesth. 2008; 100(1):50–54

[28] Amorocho MR, Sordillo A. Anesthesia for functional endoscopic sinus surgery: a review. Anesthesiol Clin. 2010; 28(3):497–504

[29] Baker AR, Baker AB. Anaesthesia for endoscopic sinus surgery. Acta Anaesthesiol Scand. 2010; 54(7):795–803

[30] Manola M, De Luca E, Moscillo L, Mastella A. Using remifentanil and sufentanil in functional endoscopic sinus surgery to improve surgical conditions. ORL J Otorhinolaryngol Relat Spec. 2005; 67(2):83–86

[31] Kleinschmidt S. Hat die kontrollierte Hypotension einen Stellenwert im Rahmen fremdblutsparender Verfahren? Anaesthesist. 2001; 50:39–42

[32] Mandal P. Isoflurane anesthesia for functional endoscopic sinus surgery. Indian J Anaesth. 2003; 47(1):37–40

[33] Boezaart AP, van der Merwe J, Coetzee A. Comparison of sodium nitroprusside- and esmolol-induced controlled hypotension for functional endoscopic sinus surgery. Can J Anaesth. 1995; 42(5, Pt 1):373–376

[34] Nair S, Collins M, Hung P, Rees G, Close D, Wormald PJ. The effect of beta-blocker premedication on the surgical field during endoscopic sinus surgery. Laryngoscope. 2004; 114(6):1042–1046

[35] Cardesín A, Pontes C, Rosell R, et al. Hypotensive anaesthesia and bleeding during endoscopic sinus surgery: an observational study. Eur Arch Otorhinolaryngol. 2014; 271(6):1505–1511

[36] Elsharnouby NM, Elsharnouby MM. Magnesium sulphate as a technique of hypotensive anaesthesia. Br J Anaesth. 2006; 96(6):727–731

[37] Nho JS, Lee SY, Kang JM, et al. Effects of maintaining a remifentanil infusion on the recovery profiles during emergence from anaesthesia and tracheal extubation. Br J Anaesth. 2009; 103(6):817–821

[38] Hogue CW, Jr, Bowdle TA, O'Leary C, et al. A multicenter evaluation of total intravenous anesthesia with remifentanil and propofol for elective inpatient surgery. Anesth Analg. 1996; 83(2):279–285

[39] Choi EM, Park WK, Choi SH, Soh S, Lee JR. Smooth emergence in men undergoing nasal surgery: the effect site concentration of remifentanil for preventing cough after sevoflurane-balanced anaesthesia. Acta Anaesthesiol Scand. 2012; 56(4):498–503

[40] Lee B, Lee JR, Na S. Targeting smooth emergence: the effect site concentration of remifentanil for preventing cough during emergence during propofol-remifentanil anaesthesia for thyroid surgery. Br J Anaesth. 2009; 102(6):775–778

[41] Ahmed MZ, Vohra A. The reinforced laryngeal mask airway (RLMA) protects the airway in patients undergoing nasal surgery–an observational study of 200 patients. Can J Anaesth. 2002; 49(8):863–866

[42] Webster AC, Morley-Forster PK, Janzen V, et al. Anesthesia for intranasal surgery: a comparison between tracheal intubation and the flexible reinforced laryngeal mask airway. Anesth Analg. 1999; 88(2):421–425

[43] Kaplan A, Crosby GJ, Bhattacharyya N. Airway protection and the laryngeal mask airway in sinus and nasal surgery. Laryngoscope. 2004; 114(4):652–655

[44] Williams PJ, Thompsett C, Bailey PM. Comparison of the reinforced laryngeal mask airway and tracheal intubation for nasal surgery. Anaesthesia. 1995; 50 (11):987–989

[45] Danielsen A, Gravningsbråten R, Olofsson J. Anaesthesia in endoscopic sinus surgery. Eur Arch Otorhinolaryngol. 2003; 260(9):481–486

[46] Wilson IG, Fell D, Robinson SL, Smith G. Cardiovascular responses to insertion of the laryngeal mask. Anaesthesia. 1992; 47(4):300–302

[47] Visser K, Hassink EA, Bonsel GJ, Moen J, Kalkman CJ. Randomized controlled trial of total intravenous anesthesia with propofol versus inhalation anesthesia with isoflurane-nitrous oxide: postoperative nausea with vomiting and economic analysis. Anesthesiology. 2001; 95 (3):616–626

[48] Apfel CC, Korttila K, Abdalla M, et al. IMPACT Investigators. A factorial trial of six interventions for the prevention of postoperative nausea and vomiting. N Engl J Med. 2004; 350(24):2441–2451

[49] Friedman M, Venkatesan TK, Lang D, Caldarelli DD. Bupivacaine for postoperative analgesia following endoscopic sinus surgery. Laryngoscope. 1996; 106(11):1382–1385

[50] Buchanan MA, Dunn GR, Macdougall GM. A prospective double-blind randomized controlled trial of the effect of topical bupivacaine on post-operative pain in bilateral nasal surgery with bilateral nasal packs inserted. J Laryngol Otol. 2005; 119(4):284–288

# 20 Postoperative Care and Complications Following Open and Endoscopic Orbital Surgery

*Saul N. Rajak, Richard G. Douglas, and Alkis J. Psaltis*

**Abstract**

Appropriate postoperative care after orbital surgery is fundamental for surgical recovery and avoidance of complications. This chapter reviews the measures that can be employed to prevent complications and manage them should they occur.

*Keywords:* postoperative care, retrobulbar hemorrhage, orbital compartment syndrome, the tight orbit, orbital emphysema, orbital infection, CSF leak

## 20.1 Introduction

Orbital surgery occurs in a confined space that contains critical neurovascular structures. Postoperative complications can be devastating as they have the potential to affect vision and very rarely life. Although some aspects of postoperative care are applicable to all orbital procedures, others are individualized according to patient factors and the surgical procedure performed. Orbital surgeons need to be cognizant of the potential for complications, monitor and manage patients appropriately in the postoperative period, and be aware of how to deal effectively with complications should they occur.

## 20.2 Observations of Vital Signs

Measurement of a patient's vital signs should be undertaken postoperatively at least every 1 to 2 hours for the first 12 hours, reducing to every 4 to 6 thereafter until discharge. Changes in such parameters may indicate the presence of active bleeding (reduced blood pressure and increased pulse), imminent bleeding (high blood pressure), infection (increased pulse, temperature, or respiratory rate), pulmonary embolus (increased respiratory rate and pulse), or postoperative pain (increased blood pressure, pulse, or respiratory rate).

## 20.3 Prevention of Postoperative Bleeding

Retrobulbar hemorrhage is the most feared complication of orbital surgery. Accumulation of blood in the confined space of the orbit can rapidly compress the optic nerve resulting in optic neuropathy that may lead to irreversible visual loss. This is sometimes referred to as orbital compartment syndrome (OCS). Endoscopic endonasal orbital procedures that create a communication between the orbit and the sinonasal cavity (such as orbital decompression) carry a very low risk of confined retrobulbar hemorrhage or compartment syndrome, as blood can exit the orbit. However, there are rare reports of compartment syndrome developing in an unconnected orbital compartment despite a sinonasal–orbital connection having been made.[1] A transorbital approach to lesions that leave the orbital bones intact carries a small but significant risk of postoperative hemorrhage, particularly if the surgery was undertaken for a vascular lesion, or if the patient is taking anticoagulant medications or has a pre-existent bleeding diathesis.

Meticulous intraoperative hemostasis minimizes the risk of retrobulbar hemorrhage. The following postoperative measures should be considered.

### 20.3.1 Blood Pressure Control

Regular monitoring of blood pressure is essential in the first 24 hours postsurgery. Raised blood pressure increases the risk of postoperative bleeding. Patients should continue antihypertensive medication on the day of surgery and during the perioperative period. Pain may be accompanied by increases in blood pressure and so should be managed with regular analgesia. Activities that acutely increase intracranial pressure, orbital pressure, and blood pressure such as strenuous exercise, lifting, stooping over, and nose blowing should be avoided in the first 2 weeks of postorbital surgery.

### 20.3.2 Pad and Dressings

The utility of postoperative ocular padding and pressure dressing has been debated in the orbital surgery literature. Although pressure dressings may assist hemostasis, they may also potentially increase the pressure of a developing hemorrhage on the optic nerve (exacerbating the tight orbit) and possibly conceal reducing vision and increasing proptosis. If a pad and/or pressure dressing is used, vision must be checked on emergence from anesthetic and every 2 to 4 hours for the first 24 hours. The patient must also be advised to immediately report increased pain or reduced vision. It is the authors' preference to use a lightly taped double pad to put gentle pressure on the orbit for 12 to 24 hours after transorbital procedures and no pad after endoscopic orbital procedures.

### 20.3.3 Surgical Drains

Increases in orbital volume by as little as 7 mL can cause significant acute changes to the optic disc morphology.[2] Drain collection volumes over 70 mL of serosanguineous fluid have been reported.[3] Despite this, most orbital surgeons use drains rarely, reserving them for prolonged cases or cases involving excision or debulking of vascular lesions. If used, a fine suction drain is generally preferred and this can almost always be removed after a period of 12 to 24 hours without fluid collection.

### 20.3.4 Hot Drinks

It has been common practice to advise patients to avoid hot drinks and baths in the first postoperative week. Hot drinks and baths may increase peripheral vasodilation. However, there is no evidence to support this practice and unless a patient is at very high risk of bleeding, these measures are probably not required.

**Table 20.1** Symptoms and signs of orbital compartment syndrome

- Reducing vision
- Orbital pain
- Periocular bruising
- Increasing proptosis
- Increased orbital tension (elicited by globe retropulsion)—"the tight orbit"
- Reduced ocular motility
- Relative afferent pupillary defect
- Increased intraocular pressure
- Loss of spontaneous venous pulsation of the optic disc

## 20.3.5 Recommencing Anticoagulation

Decisions on stopping and restarting anticoagulant and antiplatelet medications must be individualized and discussed with the patient's physicians. The risk of severe hemorrhage (requiring transfusion or surgical intervention) in patients undergoing endoscopic dacryocystorhinostomy (DCR) is 0.6%.[4] The risk in orbital surgery has not been reported, but would likely vary according to the nature of the procedure and the lesion. In general, patients with a high risk of cerebral or cardiac vascular occlusion should have anticoagulation restarted immediately postoperatively or not stopped at all, while those at low risk might restart at 5 days postoperative when the primary clot is more secure.

## 20.3.6 Detection and Management of Orbital Hemorrhage

Postoperative OCS is a surgical emergency. It can occur in the early postoperative period particularly if intraoperative hemostasis was not achieved or if there is a marked increase in blood pressure. Rarely, it can occur several days postoperatively from clot dissolution (usually in patients on aspirin). Vision can be irreversibly lost within 2 hours of the onset of hemorrhage.[5] It is recognized by the symptoms and signs summarized in ▶ Table 20.1. The management of OCS necessitates an immediate return to the operation theater and blood pressure control with head elevation until surgery commences.

Decompression of the orbit should be performed immediately upon recognition of the problem, despite the fact that there are reports of it being beneficial up to 48 hours posthemorrhage.[6] Decompression can be achieved via a lateral canthotomy and inferior ± superior canthal tendon cantholysis, orbital floor fracture, or medial orbital wall decompression.[7,8,9] If theater space is not available, both lateral canthotomy and orbital floor decompression can be conducted at the bedside under local anesthetic. ▶ Table 20.2 demonstrates the technique for performing a lateral canthotomy.

## 20.3.7 Detection and Management of Epistaxis

A minor amount of anterior and posterior nasal blood loss is expected postsurgery. The use of a nasal bolster to catch anterior bleeding is recommended. Mild to moderate epistaxis usually settles with conservative measures including blood

**Table 20.2** Lateral canthotomy for orbital hemorrhage

1. Instill topical anesthetic eyedrops and inject local anesthetic (lidocaine 2% and adrenaline) subcutaneously at the lateral canthus. Sterilize the area

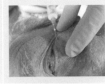

2. Lateral canthotomy: divide the upper and lower eyelid with a cut through the lateral canthus using scissors or a blade

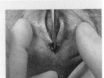

3. Lateral cantholysis: grasp the lateral edge of the lower lid with toothed forceps and with scissors directed inferomedially, divide the restricting band of lateral canthal tendon and septum. This band is "strummable" like a thick guitar string and sits between the posterior part of the lateral lower lid and the inferolateral orbital rim using blunt-tipped scissors

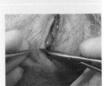

4. Once the septal band has been adequately divided, the edge of the lower lid grasped in step 4 should easily "give" and the lower lid can be easily distracted from the globe.

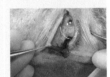

5. Divide the deeper septal fibers that separate the orbit from the preseptal tissues. Orbital hemorrhage should be released.

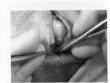

6. The optic nerve should be checked to observe vessels of normal caliber with spontaneous venous pulsation and an absence of the "winking" or "flashing" venous system that occurs under pressure

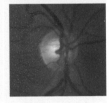

pressure control, analgesia, head elevation (without neck hyperextension), icepacks on the neck and bridge of the nose, and topical nasal vasoconstrictor sprays. If bleeding persists, packing may be required. If necessary, this should be performed, preferably under endoscopic guidance to avoid trauma to the recently operated site. If bleeding persists despite these measures, a return to theater may be required for sphenopalatine, or anterior ethmoidal artery ligation.

## 20.4 Control of Periorbital Bruising and Swelling

### 20.4.1 Head Elevation and Mobilization

Postoperative head elevation reduces periocular edema, through gravity-assisted venous drainage. A higher sitting angle would be expected to be more effective. One study has reported less facial edema in patients nursed at 90 degrees than those at

30 degrees.[10,11] Patients often find it uncomfortable to sit upright in the postoperative period and so we usually recommend that the patient be nursed at the highest comfortable angle, which is typically around 45 degrees. Gentle, early mobilization is to be encouraged to minimize the risk of deep vein thrombosis and pulmonary embolus, and to reduce periocular swelling.

## 20.4.2 Icepacks

The judicious use of icepacks acutely reduces swelling through local vasoconstriction, although there is no evidence that this alters the postoperative recovery time course.

## 20.4.3 Postoperative Corticosteroids

Oral and topical corticosteroids are widely used after endoscopic endonasal surgery, as they may reduce swelling and promote wound healing. Despite this, there is limited evidence that administration of intraoperative or postoperative corticosteroids reduces postoperative swelling following orbital surgery and no evidence of a benefit to outcomes.[12] Despite the absence of evidence, the administration of systemic steroids is recommended in patients undergoing orbital surgery with underlying inflammatory conditions such as thyroid eye disease and granulomatosis with polyangiitis.

## 20.5 Antibiotics and Infection Prevention

Orbital surgery can be divided into procedures that are confined to the orbit and those that connect the orbit to the sinonasal cavity, such as medial wall decompression, fracture repairs, and endonasal endoscopic approaches to the orbit. Theoretically, the former group is considered clean surgery, while the latter can be classified as clean-contaminated due to the extensive colonization of the nasal cavity by microbial organisms. Interestingly, the risk of infection does not seem to be higher in the latter group, at least anecdotally. Postoperative antibiotics are widely used in orbital surgery although there is currently no evidence to support this practice. Studies of antibiotics postorbital floor fracture repair did not find a significant risk of infection in patients not receiving antibiotics or those receiving them for 24 hours postoperatively. It should be noted, however, that all patients in these studies did receive preoperative antibiotics.[13,14]

Postoperative orbital inflammation occasionally does not settle despite antibiotic treatment for presumed infection. The possibility of a retained foreign body, such as gauze, neuropathies, or organic matter from traumatic injury, must be considered. The foreign body may be identified on fine-cut MRI (magnetic resonance imaging) or computed tomography (CT) scanning. Surgical exploration and foreign body excision may be required. Bone wax can also cause persistent giant cell granulomatosis, which may require surgical removal.[15]

## 20.5.1 Detection and Management of Orbital Infection

▶ Table 20.3 summarizes the clinical and laboratory findings associated with orbital infection. Orbital infection is treated

**Table 20.3** Symptoms, signs, and laboratory results in orbital infection
- Pain, erythema, warmth, swelling, and loss of function
- Purulent discharge
- Visual loss from optic nerve compromise
- Systemic symptoms such as fever and tachycardia
- Leukocytosis and elevated inflammatory markers

with intravenous antibiotics and may require incision and curettage or debriding of purulent collections.

## 20.6 Prevention of Orbital Emphysema

Orbital emphysema can complicate surgery that connects the orbit to the sinonasal cavity (▶ Fig. 20.1). This typically occurs if the patient blows his or her nose, but a "ball valve" phenomenon can occur with normal respiratory pressure. Therefore, all patients with known or possible sino-orbital communication should be instructed not to blow their nose for 2 weeks postoperatively. Orbital emphysema typically presents with rapid- or even sudden-onset proptosis and lid swelling, diplopia, crepitus, and raised intraocular pressure. It is typically a self-limiting condition that can be treated conservatively with advice to avoid nose blowing. However, very occasionally it can result in optic nerve compression and visual loss. For this reason, 15- to 30-minute visual observations should be performed in the first 24 hours after its occurrence. Vision-threatening orbital emphysema can be treated with surgical drainage, aspiration of trapped air, and palmar pressure on the globe.[16,17,18,19,20]

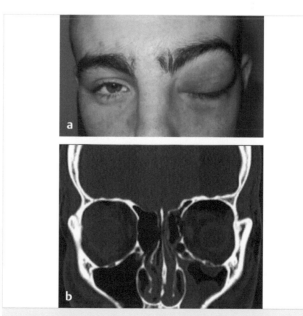

**Fig. 20.1** Orbital emphysema. **(a)** Clinical. **(b)** CT (computed tomography) scan.

## 20.7 Postoperative Irrigation and Intranasal Sprays

The benefit of postoperative high-volume irrigations for chronic rhinosinusitis is now well established and therefore may be considered postoperatively for trans-sinus orbital surgery (100- to 200-mL nasal irrigation two or three times a day for 2 weeks commencing on the day after surgery) as irrigation can facilitate the removal of crusts, clots, and debris that can serve as a source of infection and adhesion formation.[21] Endoscopic DCR does not involve significant sinus surgery and therefore low-volume nasal saline may be more appropriate to moisten the surgical site and prevent clot formation.

## 20.8 Intranasal Debridement

Intranasal debridement of crusting, dried blood, and unresorbed soluble packing materials is frequently practiced after endoscopic sinus surgery. Advocates report that this practice removes the framework for scarring, ostial stenosis, and middle turbinate lateralization, thereby improving ostial patency.[21] The indications for endoscopic orbital surgery are different to sinus surgery and therefore we do not advocate routine debridement unless endoscopic examination shows excessive crusting that may jeopardize sinus ostium patency.

## 20.9 Wound Management

Transorbital procedures may be repaired with skin and/or absorbable conjunctival sutures. The conjunctival sutures can be left to dissolve in situ, but skin sutures should be removed at 7 to 10 days postoperatively. Wound dehiscence is rare and usually occurs as a complication of increased orbital pressure from hemorrhage, pus, or emphysema or from wound infection. If orbital pressure is suspected, orbital imaging may be informative and if infection is suspected, antibiotics should be administered. The incision can then be sutured again unless continued pus drainage is anticipated.

## 20.10 Diplopia Management

Short-term diplopia is common after orbital surgery. Long-term diplopia is less common but can occur from decompression surgery or as a consequence of intraoperative extraocular muscle damage.[22] Eye patching may be required during the period of diplopia and referral to an ophthalmologist with an interest in squint surgery for nonresolving symptoms is advisable.

## 20.11 Resumption of Continuous Partial Airway Pressure

Continuous partial airway pressure (CPAP) used for the treatment of obstructive sleep apnea (OSA) applies positive pressure to the sinonasal cavity. It does not need to be stopped for trans-orbital procedures in which the orbital walls are not removed or fractured. However, the intranasal positive pressure risks orbital emphysema in procedures in which the barriers between orbit and sinus have been breached and therefore CPAP should be stopped postoperatively. There are currently no widely accepted guidelines on the timing of resumption and practice varies widely.[23] In the absence of significant risk of dangerous nocturnal apneic episodes, we advocate cessation of CPAP for 2 weeks. CPAP-specific symptoms after endoscopic DCR are common, with air regurgitation reported by 70% of patients.[24] This may contribute to poor compliance with CPAP therapy. Intolerable symptoms of air regurgitation are almost inevitable after conjunctivodacryocystorhinostomy (lacrimal bypass/Lester Jones tube surgery), and CPAP is therefore a contraindication to this surgery.[25] Detailed preoperative counseling with regards to CPAP use and its effects is mandatory in OSA patients undergoing DCR.

## 20.12 Observation for Rare Complications

### 20.12.1 Cerebrospinal Fluid Rhinorrhea

Cerebrospinal fluid (CSF) leaks are reported to occur in up to 5% of orbital surgery procedures and are usually noted intraoperatively.[26] However, they can be missed, particularly when resulting from a spiral fracture. A suspected leak should be investigated with laboratory assessment of any nasal fluid for the presence of beta-2-transferrin and high-resolution CT (with consideration of intrathecal metrizamide injection) to establish the leak site and exclude intracranial hemorrhage. Breaches of the skull base are usually noted at the time of surgery. Patients with suspected CSF leak must remain under strict neurological observation and otolaryngologic input is likely to be required for the closure and management. Unrecognized ongoing CSF leaks can result in CSF hypotension syndrome. This is characterized by postural headache, nausea, vomiting, photophobia, blurred vision, and sixth cranial nerve palsy. Persistent clear or serous nasal discharge may be noted.

### 20.12.2 Confusion

Cerebral complications occasionally occur in orbital surgery. Intracranial hemorrhage can very occasionally occur from bone trauma or bleeding of vascular emissaries during orbital surgical procedures including bony decompression and exenteration.[27,28]

Meningitis has been reported after sinus surgery and necrotizing fasciitis has been reported after both blepharoplasty and DCR, and therefore both complications are theoretically possible after orbital surgery.[29,30,31]

### 20.12.3 Epiphora

The nasolacrimal drainage system can be knowingly or inadvertently traumatized during orbital surgery. While this does not require specific postoperative care, awareness of the complication is important and referral to an ophthalmologist indicated if persistent postoperative epiphora is observed.

# References

[1] See A, Gan EC. Orbital compartment syndrome during endoscopic drainage of subperiosteal orbital abscess. Am J Otolaryngol. 2015; 36(6):828–831

[2] Akar Y, Apaydin KC, Ozel A. Acute orbital effects of retrobulbar injection on optic nerve head topography. Br J Ophthalmol. 2004; 88(12):1573–1576

[3] Fenzl CR, Golio D. The impact of suction drainage on orbital compartment syndrome after craniofacial surgery. J Craniofac Surg. 2014; 25(4):1358–1361

[4] Andrew N, Selva D. Postoperative haemorrhage in powered endoscopic dacryocystorhinostomy. Clin Experiment Ophthalmol. 2014; 42(3):262–265

[5] Hayreh SS, Kolder HE, Weingeist TA. Central retinal artery occlusion and retinal tolerance time. Ophthalmology. 1980; 87(1):75–78

[6] Soare S, Foletti JM, Gallucci A, Collet C, Guyot L, Chossegros C. Update on orbital decompression as emergency treatment of traumatic blindness. J Craniomaxillofac Surg. 2015; 43(7):1000–1003

[7] Liu D. A simplified technique of orbital decompression for severe retrobulbar hemorrhage. Am J Ophthalmol. 1993; 116(1):34–37

[8] Voss JO, Hartwig S, Doll C, Hoffmeister B, Raguse JD, Adolphs N. The "tight orbit": incidence and management of the orbital compartment syndrome. J Craniomaxillofac Surg. 2016; 44(8):1008–1014

[9] Colletti G, Fogagnolo P, Allevi F, et al. Retrobulbar hemorrhage during or after endonasal or periorbital surgery: what to do, when and how to do it. J Craniofac Surg. 2015; 26(3):897–901

[10] Ong AA, Farhood Z, Kyle AR, Patel KG. Interventions to decrease postoperative edema and ecchymosis after rhinoplasty: a systematic review of the literature. Plast Reconstr Surg. 2016; 137(5):1448–1462

[11] Stucker FJ. Prevention of post-rhinoplasty edema. Laryngoscope. 1974; 84(4):536–541

[12] Flood TR, McManners J, el-Attar A, Moos KF. Randomized prospective study of the influence of steroids on postoperative eye-opening after exploration of the orbital floor. Br J Oral Maxillofac Surg. 1999; 37(4):312–315

[13] Wladis EJ. Are post-operative oral antibiotics required after orbital floor fracture repair? Orbit. 2013; 32(1):30–32

[14] Zix J, Schaller B, Iizuka T, Lieger O. The role of postoperative prophylactic antibiotics in the treatment of facial fractures: a randomised, double-blind, placebo-controlled pilot clinical study. Part 1: orbital fractures in 62 patients. Br J Oral Maxillofac Surg. 2013; 51(4):332–336

[15] Katz SE, Rootman J. Adverse effects of bone wax in surgery of the orbit. Ophthal Plast Reconstr Surg. 1996; 12(2):121–126

[16] Chaudhry IA, Al-Amri A, Shamsi FA, Al-Rashed W. Visual recovery after evacuation of orbital emphysema. Orbit. 2007; 26(4):283–285

[17] Hunts JH, Patrinely JR, Holds JB, Anderson RL. Orbital emphysema. Staging and acute management. Ophthalmology. 1994; 101(5):960–966

[18] Silbert JE, Rudich DS, Wasserman EL, Lesser RL. Recurrent vision loss after endoscopic sinus surgery managed with palmar pressure. Ophthal Plast Reconstr Surg. 2008; 24(2):150–152

[19] Singh M, Phua VM, Sundar G. Sight-threatening orbital emphysema treated with needle decompression. Clin Experiment Ophthalmol. 2007; 35(4):386–387

[20] Tomasetti P, Jacbosen C, Gander T, Zemann W. Emergency decompression of tension retrobulbar emphysema secondary to orbital floor fracture. J Surg Case Rep. 2013; 2013(3):rjt011

[21] Rudmik L, Smith TL. Evidence-based practice: postoperative care in endoscopic sinus surgery. Otolaryngol Clin North Am. 2012; 45(5):1019–1032

[22] Mainville NP, Jordan DR. Effect of orbital decompression on diplopia in thyroid-related orbitopathy. Ophthal Plast Reconstr Surg. 2014; 30(2):137–140

[23] Cohen JC, Larrabee YC, Weinstein AL, Stewart MG. Use of continuous positive airway pressure after rhinoplasty, septoplasty, and sinus surgery: A survey of current practice patterns. Laryngoscope. 2015; 125(11):2612–2616

[24] Ali MJ, Psaltis AJ, Murphy J, Wormald PJ. Endoscopic dacryocystorhinostomy and obstructive sleep apnoea: the effects and outcomes of continuous positive airway pressure therapy. Clin Experiment Ophthalmol. 2015; 43(5):405–408

[25] Cannon PS, Madge SN, Selva D. Air regurgitation in patients on continuous positive airway pressure (CPAP) therapy following dacrocystorhinostomy with or without Lester-Jones tube insertion. Br J Ophthalmol. 2010; 94(7):891–893

[26] Limawararut V, Valenzuela AA, Sullivan TJ, et al. Cerebrospinal fluid leaks in orbital and lacrimal surgery. Surv Ophthalmol. 2008; 53(3):274–284

[27] Gonzalez LF, Bilyk JR. Intracranial arterial avulsion during orbital exenteration. Orbit. 2012; 31(3):190–193

[28] Badilla J, Dolman PJ. Intracranial hemorrhage complicating an orbital decompression. Orbit. 2008; 27(2):143–145

[29] Véber F, Gehanno P, Perrin A. Purulent meningitis after minor nasosinus surgery. Apropos of 10 cases. Ann Otolaryngol Chir Cervicofac. 1985; 102(3):163–167

[30] Matar VW, Betz P. Periorbital necrotizing fasciitis: a complication of a dacryocystorhinostomy. J Fr Ophtalmol. 2011; 34(4):258.e1–258.e5

[31] Suñer IJ, Meldrum ML, Johnson TE, Tse DT. Necrotizing fasciitis after cosmetic blepharoplasty. Am J Ophthalmol. 1999; 128(3):367–368

# Index